ARTHROSCOPIC SURGERY

ARTHROSCOPIC SURGERY

THE FOOT & ANKLE

Richard D. Ferkel, M.D.

Clinical Instructor of Orthopedic Surgery
University of California, Los Angeles, Center for Health Science

Chief of Arthroscopy
Wadsworth VA Hospital
Los Angeles, California

Attending Surgeon and Director of Fellowship
Southern California Orthopedic Institute
Van Nuys, California

Terry L. Whipple, M.D.

Editor-in-Chief

Illustrated by Susan E. Brust, M.S., C.M.I.

With 10 Contributors

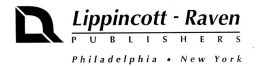

Lippincott · Raven
PUBLISHERS

Philadelphia · New York

Acquisitions Editor: James D. Ryan
Developmental Editor: Susan R. Skand
Project Editor: Ellen M. Campbell
Production Manager: Caren Erlichman
Production Coordinator: David Yurkovich
Design Coordinator: Doug Smock
Indexer: Betty Herr Hallinger
Compositor: Tapsco, Incorporated
Printer: Quebecor/Kingsport

Library of Congress Cataloging-in-Publication Data

Ferkel, Richard D.
    Arthroscopic surgery: The foot and the ankle/Richard D. Ferkel;
  illustrated by Susan E. Brust; Terry L. Whipple, editor-in-chief;
  with 10 contributors.
      p. cm.
  Includes bibliographical references and index.
  ISBN 0-397-51093-4 (alk. paper)
  1. Ankle—Endoscopic surgery. 2. Foot—Endoscopic surgery.
  I. Whipple, Terry L. II. Title.
    [DNLM: 1. Foot—surgery. 2. Arthroscopy—methods. 3. Ankle—surgery.
  WE 880F356a 1996]
  RD562.F47 1996
  617.5′84059—dc20
  DNLM/DLC
  for Library of Congress
                                           95-33702
                                              CIP

9 8 7 6 5 4 3 2 1

To my wife Michelle, and to Eric and Megan,
for their love, support, and understanding.

To Mom, Dad, and Donna

CONTRIBUTORS

Richard D. Ferkel, M.D.
Clinical Instructor of Orthopedic Surgery
University of California, Los Angeles, Center for Health Sciences

Chief of Arthroscopy
Wadsworth VA Hospital
Los Angeles, California

Attending Surgeon and Director of Fellowship
Southern California Orthopedic Institute
Van Nuys, California

James M. Glick, M.D.
Associate Clinical Professor of Orthopaedic Surgery
Senior Attending Physician
Mount Zion Hospital Campus
University of California, San Francisco

James F. Guhl, M.D.
Past President
Arthroscopic Association of North America
Professor of Orthropaedic Surgery
Medical College of Wisconsin
Chief Emeritus
Department of Orthopaedic Surgery
St. Francis Hospital
Milwaukee, Wisconsin

Richard B. Hawkins, M.D.
Burbank Hospital
Fitchburg, Massachusetts

Sevil K. Brahme, M.D.
Assistant Clinical Professor
University of California, San Diego
Staff Radiologist
Sharp Memorial Hospital
San Diego, California

John F. Orwin, M.D.
Assistant Professor
University of Wisconsin Medical School
University of Wisconsin Hospital
and Clinics
Madison, Wisconsin

Melanie Reid, R.Pt.
Formerly, Director of Physical Therapy
Health South Rehabilitation
Van Nuys, California

Mark E. Schweitzer, M.D.
Associate Professor
Department of Radiology
Thomas Jefferson University Hospital
Philadelphia, Pennsylvania

James W. Stone, M.D.
Assistant Clinical Professor
of Orthopaedic Surgery
Medical College of Wisconsin
Milwaukee, Wisconsin

Richard A. Weiss, M.D.
North Shore Orthopaedic Surgery
and Sports Medicine
Smithtown, New York

Timothy J. Zimmer, M.D.
Director, Orthopaedic Research
of Virginia
Richmond, Virginia

FOREWORD

You cannot tell this book by its cover. When I say the title *Arthroscopic Surgery: The Ankle and Foot* is misleading, it is meant to be complimentary. The potential reader might think this text is solely about arthroscopic technique; to the contrary, it is directed towards care of the patient with foot and ankle problems.

It is no easy feat to successfully write a text for all levels of students, from medical school to practicing surgeon. In my view, Dr. Ferkel has done just that. This book should be especially helpful for the experienced foot and ankle surgeon with developing arthroscopic skills, reminiscent of the introduction of arthroscopy to knee and shoulder surgeons.

In this text, basic arthroscopic surgical principles have been transported to the anatomical requirements of the smaller ankle and foot joints. Although arthroscopy is extensively discussed, the procedure itself is relegated to its proper role in patient care. The attention to detail necessary for technical success is outlined: instrumentation, room setup, the role of the assistant, surgical approaches, and various procedures. There is repeated emphasis in each chapter on the value of the medical history, differential diagnosis, disease classifications, and non-operative treatment modalities. The topics that do not need repeating or are beyond the scope of his text are handled by the extensive references. Therefore, the reader's curiosity does not remain unsatisfied or undirected.

This text could be compiled only by an experience practitioner and clinical researcher. Dr. Ferkel has been able to assemble this information through years of clinical practice, careful study of the literature and his own results, scientific presentations, and publications. His knowledge of arthroscopy is demonstrated by systematic documentation, 21-point anatomical examination and the regular use of videotape as a permanent record. His clinical expertise surfaces in the discussion of surgical indications, procedural limitations, and today's requirement for cost effectiveness. His conservative approach to arthroscopy is reflected by the three percent incidence of arthroscopic procedures in the 4000 cases seen at his institution.

The clinical reports are extensive. Dr. Ferkel presents information from the literature and his own original series reports, which he made the effort to update for this publication. In addition, he makes available to the reader the extensive case experience from his practice group, the Southern California Orthopedic Institute. He is open in his discussion of surgical complications, their avoidance and management. I especially appreciate that after any comprehensive listing of options, he always states his preference and rationale. This method of presentation brings the reader into a dialogue with the author.

The illustrative drawings with correlation between lesions and physical exam are particularly helpful. It is not meant to be demeaning to say that one can read some sections just by looking at pictures. The detailed illustrations of the various portals and diagnostic zones are so good, they should be ready references in surgical suites everywhere.

Arthroscopic Surgery: The Foot and Ankle deals with contemporary issues and controversy in arthroscopy: the adjunct use in acute fractures, ankle arthrodesis, subtalar and great toe surgery, rehabilitation, and potential for the laser. An algorithm is presented on the treatment of chronic ankle pain. His arthroscopic experience has resulted in some changes in terminology: from chronic post ankle sprain pain to anterolateral impingement of the ankle.

The quality of this textbook is a reflection of the high level of the practice of orthopedic surgery at the Southern California Orthopedic Institute. We are indebted to Dr. Ferkel for presenting a prudent and judicious use of arthroscopy in the management of patients with foot and ankle problems. He has done us the service of placing all this information in one place, a ready reference on foot and ankle surgery.

Lanny L. Johnson, M.D.
Clinical Professor
Department of Surgery
College of Human Medicine
Michigan State University
East Lansing, Michigan

PREFACE

*I*n June 1983, I completed a sports medicine fellowship at the Southern California Orthopedic Institute (SCOI) and was asked to join the group. At that point, the five orthopedic surgeons in the group were primarily knee surgeons and were starting to develop a bigger interest in the shoulder. Because they felt uncomfortable with the treatment of foot and ankle problems, I was asked to travel around the country and learn more about these disorders. It was thought that, as my sports medicine practice grew, I could fill the extra time seeing patients with foot and ankle problems.

Concurrent to this, operative knee arthroscopy was becoming more popular, and numerous courses were being held around the country to teach these skills. After one of these seminars, my partner, Jim Fox, speculated, "Someday ankle arthroscopy will be big, and you better get busy learning how to do it." Since that time, arthroscopy of the foot and ankle has become an integral part of orthopedic care.

In 1989, Terry Whipple invited me to write a monograph on arthroscopy of the foot and ankle. Although I had hoped to complete this project in 2 years, it has taken much longer. This book is not intended as just a technical manual on how to do procedures. Instead, I tried to incorporate what I have learned as both a sports medicine and foot and ankle surgeon to give the reader an integrated approach to these problems. To perform foot and ankle arthroscopy successfully, a surgeon must understand anatomy, biomechanics, and physiology, as well as the technical aspects of these procedures. Section I of *Arthroscopic Surgery: The Foot and Ankle* considers preoperative evaluation, instrumentation, surgical environment, and correlative surgical anatomy. Once the surgeon synthesizes this information, the diagnostic arthroscopic examination can be undertaken. Section II discusses the various pathologic conditions that are amenable to arthroscopic surgery; newer techniques, such as subtalar and great toe arthroscopy; and rehabilitation, complications, and future developments.

It is fortunate that this book was not completed in 1991. Foot and ankle arthroscopy has changed dramatically during the past 5 years. In the future, we must continue to "push the envelope," to be bold in developing newer, better arthroscopic methods of treating foot and ankle problems. We must not be afraid of failure but rather must be excited by the challenge to continue improving the quality of care to our patients.

—*R.D.F.*

ACKNOWLEDGMENTS

Many people have contributed to the successful completion of this text. I would like to thank Terry Whipple and Lippincott–Raven Publishers for their encouragement, help, and great patience. My partners at Southern California Orthopedic Institute—especially James M. Fox, Wilson Del Pizzo, Marc J. Friedman, Stephen J. Snyder, and Ronald P. Karzel—have supported all my efforts throughout the years.

Susan Brust spent countless hours developing the illustrations with me. Her drawings make the text come alive with incredible accuracy, precision and beauty.

Arthroscopic Surgery: The Foot and Ankle would never have been completed without the help of Eleanor O'Brien at Southern California Orthopedic Research and Education (SCORE). She was my manuscript typist and second conscience, even though she will not miss the roar of jet engines that permeated my dictations. The three Chrises and one Lois at SCORE Media Center have spent tireless hours shooting pictures of radiographs and surgical procedures, as well as locating hundreds of surgical tapes.

Many people at Valley Presbyterian Hospital have also given generously of their time, including Robert Williams, Grace Sussman, RN, and Drs. Dennis Kasimian, Judy Rose, and Greg Applegate. My secretary, Judy Koransky, and my orthopedic physician assistant, Ric Campbell, have both helped me get through this project and still continue to practice medicine.

I wish to acknowledge Drs. Ron Smith, Roger Mann, Mike Coughlin, and William Hamilton for believing in the importance of arthroscopy in the treatment of foot and ankle disorders. Finally, I thank Jim Guhl for sharing his knowledge and showing me the way.

CONTENTS

ARTHROSCOPIC SURGERY

Arthroscopic Surgery: The Foot and Ankle,
by Richard D. Ferkel.
Lippincott-Raven Publishers, Philadelphia © 1996.

Introduction

*A*rthroscopy has revolutionized the practice of orthopaedic surgery since the mid-1970s. After a long history of sporadic attempts at arthroscopy, technological breakthroughs in Japan and several surgical pioneers in North America launched widespread interest in percutaneous joint surgery.

In 1918, Takagi initiated efforts at endoscopic examination of cadaver knees at the University of Tokyo, using a number 22 French Cystoscope.[1] Bircher advanced the technique in 1921 by using gaseous distention of the knee.[2] In the United States, Kreuscher reported clinical results in diagnostic knee arthroscopy for meniscus disorders in 1925.[3] The large diameter of the cystoscope limited its utility, but in 1931 Takagi developed an arthroscope 3.5 mm in diameter that incorporated a lamp and magnifying optics and provided a clearer visual field. With this device, he compiled unprecedented clinical experience in endoscopic examination of the knee.

In New York, Burman made significant arthroscopic advances. In 1931, he reported using a scope of his own design to examine 100 cadaver knee joints, but he extended his examinations to 25 shoulders, 20 hips, 15 elbows, 3 ankles, and 6 wrists.[4] His arthroscope, used also by colleagues Finkelstein and Mayer in clinical applications, incorporated channels for fluid or gas distention of the joint.[5]

Arthroscopy of the knee was elegantly and convincingly demonstrated by endoscopic photography in Watanabe's *Atlas of Arthroscopy,* published in 1969.[1] Only then did the technique begin to gain clinical credibility and acceptance. Watanabe was a protege of Takagi at the University of Tokyo. He attracted the attention and enthusiasm of several North American surgeons—notably S. Ward Casscells of Wilmington, Delaware; Robert W. Jackson of Toronto, Canada; John Joyce of Philadelphia, Pennsylvania; and Richard O'Connor of West Covina, California. Using the improved Watanabe No. 21 arthroscope with an incandescent bulb at the tip, these surgeons established the application of Watanabe's techniques for knee arthroscopy in the United States and Canada. In various publications, they reported their experience with the numerous advantages of arthroscopy for diagnostic purposes, as well as for early arthroscopic surgery in the knee.[6–10]

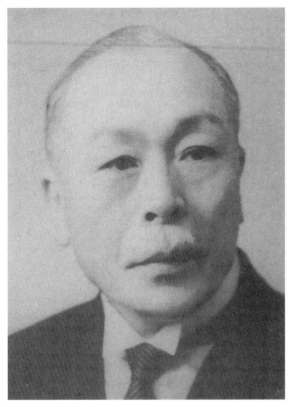

Professor Takagi, Tokyo, Japan

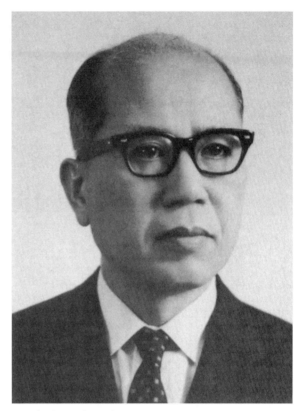

Masaki Watanabe, Tokyo, Japan

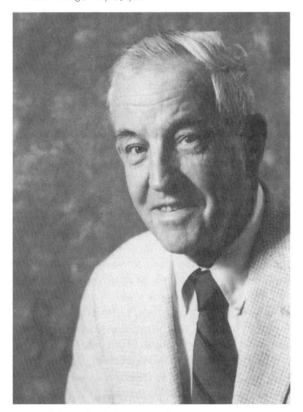

S. Ward Casscells, Wilmington, Delaware

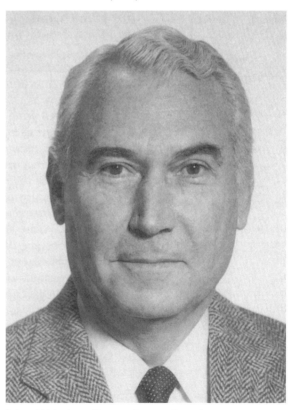

Robert W. Jackson, Toronto, Ontario, Canada

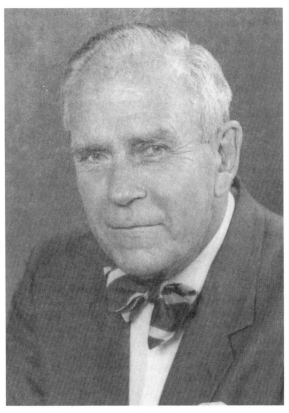

John J. Joyce, III, Philadelphia, Pennsylvania

The success of increasing numbers of surgeons with arthroscopic procedures inspired John Joyce to organize the International Arthroscopy Association in 1974 at a meeting in Philadelphia. The development of fiberoptic technology led to further improvement in arthroscope designs, providing better illumination and more durable instruments. O'Connor began to devise surgical techniques for the knee through an operating arthroscope that incorporated a channel for accessory instruments.[11] In the decade that followed, hundreds of orthopaedic surgeons around the world assimilated arthroscopy into their routine practices. Power instruments and miniaturized closed-circuit television cameras were developed for use in arthroscopic surgery.

Other joints began to be exposed by the magnification and illumination provided by arthroscopy. The improved precision and reduced morbidity of surgical procedures performed under arthroscopic control heralded a new era in orthopaedics. Minimally invasive surgical techniques have been responsible for earlier definitive treatment of many joint disorders, with the additional advantages of reduced cost and faster recuperation.

Arthroscopy has become an integral part of modern orthopaedic surgery. However, innovative arthroscopic procedures can be most successfully employed when practiced with a firm understanding of their subtle refinements, their limitations, and their risks. This text was inspired by the need for a comprehensive discourse on arthroscopy that is of practical clinical value. It should be a tribute to those pioneering surgeons who dared to do things a little bit differently . . . a little bit better.

REFERENCES

1. Watanabe M, Takeda S, Ikeuchi H. Atlas of arthroscopy. 2nd ed. Tokyo: Igakui-Shoin, 1969.
2. Bircher E. Die Arthroendoskopie. Zentralbl Chir 1921;14:1460.
3. Kreuscher PH. Semilunar cartilage disease, a plan for early recognition by means of the arthroscope and early treatment of this condition. Illinois Medical Journal 1925;47:290.
4. Burman MS. Arthroscopy, a direct visualization of joints: an experimental cadaver study. J Bone Joint Surg [Am] 1931;13(4):669.
5. Finkelstein H, Mayer L. The arthroscope, a new method of examining joints. J Bone Joint Surg [Am] 1931;13:583.
6. Joyce JJ III. History of arthroscopy. In: O'Connor RL, ed. Arthroscopy. Kalamazoo: Upjohn, 1977:11.
7. Casscells SW. Arthroscopy of the knee joint, a review of 150 cases. J Bone Joint Surg [Am] 1971;53:287.
8. Jackson RW, Abe I. The role of arthroscopy in the management of disorders of the knee: an analysis of 200 consecutive examinations. J Bone Joint Surg [Br] 1972;54:310.
9. O'Connor RL. The arthroscope in the management of crystal-induced synovitis of the knee. J Bone Joint Surg [Am] 1973;55:1443.
10. O'Connor RL. Arthroscopy in the diagnosis and treatment of acute ligament injuries of the knee. J Bone Joint Surg [Am] 1974;56(2):333.
11. Watanabe M, Bechtol RC, Nottage WM. History of arthroscopic surgery. In: Shahriaree H, ed. O'Connor textbook of arthroscopic surgery. Philadelphia: JB Lippincott, 1984:1.

Section One

Basics of Ankle Arthroscopy

Arthroscopic Surgery: The Foot and Ankle,
by Richard D. Ferkel.
Lippincott-Raven Publishers, Philadelphia © 1996.

1

Historical Developments

Richard D. Ferkel

*I*nterest in ankle arthroscopy has steadily increased following successful clinical experience with arthroscopy of the knee and shoulder. This rapid rise in the popularity of foot and ankle arthroscopy is partly because other noninvasive techniques cannot adequately diagnose disorders in this joint, particularly soft-tissue lesions. The advantages of arthroscopy in the foot and ankle are similar to those for other joints, including minimal incisions, outpatient surgery, decreased surgical morbidity, faster recovery, and earlier return to functional activities than with open surgical procedures. As surgical experience increases and technology and instrumentation improve, the diagnostic and surgical indications for foot and ankle arthroscopy are increasing.

The history of foot and ankle arthroscopy is relatively short, and there is a paucity of historical documentation. In 1931, Burman, from the Hospital for Joint Diseases, reported on his arthroscopic investigation on small joints in cadavers.[1] He used an endoscope 3.0 mm in diameter; the total outside diameter of the sheath was 4.0 mm. Due to the size of the arthroscope used, only the shoulder and elbow joints were accessible for examination in living patients. After visualizing the ankle in a cadaver, he was quite pessimistic, stating that the ankle joint was unsuitable for arthroscopy because the joint space was too narrow, the joint surface could not be manually separated, and a posterior puncture was not feasible.

In 1939, Takagi described six arthroscopic procedures in joints other than the knee: four hip, one shoulder, and one ankle (flail joint). He worked extensively on designing different types of instrumentation and used a #11 arthroscope with a diameter of 2.7 mm.[2,3] For many years, Watanabe attempted to develop an arthroscope of extremely small gauge to meet small joint requirements and improve picture quality. All efforts were unsuccessful until 1968, when a new light-transmitting material, Selfoc, was developed jointly by the Nippon Sheet Glass Company, Osaka, and the Nippon Electric Company, Tokyo. Selfoc, a brand name meaning self-focusing, was first developed as a laser beam-transmitting material. Using this material, Watanabe in 1970 developed an arthroscope for small joints with a Selfoc glass rod, and ultimately produced a 1.7-mm arthroscope

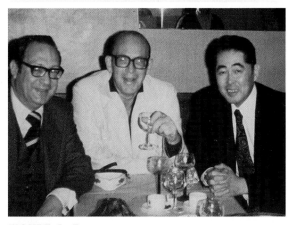

FIGURE 1-1.

Dr. James Guhl (*left*), Dr. Richard O'Connor, and Dr. Hiroshi Ikeuchi (*right*) pioneered the use of arthroscopy, with Ikeuchi and Guhl leading the way in arthroscopy of the ankle. (Courtesy of James F. Guhl, MD.)

many, also described his experience with arthroscopy of the ankle in 1978.[7] In the 1980s, several investigators reported their experience with arthroscopy of the ankle[8-12] (Fig. 1-1).

As experience with ankle arthroscopy increased, the indications evolved to include more technically demanding procedures. To operate in the central and posterior ankle, some type of distraction device was necessary. Skeletal distraction was tried in the early 1980s using external fixation devices and the Henning distractor.[13] In 1987, Guhl introduced a skeletal distraction device with pins in the tibia and calcaneus. Simultaneously, small-joint arthroscopes and instrumentation were developed (Fig. 1-2). The combination of skeletal distraction and smaller instrumentation made visualization easier, safer, and more complete. Although skeletal (invasive) distraction has been shown to be effective, there are potential risks. In 1988, Yates and Grana described their technique for noninvasive distraction[14] (Fig. 1-3). Since then, a number of straps have been developed that use a clove hitch-type apparatus to grasp the foot and heel and allow a force to be attached.

In 1988, the first textbook on ankle arthroscopy, by James Guhl, discussed the current status of both diagnostic and therapeutic uses.[13] With the advent of better small-joint arthroscopes and instrumentation, and the introduction of more efficient noninvasive distraction devices, ankle arthroscopy has developed to the current state presented in this text. Numerous

with a 55° to 70° viewing angle.[4] Watanabe named his #24 arthroscope the Selfoscope, and between 1970 and 1972 he examined 28 ankles and three metatarsophalangeal joints of the foot. In 1972, he published his experience, describing the anteromedial, anterolateral, and posterolateral portals and the arthroscopic findings in the ankle.

Further reports on ankle arthroscopy by Chen[5] and Ikeuchi[6] emphasized the techniques as well as indications and complications. Plank, from Ger-

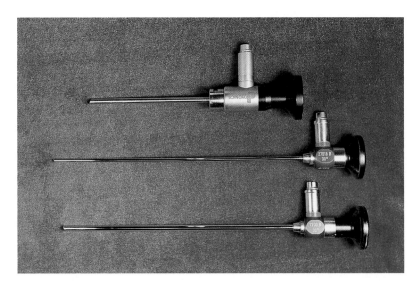

FIGURE 1-2.

Standard 4.0-mm 30° arthroscopes used in the knee and shoulder, compared with a customized short 4.0-mm 30° arthroscope used in the early phases of ankle arthroscopy by the author.

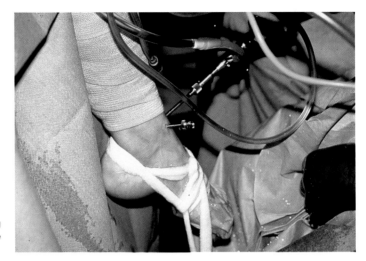

FIGURE 1-3.
Yates-Grana method of noninvasive distraction using a Kerlex loop wrapped around the patient's ankle and foot. (Courtesy of Carlin Yates, MD.)

symposia and courses have been offered to teach the orthopedist current techniques and methods.

ADVANTAGES AND DISADVANTAGES

Arthroscopy of the foot and ankle allows direct visualization of all intraarticular structures without the need for an extensive surgical approach or a malleolar osteotomy. Direct inspection of the ankle permits the best assessment of articular surface changes and pathologic conditions. In addition, the surrounding synovial and ligamentous structures can be clearly assessed using an arthroscopic approach. Intraoperative stress testing can be done while visualizing the specific sites of laxity. A multitude of surgical procedures may be performed using arthroscopic techniques, including biopsy, debridement, synovectomy, loose body removal, and "plastic" procedures. The postoperative advantages have been mentioned above.

Disadvantages of foot and ankle arthroscopy are similar to those of arthroscopy of other joints. These include the potential for complications (see Chap. 15), the need for special equipment and operating personnel, a high likelihood for equipment failure, and expense.

INDICATIONS

Foot and ankle arthroscopy is a valuable adjuvant to the diagnosis and treatment of certain disorders of the foot and ankle, and the indications for this proce-

dure continue to increase. The diagnostic indications include unexplained pain, swelling, stiffness, instability, hemarthrosis, locking, and popping. The therapeutic indications for foot and ankle arthroscopy include articular injury, soft-tissue injury, bony impingement, arthrofibrosis, fracture, synovitis, loose

TABLE 1-1.
PREOPERATIVE DIAGNOSES

Osteochondral lesion of talus	127 (23.5%)
Impingement	115 (21.3%)
Chondromalacia	43 (7.9%)
Instability	39 (7.2%)
Degenerative joint disease	39 (7.2%)
Acute fracture	35 (6.5%)
Fibrosis	26 (4.8%)
Adhesions	25 (4.6%)
Loose bodies	20 (3.7%)
Osteophyte(s)	19 (3.5%)
Synovitis	18 (3.3%)
Ossicles	14 (2.6%)
Torn ATFL	5 (0.9%)
Pain, unknown etiology	5 (0.9%)
Cyst	4 (0.7%)
Chondral fracture	3 (0.7%)
Osteophyte & loose body	2 (0.4%)
Subluxation of peroneal tendon	1 (0.2%)
Torn peroneal tendon	1 (0.2%)
Total	541

TABLE 1-2.

PRIMARY PROCEDURES

Debride lateral gutter	118 (21.8%)
Excision OLT/TM drilling	105 (19.4%)
Chondroplasty	72 (13.3%)
Excision of scar bands	37 (6.8%)
Removal of loose bodies	31 (5.7%)
Excision of fracture	29 (5.3%)
Diagnostic arthroscopy	27 (5.0%)
Synovectomy	23 (4.3%)
Excision of osteophyte(s)	23 (4.3%)
Transmalleolar drilling OLT	18 (3.3%)
Lysis adhesions	17 (3.1%)
Removal of ossicle(s)	14 (2.6%)
Arthrodesis	14 (2.6%)
Pin fracture	8 (1.5%)
Stabilization	3 (0.6%)
Cyst	2 (0.4%)
Total	541

bodies, osteophytes, and osteochondral defects. Depending on the patient and the specific condition involved, arthroscopy may also be indicated in ankle stabilization and arthrodesis.

Despite the advantages of direct visualization of the foot and ankle joints, arthroscopy should not take the place of careful conservative management. This includes the use of physiotherapy, ankle supports, anti-inflammatories, injections, and cast immobilization when indicated. With good conservative care, most foot and ankle conditions resolve without further treatment. Arthroscopy should also not preempt the use of carefully selected diagnostic procedures and good clinical judgment.

CONTRAINDICATIONS

The relative contraindications for foot and ankle arthroscopy include moderate degenerative joint disease with restricted range of motion, a significantly reduced joint space, severe edema, and tenuous vascular status. The absolute contraindications for foot and ankle arthroscopy include localized soft-tissue infection and severe degenerative joint disease. With severe joint space narrowing, it is difficult to achieve successful distraction and adequate range of motion for joint visualization. A localized soft-tissue infection is an absolute contraindication because of the potential for dissemination of localized infection intraarticularly and, thus, development of septic arthritis. However, if septic arthritis is already present, foot and ankle arthroscopy is indicated, as it is a useful tool for drainage, debridement, and lavage of the joint.

PREFERRED TREATMENT

Using the techniques that appear in the following chapters, about 541 cases of foot and ankle arthroscopy have been performed from 1984 through 1994. The primary preoperative diagnoses for these cases are listed in Table 1-1, and the primary procedure performed is listed in Table 1-2.

REFERENCES

1. Burman MS. Arthroscopy or the direct visualization of joints. J Bone Joint Surg 1931;13:669.
2. Takagi K. The arthroscope. J Jap Orthop Assn 1939a;14:359.
3. Takagi K. The arthroscope: the second report. J Jap Orthop Assn 1939b;14:441.
4. Watanabe M, Takeda S, Ikeuchi H, Sakakibara J. Development of the Selfoc arthroscope. J Jap Orthop Assn 1972;46:154.
5. Chen YC. Clinical and cadaver studies on the ankle joint arthroscopy. J Jap Orthop Assn 1976;50:631.
6. Ikeuchi H. Arthroscopy of the ankle joint. Presented at International Arthroscopy Association Meeting, 1977.
7. Plank E. Die Arthroskopie des oberen sprunggelenkes. Helfe sur Unfallheinkunde 131:245, 1978.
8. Andrews JR, Previte WJ, Carson WG. Arthroscopy of the ankle: technique and normal anatomy. Foot Ankle 1985;6:29.
9. Drez D, Guhl JF, Gollehon DL. Ankle arthroscopy: technique and indications. Foot Ankle 1981;2:138.
10. Parisien JS. Diagnostic and operative arthroscopy of the ankle: technique and indications. Bull Hosp Jt Dis Orthop Inst 1985;45:38.
11. Johnson LL. Arthroscopic surgery: principles and practice, 3d ed. St. Louis: CV Mosby, 1986:1517.

12. Ferkel RD, Fischer SP. Progress in ankle arthroscopy. Clin Orthop 1989;240:210.
13. Guhl JF. Ankle arthroscopy: pathology and surgical techniques. Thorofare, NJ: Slack, 1988.
14. Yates CK, Grana WA. A simple distraction technique for ankle arthroscopy. Arthroscopy 1988;4:103.

BIBLIOGRAPHY

Lundeen GW. Historical perspectives of ankle arthroscopy. J Foot Surg 1987;26:3.
Watanabe M. Arthroscopy of small joints. Tokyo: Igaku-Shoin, 1985.

Arthroscopic Surgery: The Foot and Ankle,
by Richard D. Ferkel.
Lippincott-Raven Publishers, Philadelphia © 1996.

2

Preoperative Evaluation and Imaging

Richard D. Ferkel, Mark Schweitzer, and Sevil K. Brahme

*T*he ankle and foot are complex structures composed of multiple joints and anatomic structures. Evaluation of the ankle and foot requires a thorough knowledge of the intra- and extraarticular anatomy, normal variants, kinesiology, and imaging appearance. It is important to be able to separate normal from abnormal complaints and findings, and to understand how the ankle and foot relate to the rest of the body.

The most important methods of evaluation are a careful history and a physical examination. Plain radiographs are then obtained and a preliminary diagnosis is made. Sometimes the diagnosis is not obvious, and various etiologies must be considered in the differential diagnosis. In these cases, additional diagnostic tests may be necessary. Many different tests are useful in the ankle and foot, but they must be used judiciously and a "shotgun" approach avoided (Table 2-1). A keen understanding of the indications and limitations of each test is mandatory for cost-effectiveness; they vary from case to case.

HISTORY

The most common complaints or symptoms patients note in the ankle and foot include one or more of the following: pain, swelling, locking, catching, grinding, loss of motion, giving way, deformity, numbness, or tingling. It is important to note when the pain started and how long the pain has been present. If an accident or injury was involved, the mechanism of injury must be identified. The patient should be asked what brings on the symptoms, how long they last, and what relieves them. Sometimes ankle and foot symptomatology is associated with symptoms in other areas of the body, and this should be sought. If the patient is on medication or using braces, supports, or orthotics, this should be noted in relation to his or her complaints.

A history of current shoe wear is important, because often new shoes

TABLE 2-1.
DIAGNOSTIC TESTING OF THE FOOT AND ANKLE

- History
- Physical examination
- Plain x-rays
- Harris mat imprints
- Gait analysis
- Selective injections
- Fluoroscopic examination
- Arthrography
- Technetium-99 and gallium bone scan
- CT
- MRI
- Cine-MRI
- Arthroscopy

are associated with certain types of ankle and foot complaints, or can contribute to the symptoms with certain activities. A complete medical history is necessary, because some ankle and foot conditions are related to systemic diseases or conditions in other parts of the body. Moreover, the family history may detect certain congenital abnormalities that cause similar complaints from generation to generation.

The most important complaint in the ankle and foot is pain. Localizing the pain to a specific area helps to narrow the diagnosis. Acute pain must be differentiated from chronic pain. Using the questions mentioned above, a differential diagnosis can be developed, and in many cases a definitive diagnosis made. A detailed differential diagnosis of pain in the ankle and foot is beyond the scope of this chapter, and the reader is referred elsewhere for a detailed list.[1]

Pain, mechanical blockage, muscle/tendon problems, scarring at the joint, and nerve injury can all cause loss of motion. In addition, swelling can be either localized or generalized, painful or nonpainful, and related to activity.

Locking can be due to acute pain, swelling, loose bodies, tendon subluxation, ligamentous injury, or osteoarthritic formation. Although "locking" and "catching" represent different sensations and are usually caused by different pathologies, the patient may use the terms interchangeably.

Patients often complain of popping around the joint, midfoot, or forefoot. These sounds are usually normal but must be investigated if they continue or suggest intraarticular damage. It is not uncommon for the peroneal tendons to click or pop, particularly in hyperlax patients, or for the extensor tendons to cause similar problems. In a dancer, however, persistent popping or catching on the medial side of the foot may suggest a tenosynovitis of the flexor hallucis longus or "hallux saltans". Deformities about the ankle and foot are usually congenital, insidious, or traumatic in origin. Only when the patient becomes symptomatic is the deformity noted, although it may have been present for a long time. Such is the case with pain over "pump bumps" or in the area of the accessory navicular, and occasionally over the base of the fifth metatarsal.

Numbness and tingling may represent either localized nerve entrapment or referred pain from a nerve injury more proximally or along the spine.

PHYSICAL EXAMINATION

Standing Examination

To avoid overlooking pertinent findings, the physical examination of the ankle and foot is both tedious and demanding. Each examiner may develop a specific routine, and the exact sequence of the examination is not critical. However, each area must be carefully evaluated and the entire examination must be integrated with the history. According to Mann and Coughlin, the examiner must consider the foot and ankle from three different points of view: first, as parts of the entire body; second, as important constituents of the locomotor system; and third, as relatively recent evolutionary acquisitions and, thus, subject to various individual anatomic and functional variations.[2]

Every ankle and foot examination should include inspection, palpation, and manipulation. The sequence varies for walking, standing, or sitting, and also varies with and without shoes.

The initial examination should include an assessment of the patient's gait with and without shoes, noting any limp, asymmetry of the arm swing, degree of toeing in and out, and the amount of excessive pronation or supination. The gait should be analyzed as to normal amount of stance and swing phase; the phase in which the gait abnormalities occur should be noted.

The patient's shoes should be inspected for the

type worn, asymmetry of wear, and any pads, lifts, or orthotics present. Walking should be assessed, as well as the ability to go up on tiptoes and heels while standing and walking, as well as hopping and squatting. Then the shape of the foot is evaluated. Usually the dorsum of the foot makes a dome, secondary to the medial longitudinal arch (Fig. 2-1). The arch can be unusually high (pes cavus) or diminished (pes planus; Fig. 2-2).

The alignment of the calf to the hindfoot is also carefully evaluated. Excessive hindfoot valgus with prominence of the medial part of the foot may suggest rupture of the posterior tibial tendon. This can be confirmed by the presence of a positive "too many toe" sign and inability of the patient to go up on his or her tiptoes on the affected side (see Fig. 2-2C). The windlass action of the foot is also evaluated. Normally, dorsiflexion in the toes increases the tension of the plantar aponeurosis, which causes the longitudinal arch to rise. Failure of the longitudinal arch to rise suggests prolonged pes planus, with abnormal stretching and elongation of the plantar aponeurosis (Fig. 2-3).

With the patient standing, a careful assessment is made of the alignment of the hip to the knees to the ankle. A patient with "malicious malalignment" has a combination of abnormalities that contribute to pain about the hip, knee, and ankle (Fig. 2-4). When appropriate, pelvic tilt and lower back abnormalities should also be assessed.

Seated Examination

Once the patient has been carefully evaluated in the standing position, he or she is then examined seated.

Ankle

The ankle is initially evaluated visually for swelling or edema. The examiner should note whether the swelling appears to be intra- or extraarticular and whether it is anterior, posterior, medial, or lateral.

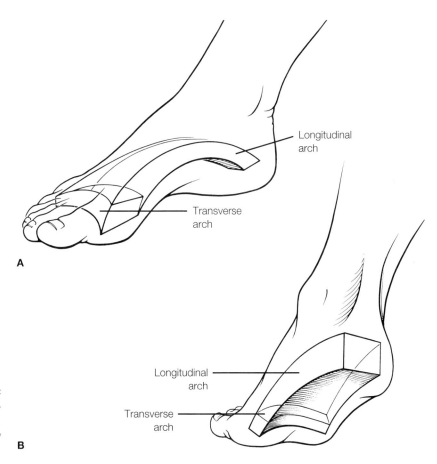

FIGURE 2-1.
Longitudinal arch. (**A**) Lateral view of medial longitudinal arch. (**B**) Posterior view of medial longitudinal arch. Note the transverse arch provided by the metatarsal heads.

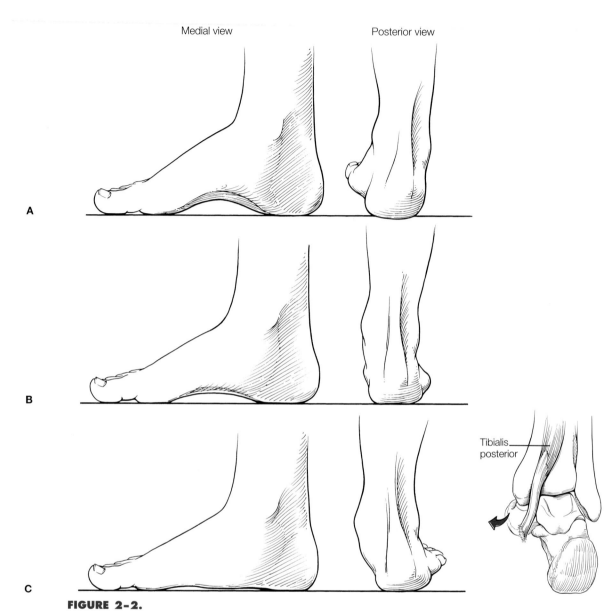

FIGURE 2-2.

Arch types. (**A**) Cavus foot, with elevation of the medial longitudinal arch and a slight hindfoot varus. (**B**) Normal arch. (**C**) Pes planus, with loss of the medial longitudinal arch and hindfoot valgus. From the posterior view, the "too many toe" sign can be noted secondary to a rupture of the posterior tibial tendon.

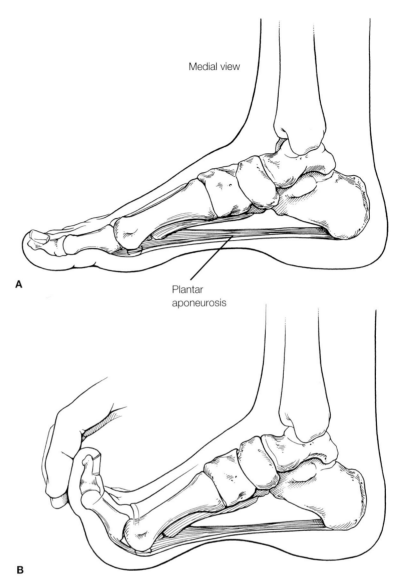

Medial view

Plantar
aponeurosis

A

FIGURE 2-3.
Windlass mechanism. (**A**) Normal position
of plantar aponeurosis. (**B**) Dorsiflexion with
the toes increases the tension on the plantar
aponeurosis, which causes the longitudinal
arch to rise.

B

Palpation should be done carefully to detect areas of specific pain about the ankle. After a chronic ankle sprain, there is sometimes pain along the lateral portion of the ankle and foot. It is important to pinpoint the exact location of the pain, including whether it is at the syndesmosis, over the lateral gutter and anterior talofibular ligament, or at the sinus tarsi (Fig. 2-5). Sometimes there is pain in all areas. Posterior ankle pain is sometimes difficult to elicit on examination, and a high index of suspicion is necessary to rule out posteromedial osteochondral lesions and to differentiate them from injuries to the Stieda process or the os trigonum. Attachments of all the ligaments about the ankle should be carefully palpated, including the deltoid, the anterior and posterior inferior tibiofibular ligaments, the anterior and posterior talofibular ligaments, and the calcaneofibular ligaments.

Range of Motion

The range of motion of the ankle joint is assessed passively and actively (Fig. 2-6*A*). It is important to compare one side to the other to detect subtle losses in motion and to determine whether an abnormality exists. In the elderly, physiologic limitation of plantarflexion may be present; it is usually of no clinical significance.[3] However, limitation of any dorsiflex-

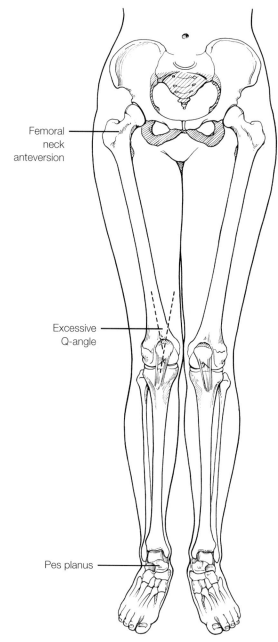

FIGURE 2-4.
''Malicious malalignment'' syndrome. The combination of increased Q-angles of the knee, hindfoot and forefoot valgus, and femoral neck anteversion contribute to this problem.

Femoral neck anteversion

Excessive Q-angle

Pes planus

ion is usually significant. Loss of dorsiflexion of more than 10° should be assessed with the knee in both extension and flexion. If dorsiflexion in the ankle is significantly increased by flexion in the knee, a shortened gastrocnemius is diagnosed because this muscle crosses the knee joint, whereas the soleus does not. In this case, flexing the knee should relax the tight gastrocnemius and allow more ankle dorsiflexion. If knee flexion does not improve dorsiflexion, it may be due to contracture of the soleus or gastrocnemius, or both. Ankle dorsiflexion can also be limited secondary to arthrofibrosis, posterior ankle capsular contraction, previous trauma, and osteophytes of the distal tibia and talus (see Fig. 2-6*B*). Ankle plantarflexion can be limited by a ruptured Achilles tendon, arthrofibrosis, and rupture of the posterior tibial tendon (see Fig. 2-6*C*).

The dorsum of the foot fits into a socket or mortise formed superiorly by the tibia and laterally by the fibula. Because the talus is wider anteriorly, it is held tightly between the malleoli when the ankle is dorsiflexed. However, when the ankle is plantarflexed, the narrower posterior aspect lies between the malleoli, and there is some mild degree of lateral mobility (Fig. 2-7). Dorsiflexion may be diminished or restricted when the wider anterior part of the talus no longer fits easily into the mortise. This is the case when the intermalleolar distance has been narrowed secondary to persistent equinus of the foot or after fractures or other trauma. Dorsiflexion can also be restricted with incongruity of the mortise after trauma (Fig. 2-8). Moreover, active dorsiflexion may be limited by weakness of the extensor tendons and, in some cases, a ruptured anterior tibial tendon may be missed if a careful assessment of ankle dorsiflexion by the extensor hallucis longus is not made.

Ligament Testing

The anterior talofibular ligament is best tested with the foot in a plantarflexed position. In this position, inversion stress testing of the hindfoot will demonstrate any laxity present in the anterior talofibular ligament (Fig. 2-9). When the foot is dorsiflexed, the calcaneofibular ligament is placed on stretch, and with inversion stress testing, the laxity of this ligament may be noted. With a tear of both the anterior talofibular and calcaneofibular

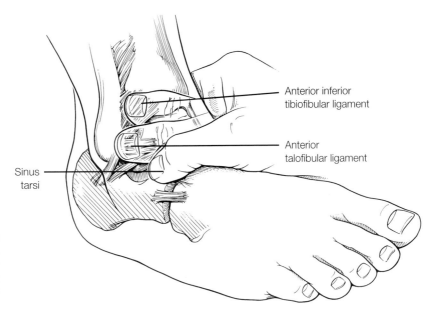

Anterior inferior
tibiofibular ligament

Anterior
talofibular ligament

Sinus
tarsi

FIGURE 2-5.
Pain in the lateral aspect of the ankle can cause confusion as to its origin. The pain can occur at the syndesmosis (*top thumb*), the anterior talofibular ligament (*middle thumb*), or the subtalar joint (*lower thumb*).

ligaments, a "double ligament tear," talar tilt will occur in dorsi- and plantarflexion (see Fig. 2-9).

The anterior drawer test is an important test for ligamentous laxity and is performed with the ankle held at 90° and the calcaneus pulled anteriorly and slightly internally, while the examiner's other hand holds the distal tibia (Fig. 2-10). An appreciation for the amount of forward motion of the talus in relation to the tibia and talus is important. Anterior motion of more than 3 to 4 mm usually indicates laxity and injury in the anterior talofibular ligament. An increased anterior drawer suggests a double ligament tear (see Fig. 2-10).

It is always important with inversion stress testing and anterior drawer testing to compare the findings with the asymptomatic opposite side. Mann and Coughlin have noted a variation of the anterior drawer sign that may be useful to determine how much internal rotation occurs when the lateral aspect of the foot is grasped with one hand and the other hand is placed on the distal tibia, while palpating the articulation between the lateral articular surface of the talus and the anterior aspect of the distal fibula.[2] This is done with the ankle in neutral position. Pulling forward on the forefoot while internally rotating sometimes demonstrates a rotatory laxity as a result of an injury to the anterior talofibular ligament.

Injuries to the syndesmosis are often underestimated or overlooked by orthopedists and nonorthopedists alike. Although not entirely clear, the mechanism of injury appears to be primarily an external rotation injury, although hyperdorsiflexion has been reported to lead to tears of the syndesmosis as well. Diagnosis is made by palpating directly over the syndesmosis more proximally along the interosseous membrane. The "squeeze test" is performed by compressing the fibula to the tibia above the midportion of the calf; the test is considered positive when proximal compression produces distal pain in the area of the torn interosseous membrane and syndesmotic ligament (Fig. 2-11). The "external rotation stress test" is also useful in diagnosing syndesmotic ankle sprains and is performed by applying external rotational stress to the foot and ankle with the knee bent in 90° of flexion and the ankle in neutral position (Fig. 2-12). A positive test produces pain over the anterior or posterior inferior tibiofibular ligament(s) and over the interosseous membrane. The third test is displacement of the fibula at the syndesmosis itself. The fibula sits in a groove on the lateral border of the tibia, but the anterior lip of the tibial groove is more prominent than the posterior lip. Therefore, even in a normal ankle, anterior fibular displacement is difficult, but posterior displacement

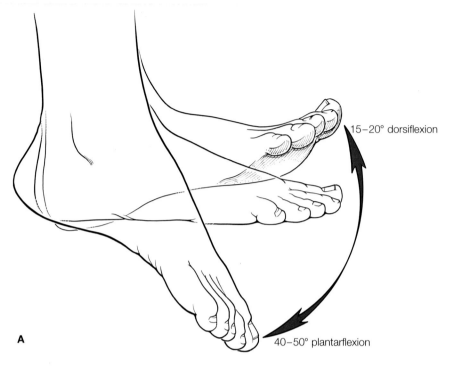

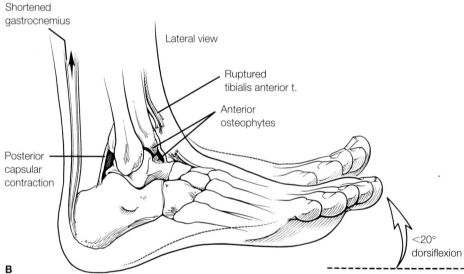

FIGURE 2-6.

Ankle range of motion. (**A**) Dorsiflexion and plantarflexion of the ankle. (**B**) Loss of dorsiflexion secondary to anterior osteophytes, posterior capsular contraction, shortened gastrocnemius, or ruptured anterior tibial tendon. (**C**) Loss of plantarflexion secondary to ruptured posterior tibialis or Achilles, or arthrofibrosis of the ankle.

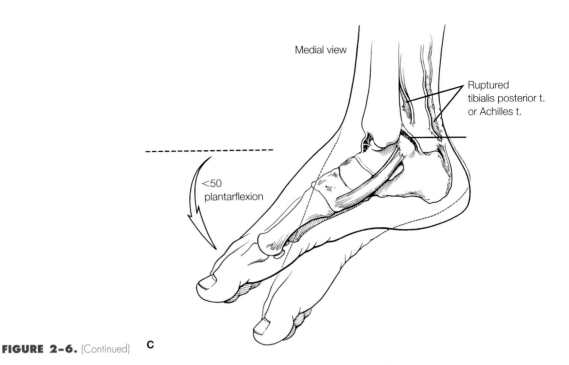

FIGURE 2-6. (Continued) **C**

can often be palpated. In the ankle with an injured syndesmosis, this posterior displacement may be increased and can elicit pain.

Muscle function about the ankle should be carefully assessed. It is important to determine the strength of each muscle and to palpate the tendon to ensure one muscle is not compensating for another. Usually this is fairly easy, except in cases of injuries to the anterior and posterior tibial tendons. A strong extensor hallucis longus can com-

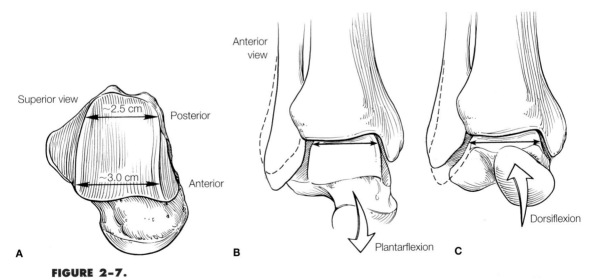

FIGURE 2-7.
Ankle excursion. (**A**) The width of the talus. The anterior talus is wider than the posterior portion. (**B**) When the ankle is plantarflexed, the narrower posterior talus lies between the malleoli, and some degree of lateral mobility exists. (**C**) With ankle dorsiflexion, the talus is held tightly between the malleoli.

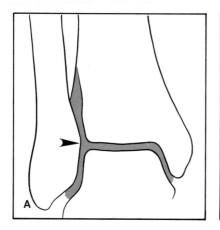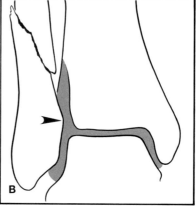

FIGURE 2-8.
Ankle mortise incongruity. (**A**) Normal ankle mortise. (**B**) After a fracture, there is a widened medial clear-space and shortening of the lateral malleolus, recognized radiologically as a stepoff in the alignment of the subchondral plates of the tibia and of the lateral malleolus.

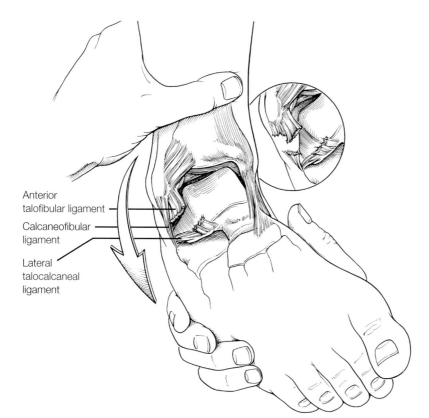

Anterior talofibular ligament

Calcaneofibular ligament

Lateral talocalcaneal ligament

FIGURE 2-9.
Inversion stress test. A single ligament tear allows increased talar tilt (*inset*). A double ligament tear leads to significant talar tilt with inversion stress.

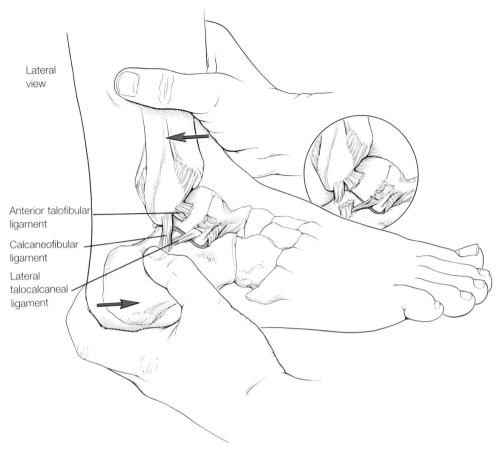

Lateral
view

Anterior talofibular
ligament

Calcaneofibular
ligament

Lateral
talocalcaneal
ligament

FIGURE 2-10.
Anterior drawer test. With the tibia secured, the heel is pulled forward and internally rotated. Note the subluxation of the talus anteriorly on the distal tibia (*inset*). A double ligament tear leads to increased anterior excursion of the talus on the tibia.

pensate for the anterior tibial tendon, and this tendon action must be eliminated to assess the anterior tibial tendon accurately.

Heel and Heel Cord

Varus or valgus deformities of the heel should be noted. The most common cause of heel pain is plantar fasciitis, which will elicit point tenderness along the medial calcaneal tuberosity (Fig. 2-13*A*). This pain can be due to multiple causes, including systemic diseases such as rheumatoid arthritis or Reiter syndrome, or nerve entrapment (see Fig. 2-13*B*). Tenderness in the retrocalcaneal bursa can be associated with inflammation of the Achilles tendon or isolated

bursal inflammation posterior to the ankle joint. Heel cord shortening was discussed in the ankle section. However, Achilles tendon problems are common and can be classified as inflammation of the peritenon, tendinosis, or partial or complete tears. A nodular thickening may be present in patients with chronic tendinosis or partial Achilles tears. Ruptures of the Achilles tendon are usually obvious and confirmed by a positive Thompson test. Tenderness along the painful thickening of the posterior-superior portion of the os calcis overlying the Achilles tendon is often found, especially in females ("pump bumps"), and is associated with palpable soft-tissue thickening. Achilles tendon pain must be differentiated from ankle pain and synovitis.

verse tarsal joint, in the other, and bringing the subtalar joint into both inversion and eversion (Fig. 2-14). The most accurate method of determining subtalar motion is to place the patient prone and flex the knee to 135°.[2] If motion is limited and considerable pain occurs on passive motion along with spasm, subtalar pathology should be suspected. Usually this is associated with tenderness along the sinus tarsi and posterior talocalcaneal joint, and occasionally tenderness along the medial portion of the subtalar joint. If loss of subtalar motion is detected, the examiner should consider the possibility of an arthritic process in the subtalar joint, peroneal spastic flatfoot, or an anatomic abnormality such as tarsal coalition.

Muscle function about the subtalar joint should also be carefully assessed. Posterior tibial tendon function may be difficult to differentiate from the anterior tibial tendon when checking inversion. The posterior tibial tendon can usually be assessed by palpation with the patient actively inverting the foot in plantarflexion. The tendon can also be checked by placing the foot into an everted position and then asking the patient to invert against some resistance (Fig. 2-15). Weakness of the peroneal tendons may be confusing because the peroneal brevis muscle everts the foot and the peroneal longus brings about plantarflexion of the medial border of the foot but can only weakly evert the foot. To test the peroneal longus, the patient should plantarflex the medial side of the foot and the examiner should resist beneath the first metatarsal head.

Tendinitis of the flexor hallucis longus tendon behind the medial malleolus is so common in dancers that it is known as "dancer's tendinitis." This condition can be misdiagnosed as Achilles or posterior tibial tendinitis if the examiner is not careful to find the exact location of the pain. The flexor hallucis longus tendon is injured as it passes through the fibro-osseous tunnel from the posterior aspect of the talus to the level of the sustentaculum tali, and acts like a rope through a pulley. When injured, it begins to bind and a nodular partial tear may be present, causing triggering of the big toe or so-called "hallux saltans"[5] (Fig. 2-16).

Transverse Tarsal Joint

The motion of the transverse tarsal joint can be determined by holding the calcaneus in line with the long axis of the tibia and the forefoot parallel to

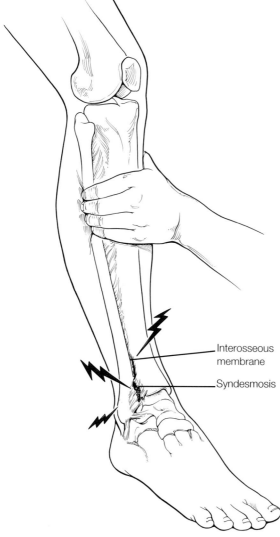

Interosseous membrane

Syndesmosis

FIGURE 2-11.
The squeeze test is performed by compressing the fibula to the tibia at the midportion of the calf. With a tear of the interosseous membrane and syndesmotic ligament, pain occurs in the region distally.

Subtalar Joint

The subtalar joint can be a difficult area to examine and diagnose. The range of motion of the subtalar joint varies, but Isman and Inman, in a series of feet in cadaver specimens, found a minimum of 20° and a maximum of 60° motion.[4] Subtalar motion is tested by holding the calcaneus in one hand and the forefoot, including the trans-

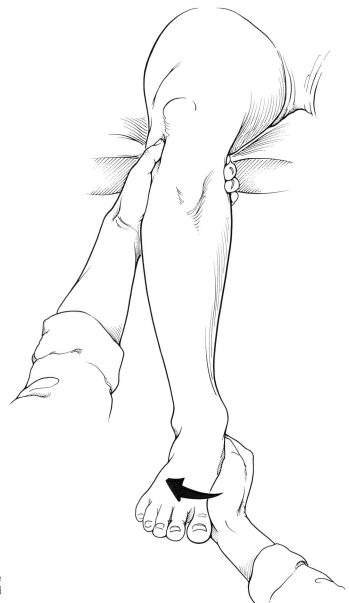

FIGURE 2-12.
The external rotation stress test produces pain over the anterior and posterior inferior tibiofibular ligaments and the interosseous membrane when positive.

the floor. Abduction and adduction are then determined and noted. There should be twice as much adduction as abduction of the forefoot. In conditions such as rupture of the posterior tibial tendon or degenerative arthritis of the midtarsal joints, a neutral position cannot be achieved because the foot is constantly maintained in a chronically abducted position. Involvement at one or more of the midtarsal joints is not uncommon and is isolated by local joint

pain and tenderness. Charcot disorder of the foot may also start in this area with palpable bony thickening.

Metatarsophalangeal Joints

Pain over the metatarsophalangeal joint of the great toe is usually due to either degenerative arthritis or a bunion-type deformity. The joint

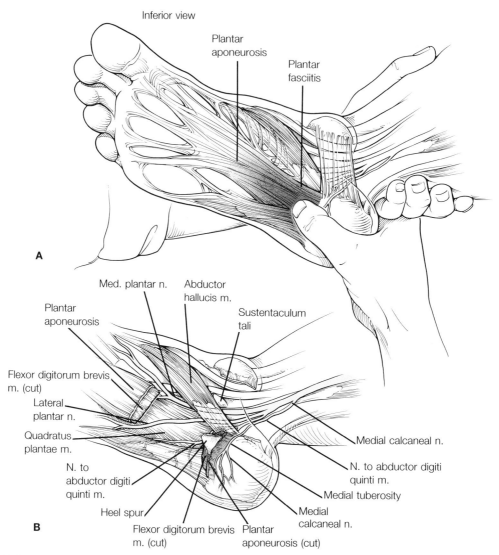

Inferior view

Plantar aponeurosis

Plantar fasciitis

A

Med. plantar n.

Abductor hallucis m.

Plantar aponeurosis

Sustentaculum tali

Flexor digitorum brevis m. (cut)

Lateral plantar n.

Quadratus plantae m.

N. to abductor digiti quinti m.

Heel spur

B

Flexor digitorum brevis m. (cut)

Plantar aponeurosis (cut)

Medial calcaneal n.

N. to abductor digiti quinti m.

Medial tuberosity

Medial calcaneal n.

Medial calcaneal n.

FIGURE 2-13.

Plantar fasciitis. (**A**) Palpation of the plantar fascia at the medial calcaneal tuberosity often elicits pain. (**B**) There are numerous causes for plantar heel pain, including entrapment of the medial or lateral plantar nerves; rarely is a calcaneal spur the source of pain.

should be palpated carefully for the presence of not only pain, but also synovitis or instability. The metatarsophalangeal joints of toes two through five should also be examined. Synovitis is often present in either the second or third metatarsophalangeal joints, and a Lachman-type maneuver at the metatarsophalangeal joint will demonstrate instability indicative of disruption of the plantar plate mechanism. The medial and lateral sesamoids should also be carefully checked beneath the first metatarsal head to rule out inflammation or fracture. Motion of the metatarsophalangeal joints is measured by placing the ankle at 90° and having the patient actively dorsi- and plantarflex at these joints and at the interphalangeal joints. Normal

(text continues on page 29)

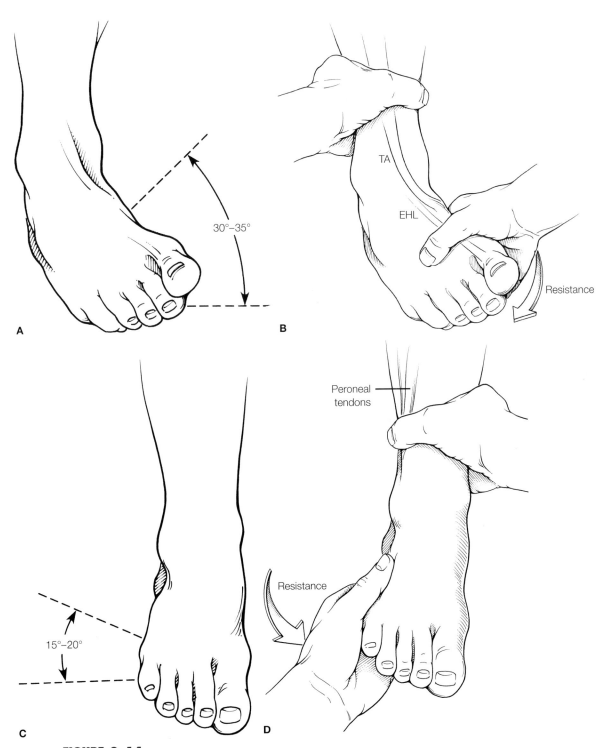

FIGURE 2-14.
Subtalar motion. (**A**) Inversion motion. (**B**) Inversion testing against resistance. (**C**) Eversion motion. (**D**) Eversion testing against resistance.

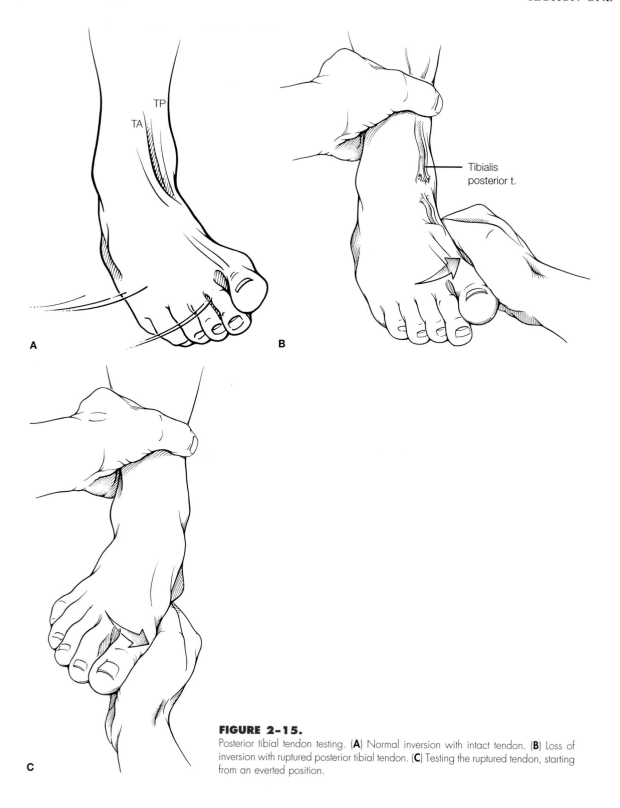

TP

TA

A

Tibialis posterior t.

B

C

FIGURE 2-15.
Posterior tibial tendon testing. (**A**) Normal inversion with intact tendon. (**B**) Loss of inversion with ruptured posterior tibial tendon. (**C**) Testing the ruptured tendon, starting from an everted position.

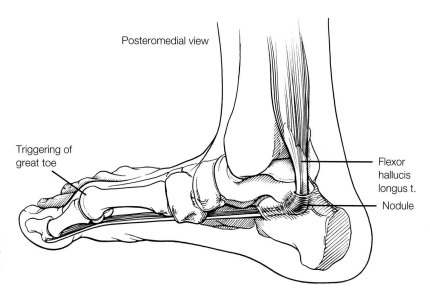

Posteromedial view

Triggering of
great toe

Flexor
hallucis
longus t.

Nodule

FIGURE 2-16.
Hallux saltans can develop from tendinitis of the flexor hallucis longus as it passes through the fibro-osseous tunnel on the medial side of the foot.

motion is 70° extension and 45° flexion (Fig. 2-17). Because there is much individual variability in motion, it is important to compare the normal to the abnormal side. Loss of motion of the great toe metatarsophalangeal joint is usually associated with degenerative joint disease and osteophyte formation, either traumatic or idiopathic in origin. Loss of motion of the interphalangeal joints may be secondary to synovitis, degenerative joint disease, Freiberg infarction, or instability.

The second metatarsal is relatively immobile and is usually the longest metatarsal. Therefore, if there is an abnormality of the first metatarsophalangeal joint such as a significant hallux valgus deformity or as a result of bunion surgery that produces shortening, dorsiflexion, or instability of the first metatarsophalangeal joint, a painful diffuse callus may develop beneath the second metatarsal. In contrast, the fourth metatarsal is the most mobile and is rarely associated with any significant pathologic condition.

Referred Pain

When examining the foot and ankle, all other joints in the lower extremity should also be carefully evaluated with a complete examination. Pathology in the lumbar back, hip, or knee may refer pain to the foot or ankle region. Symptoms of pain, numbness, weakness, and swelling can all be due to causes outside of the foot and ankle (Fig. 2-18).

RADIOLOGIC IMAGING

After a careful history and physical examination, radiologic evaluation is critical to the proper diagnosis and treatment of ankle and foot disorders. Over the

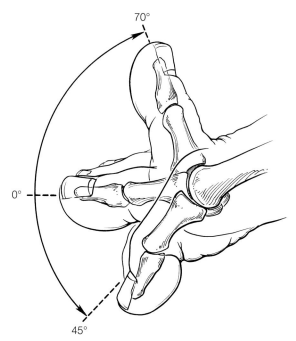

70°

0°

45°

FIGURE 2-17.
Extension and flexion of the great toe. With degenerative joint disease of this joint, motion is lost in both planes.

last 10 to 15 years, newer imaging techniques have given us the opportunity to better understand numerous pathologic disorders and sometimes to diagnose previously unknown conditions.[6]

Routine Radiography

At least two orthogonal radiographs should be performed. The anterior/posterior (AP) radiograph is the best overview of the ankle and is particularly valuable to verify that an intact distal tibiofibular joint is present (Fig. 2-19*A*). On the lateral view, the articular space between the talus and tibia is seen, as well as the articulation of the talus with the navicular and calcaneus (see Fig. 2-19*B*).

The ankle mortise is best evaluated by having the patient recumbent with the leg and foot rotated internally 20° or 30° (see Fig. 2-19*C*). If the radiograph is properly performed, the medial and lateral clear-spaces and the distal tibiofibular syndesmosis can be well seen and measured. The medial clear-space is the distance in millimeters between a line drawn tangentially to the medial articular margin of the talus and one drawn tangentially to the articular margin of the medial malleolus. The distance defines the integrity of the ankle mortise and is normally 2 to 3 mm. A medial clear-space of more than 3 to 4 mm is associated with ankle fractures or syndesmotic injuries in which the talus shifts laterally. This finding also indicates a rupture of the deltoid ligament.

Less common projections include the Harris-Beath view or the axial view of the calcaneus. This is useful for evaluating subtle calcaneal fractures, injuries to the subtalar joint, and talocalcaneal coalitions. The Broden view is helpful in visualizing the posterior facet of the subtalar, talofibular, and tibiofibular joints. Different portions of the subtalar joint can be seen depending on the tube angle. The Cobey view, used to evaluate the position of the calcaneus relative to the tibial axis and the ankle joint, is particularly helpful in looking at varus and valgus alignment.[7]

Weight-bearing AP and lateral views of the foot are routinely taken to evaluate foot disorders, and oblique x-rays are often helpful to better demonstrate the sinus tarsi, calcaneocuboid, and tarsometatarsal arrangements.

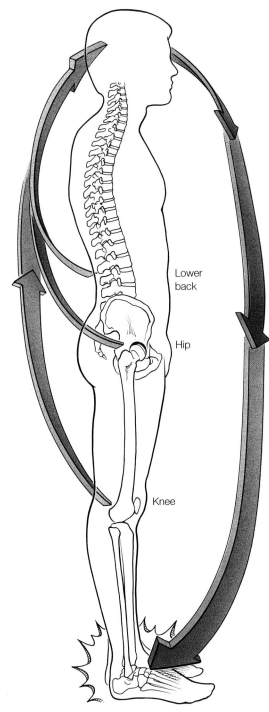

FIGURE 2-18.
Pain in the foot can be referred from the back, hip, or knee.

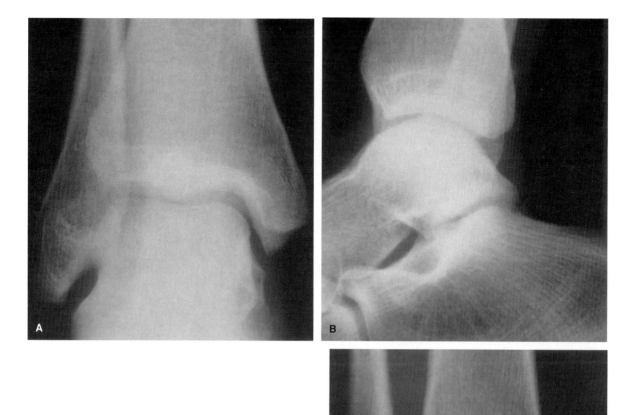

FIGURE 2-19.

Normal ankle x-rays. (**A**) Anterior/posterior view of the ankle. The medial clear-space is well seen with overlap of the fibula with the distal tibia and talus. (**B**) Lateral view of the ankle. Both the distal anterior and posterior portions of the tibia can clearly be seen, as can the space between the distal tibia and talus and subtalar joint. (**C**) Mortise view of the ankle. Normally, the medial clear-space measures 2 mm, as does the tibiofibular syndesmosis. The zone of rarefaction in the talus shows the posterior facet of the subtalar joint.

Stress Radiographs

Stress x-rays are used to evaluate ligamentous integrity about the ankle and subtalar regions. These x-rays may be done manually by the physician or an experienced assistant, or by a mechanical device or jig. Comparison x-rays are essential because there is a large variation in normal ligamentous laxity. To generate a reproducible amount of stress, the Telos device should be used[8] (Fig. 2-20). Its advantages include:

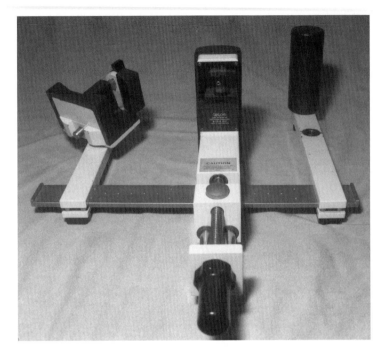

FIGURE 2-20.
Telos pressure bar with LED digital readout. Force is applied by rotating the handle of the shaft up to 20 kilopounds.

1. No radiation exposure to the examining physician
2. Reproducible patient motion
3. Gradual and accurate application of stress, which avoids muscle splinting
4. Reproducible fixation in 18° internal rotation to approximate the mortise view during stress.

Stress views are most useful for evaluating the lateral ligament complex. Plantarflexion/inversion stress is a better indicator of the integrity of the anterior talofibular ligament; dorsiflexion/inversion stress is best for testing the calcaneofibular ligament.[8] Sauser and coworkers, using the Telos device, found that a talar tilt of 10° or more was associated with a lateral ligament injury in 99% of cases.[9] Normal values for talar tilt reportedly range from 5° to 23°.[10] Chrisman and Snook noted when comparing both ankles that a difference of more than 10° was significant when measuring the anterior talofibular and calcaneofibular ligaments[11] (Fig. 2-21).

The anterior drawer stress test specifically tests the integrity of the anterior talofibular ligament and is the most reliable indicator of injury to it. Gould and colleagues found that an increase of 4 mm indicated instability in the anterior drawer test.[12] However, Laurin and associates considered an increase of more than 9 mm to be abnormal.[13] Overall values of up to 5 mm separation between the talus and distal tibia are considered normal, values of 5 to 10 mm are probably abnormal, and values over 10 mm are grossly abnormal. These measurements are best performed at the posterior aspect of the talar articular surface (Fig. 2-22).

Subtalar instability can also be tested with the Telos device. Although this is more difficult to diagnose, the stress x-ray can detect laxity in the joint when done properly (Fig. 2-23).

Tomography

In tomography, a focal point for each image is established and the structures anterior and posterior to this fulcrum are blurred out of focus by the movement of the x-ray tube and film in tandem. The tube and film can move in several different motions to optimize detail in different planes. Tomograms can be unidirectional (linear tomography) or pluridirectional (complex). The main indications for tomography include evaluations for nonunions, most arthrodeses, and occasionally Lisfranc fracture-dislocations. Infrequently they are used to evaluate osteochondral fractures of the talus, navicu-

(text continues on page 35)

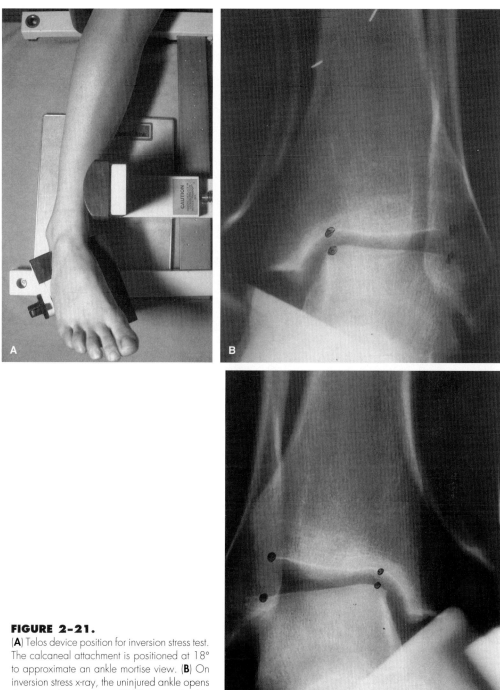

FIGURE 2-21.

(**A**) Telos device position for inversion stress test. The calcaneal attachment is positioned at 18° to approximate an ankle mortise view. (**B**) On inversion stress x-ray, the uninjured ankle opens 4 mm on the stress test. (**C**) The injured ankle opens 11 mm with the inversion stress test, indicating ankle instability.

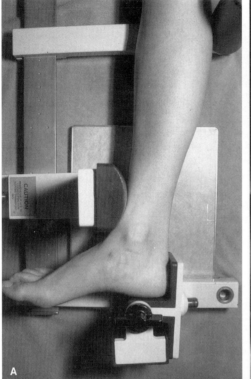

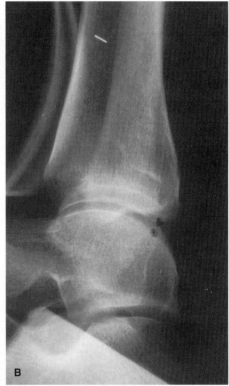

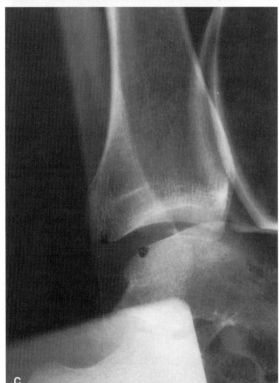

FIGURE 2-22.

(**A**) Telos device position for the anterior drawer stress test. Force is applied in a posterior direction on the distal tibia while the heel and foot are secured. (**B**) Anterior drawer test on the uninjured ankle shows minimal widening of the posterior tibial talar joint space. (**C**) The injured ankle demonstrates 10 mm of anterior displacement with anterior drawer.

often performed as part of the procedure for identifying very small bodies and for precise localization.[16]

Arthrography can be useful preoperatively when arthrodesis is considered. After joint opacification, a local anesthetic is injected. The patient's response to the anesthetic may help determine the surgical approach. It is important to observe for communication between joints, particularly the ankle and posterior subtalar joint. This occurs in 20% of normal patients, and more often with articular disease.[17] Arthrography may also be useful in the evaluation of the integrity of the ankle ligaments, but frequent false-negative examinations occur (Fig. 2-24). Because of this, magnetic resonance imaging (MRI) is now preferred to evaluate ligamentous disruption.[18]

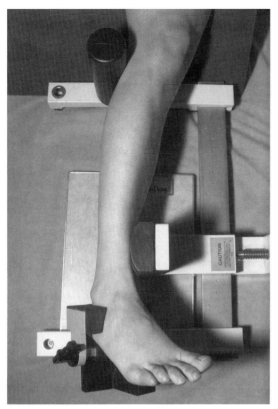

FIGURE 2-23.
Telos device positioning for the subtalar stress test. A different foot piece is secured around the heel.

lar stress fractures, calcaneal fractures, and subtalar arthritis. The disadvantages of tomography include high radiation exposure and an inaccurate picture of the structures not exactly perpendicular to the plane of the tube motion. More recently, tomography has been almost entirely replaced by computed tomography (CT). Sometimes it may be necessary to image in a tomographic plane unavailable in CT, although with recent advances in CT (spiral CT), extremely thin sections can be reconstructed in any plane.[14]

Fluoroscopy and Arthrography

Fluoroscopy may be used for optimal positioning of the stress x-rays and for looking at loose bodies. In the evaluation of loose bodies only, a small amount of positive or often negative (air) contrast is used.[15] CT is also

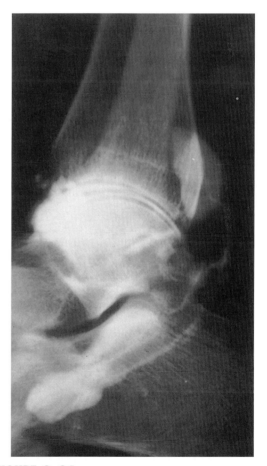

FIGURE 2-24.
Sagittal arthrogram of the ankle demonstrates a filling defect within the posterior capsule, representing a hyperplastic synovial nodule of pigmented villonodular synovitis.

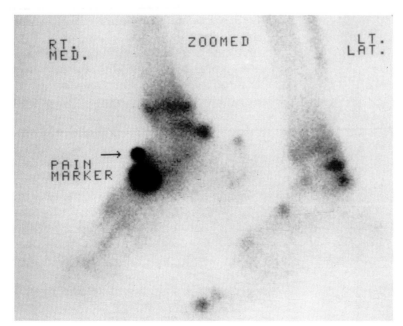

FIGURE 2-25.
Technetium-99 phosphate bone scan in a patient with a stress fracture of the navicular.

Nuclear Medicine

Although the use of nuclear medicine for the diagnosis of ankle pathology has decreased with the widespread use of CT and MRI, scintigraphy continues to play a role because of its relatively low cost and exceptional sensitivity.[19] The most commonly used radiopharmaceutical for bone imaging is a technetium-99 phosphate compound methyl diphosphonate. After intravenous injection, the phosphate compound appears to absorb into the hydroxyapatite crystal within the bone matrix. Imaging can be performed as a routine bone scan or as a three-phase examination. In the first phase (perfusion), imaging is performed during injection of the isotope. The second phase (venous pool) is obtained 60 to 90 seconds after the injection. The third phase is usually performed 3 to 4 hours after the injection. Some authors have added a fourth phase at 24 hours to increase the specificity.

Enthesopathy (bony proliferation at ligamentous insertions) can be a type of stress syndrome. Bone scans are particularly sensitive at detecting stress fractures, and a grading system can sometimes be used[20] (Fig. 2-25). Bone scintigraphy is a sensitive tool for

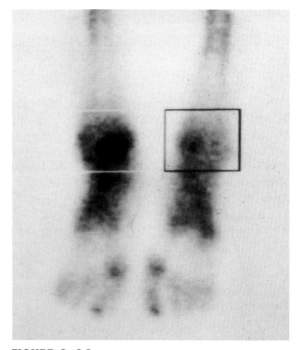

FIGURE 2-26.
Technetium-99 phosphate bone scan demonstrating increased uptake along the medial dome of the talus in a patient with an osteochondral lesion of the talus.

evaluating the early stages of bone production of any etiology.[21] Bone scans are also useful in evaluating subtle or occult trauma and such complications as delayed union, reflex sympathetic dystrophy, and metastatic disease[22] (Fig. 2-26). The three-phase bone scan is used in patients with avascular necrosis, to evaluate both hyperemia within primary bone tumors and reflex sympathetic dystrophy, and is critical in assessing inflammatory conditions of the soft tissue and bone. For most of these indications, MRI is preferred at present because the specificity of bone scintigraphy is quite limited.

Additional scintigraphic procedures used in identifying soft-tissue abscesses and osteomyelitis are gallium-67 citrate and indium-111 white cell scans. When correlated with three-phase images, these tests help differentiate osteomyelitis from cellulitis. Indium-111 white blood cell imaging appears to be the superior technique, although in some chronic bone infections gallium imaging may be positive when the indium scan is negative.[23] However, when the cost of multiple scintigraphic studies and the added time necessary are considered, MRI may be the procedure of choice in evaluating osteomyelitis, particularly in patients with underlying neuropathic disease.

Ultrasound

Ultrasound has limited application in the examination of the foot and ankle. It is ideal in characterizing cystic masses or in patients unwilling or unable to have an MRI examination. In addition, three-dimensional localization, information as to mass affecting adjacent structures, and some nonspecific tissue characterizations can be seen.[24] It may also be used as a quick, inexpensive test to evaluate the Achilles tendon, the thickness of the heel fat pad, and foreign bodies.[24]

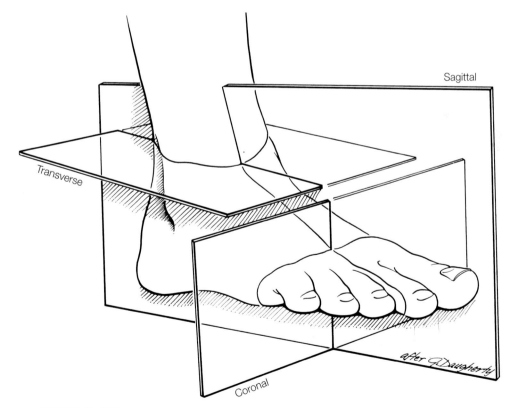

FIGURE 2-27.
Sectional plane drawing illustrating the lines of axis for the coronal, transverse (axial), and sagittal views.

Computed Tomography

The complex osseous anatomy of the ankle and foot lends itself to cross-sectional imaging by CT. To understand CT imaging, it is critical to understand how the sectional planes for scans are performed. Most images are produced in one or more of the following orthogonal planes: coronal, transverse (axial), or sagittal. The coronal view is perpendicular to the plantar surface of the foot, whereas the transverse or axial plane is parallel to the plantar surface of the foot and ankle (Fig. 2-27).

CT produces images based on tissue density secondary to differences in radiation and absorption. It

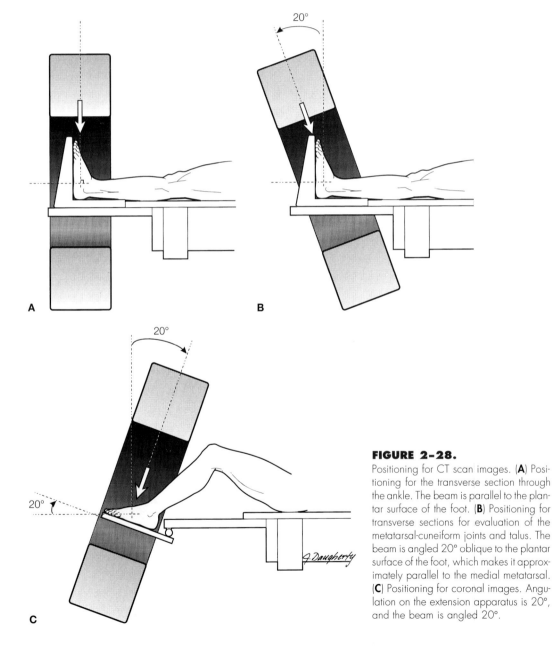

FIGURE 2-28.

Positioning for CT scan images. (**A**) Positioning for the transverse section through the ankle. The beam is parallel to the plantar surface of the foot. (**B**) Positioning for transverse sections for evaluation of the metatarsal-cuneiform joints and talus. The beam is angled 20° oblique to the plantar surface of the foot, which makes it approximately parallel to the medial metatarsal. (**C**) Positioning for coronal images. Angulation on the extension apparatus is 20°, and the beam is angled 20°.

is superior to MRI in evaluating joint surfaces and the cortical outlines of individual bones. The indications for CT include evaluation for osteochondral lesions, loose bodies, subtalar and ankle arthritis, tarsal coalition, and all fractures involving the hindfoot. Peroneal tendons can also be well seen on transverse images, and CT is particularly well suited for evaluating shallow fibular grooves in patients with peroneal subluxation.

The disadvantages of CT scanning include its high radiation dosage, its inability to image directly in various planes, and its lower spatial resolution compared with conventional radiography and tomography.

Positioning for CT scanning is very important[25] (Fig. 2-28). Symmetry between the two extremities must be maintained, and the plantar aspects of the feet should be pressed against the flat surface with a mild amount of pressure, simulating weight bearing. The sequence of sections is from the posterior surface of the talus to the body of the navicular when the hindfoot is scanned. The slice interval is usually 3 to 5 mm, but many scanners can image in segments as low as 1 mm. The slice thickness varies but is generally 3 mm. Usually both feet can be done to determine asymmetry, although image quality is slightly better if only one foot is scanned.[26]

CT is often used to evaluate ankle trauma. It is useful in documenting the extent of fractures and the number of principal fracture fragments. Two planes should usually be performed, but if

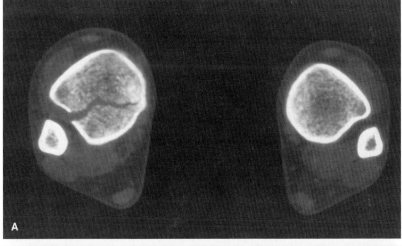

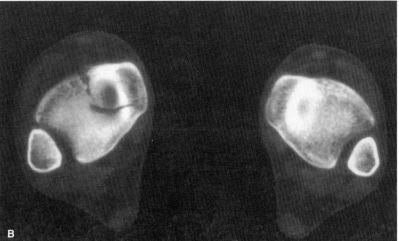

FIGURE 2-29.
Triplane fracture of the ankle. (**A**) Transverse fracture through the distal tibia. (**B**) Fracture with rotation and mild displacement through the medial portion of the tibia.

the patient cannot be positioned for the second plane, then thin (preferably 1-mm) images in one plane are performed with reconstruction in the second or third plane. Different planes are optimal to evaluate different areas of the foot and ankle.[27-29] In the tibia, pilon fractures need detailed evaluation because precise anatomic reduction is necessary to prevent or decrease posttraumatic degenerative arthritis.[30] In children, the complex epiphyseal injury of the triplane fracture is well evaluated by CT in the coronal and transaxial planes with sagittal reconstructions[31] (Fig. 2-29). CT can also be useful for evaluating loose bodies, osseous union, and pseudarthrosis, as well as osteochondral lesions of the talus, posttraumatic degenerative changes, and heterotopic bone formation[29] (Fig. 2-30). Currently, most evaluations of bone and soft-tissue tumors are performed with MRI, but CT continues to play a role (Fig. 2-31). CT is helpful for evaluating tarsal coalition and bone bridging. Joint space narrowing, sclerosis, and irregularity imply fi-

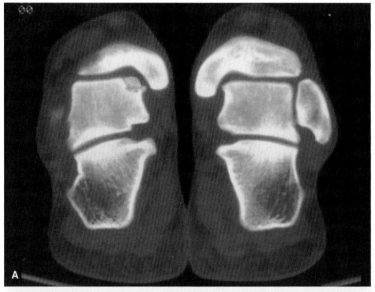

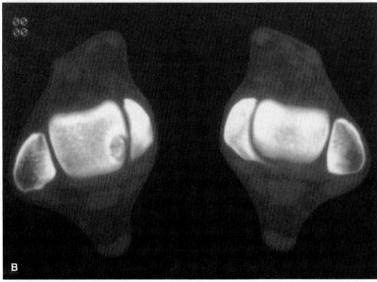

FIGURE 2-30.
Osteochondral lesion of the medial dome of the talus. (**A**) Bilateral coronal images demonstrating stage III lesion with lucency surrounding the lesion on the left. (**B**) Bilateral transverse (axial) images showing the posteromedial extent of the lesion on the left with a sclerotic line surrounding it.

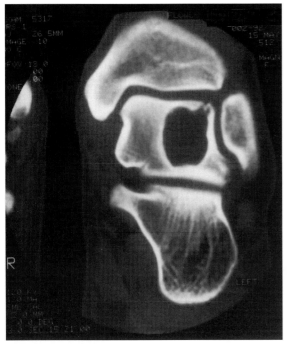

FIGURE 2-31.
Coronal CT scan in a patient with an interosseous ganglion of the talus. Note the communication into the ankle joint.

brous or cartilaginous union, which may be better evaluated with MRI.[32]

CT scans are particularly useful in evaluating osteochondral lesions of the talus. By examining both the coronal and transverse planes, the size and

TABLE 2-2.
PREFERRED MRI TECHNIQUES

AREA OF PATHOLOGY	PLANE	TE-WEIGHT
Achilles	Sagittal, axial	T2
Tibialis posterior, flexor hallucis longus, peroneal brevis	Modified coronal oblique, axial	T2
Anterolateral impingement	Axial, coronal	T2
Ankle ligaments	Axial, coronal	T1, T2
Soft tissue	Coronal, sagittal*	T1, T2
Bone	Coronal, axial	T1, T2†

(With permission from Ferkel RD, Flannigan BD, Elkins BS. Magnetic resonance imaging of the foot and ankle: correlation of normal anatomy with pathologic conditions. Foot Ankle 1991;11:289.)
* The type of view depends somewhat on the location of the lesion.
† Views should always be done at two planes 90° to each other, such as the coronal and sagittal or the coronal and axial.

location of the lesion can be assessed, both in the AP and medial/lateral directions. A staging system for osteochondral lesions developed by the author is discussed in Chapter 8.

Magnetic Resonance Imaging

Routine radiographic techniques depend on x-ray attenuation, which is secondary to the electron density of tissues. The magnetic resonance phenomenon involves an atomic nucleus. Those imaged are usually hydrogen nuclei, which consist of a single proton and are most abundant in water. A strong magnetic field is used to align these protons uniformly. Frequency pulses are then applied that change the orientation of the aligned protons. After the pulse, the protons relax back to their initial state. This relaxation process may be described by two time characteristics: T1 and T2. In the images we can emphasize either of these two characteristics by altering two variables: TE and TR. Images with short TE and

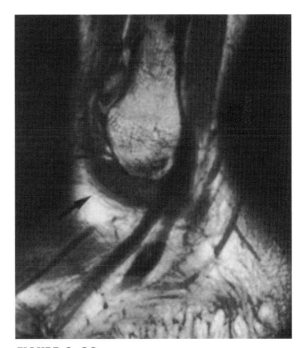

FIGURE 2-32.
Soft-tissue impingement. A sagittal T1-weighted image demonstrates a low-signal-density mass in the anterolateral gutter (*arrow*), consistent with soft-tissue impingement.

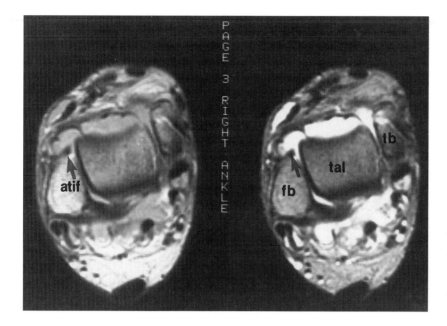

FIGURE 2-33.

Acute tear of the anterior tibiofibular ligament. These T2-weighted double-echo axial images demonstrate a ruptured left anterior tibiofibular ligament and an extensive amount of fluid. (*atif,* anterior tibiofibular ligament; *fb,* fibula; *tal,* talus; *tb,* tibia.)

TR are relatively T1-weighted; those with long TE and TR are T2-weighted. The third type of image is a ''balanced'' or intermediate-weighted image with a long TR and a short TE.

The characteristics just described apply to the most commonly used sequence, or the spin echo technique. There are many other sequences, including gradient echo and stir imaging.

The advantages of MRI include lack of ionizing radiation, the ability to scan clearly in a multiplanar fashion, and the ability to distinguish fat, ligaments, tendons, bone marrow, and fluid. Excellent resolu-

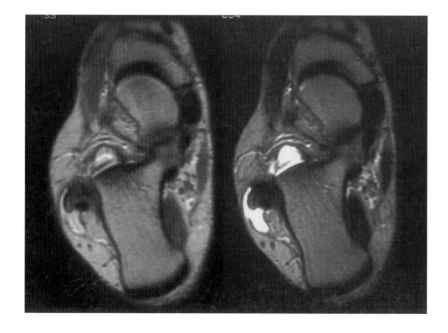

FIGURE 2-34.

Axial dual spin-echo image demonstrates a longitudinal tear of the peroneal brevis tendon, which is split into medial and lateral segments. The peroneus longus tendon is intact.

tion of the ankle, subtalar joint, and foot and surrounding soft tissue can be obtained.

MRI is indicated in the evaluation of bone and soft-tissue tumors, ischemic necrosis, infection, ligament and tendon injury, and postoperative complications.

The patient is placed either supine or prone with the feet together, parallel to one another. To perform simultaneous images of both feet, the head coil is usually used. A positioning device holds both feet so the plantar aspects are perpendicular to the plane of the table. Images are per-

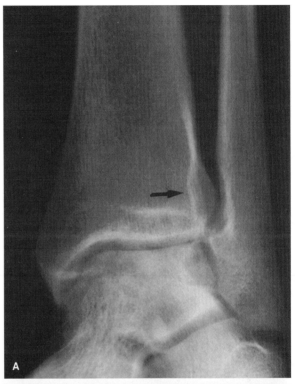

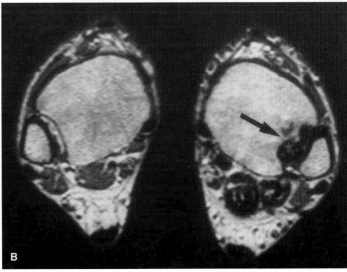

FIGURE 2-35.
Pigmented villonodular synovitis of the ankle. (**A**) Oblique x-ray showing erosion in the syndesmosis of the ankle. (**B**) Axial spin-echo images of both ankles demonstrate on the right a well-circumscribed low-signal lesion in the area of the syndesmosis and tibiofibular ligament (*arrow*), suggestive of pigmented villonodular synovitis.

formed, preferably on a 1.5-tesla MR imager. The slice thickness is usually 3 to 5 mm, with an interslice gap of 1 to 1.5 mm. Continuous imaging may be required for subtle pathology but is not routinely indicated. Imaging of only one foot or ankle is usually performed using an extremity coil; this yields higher-resolution images than when both feet are imaged together.

MRI provides dramatic tissue contrast. The pulse sequence selected for imaging influences the appearance of individual tissues; that is, fluid exhibits a low intensity on a T1-weighted image and a very high T2-weighted image. Table 2-2 illustrates the preferred MRI techniques for the tissues of the foot and ankle.

MRI is very useful in the diagnosis of numerous

pathologic conditions of the ankle and foot. The reader is referred to other sources for a detailed study of foot and ankle MRI.[33,34] At present there is controversy over whether CT or MRI is the study of choice in evaluating osteochondritis dissecans (osteochondral lesions of the talus). Although CT is more useful in preoperative planning, MRI may be more accurate in detecting cartilage healing or preoperative cartilaginous communications into the subchondral bone. In addition, MRI is useful in the diagnosis of soft-tissue impingement of the ankle, as well as tears of the ankle ligaments (Figs. 2-32 and 2-33). Injuries to the tendons, especially the Achilles, peroneals, posterior tibialis, and flexors, are also well seen on MRI (Fig. 2-34).

One of the earliest uses of MRI was in the diagnosis of avascular necrosis. Four patterns were described that were thought to represent pathologic stages.[35,36] MRI, after routine radiography, should be the imaging modality used to evaluate infection.[37,38] One of the most important roles of MRI is in the evaluation of bony and soft-tissue tumors; the reader is referred elsewhere for in-depth discussions of tumor applications (Figs. 2-35 and 2-36).

Kinematic MRI

Kinematic MRI studies appear particularly useful in evaluating bony and soft-tissue impingement, peroneal subluxation, and conditions of the subtalar joint. Further research is necessary to define the utility of this new application of MRI.

REFERENCES

1. French's index of differential diagnosis. Littleton, MA: PSB Publishing Co., 1985.
2. Mann RA, Coughlin MJ. Surgery of the foot and ankle, 6th ed. St. Louis: Mosby Yearbook, 1993.
3. Jahss MH. Examination. In Jahss MH, ed. Disorders of the foot and ankle: medical and surgical management. Philadelphia: WB Saunders, 1991:35.
4. Isman RE, Inman VT. Anthropometric studies of the human foot and ankle. Bull Prosthet Res 1969;10–11:97.
5. Hamilton WG. Tendinitis about the ankle joint in classical ballet dancers: "dancer's tendinitis." J Sports Med 1977;5:84.

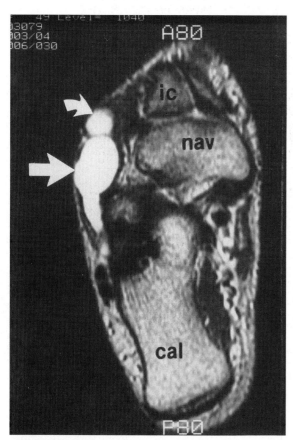

FIGURE 2-36.
The axial T2-weighted image demonstrates a ganglion cyst on the dorsolateral surface of the foot associated with the extensor digitorum brevis muscle. (*IC*, intermediate cuneiform; *nav*, navicular; *cal*, calcaneus.)

6. Ferkel RD. Radiologic imaging techniques. In Guhl JF, ed. Foot and ankle arthroscopy. Thorofare, NJ: Slack, 1994.

7. Sartoris DJ, Resnick D. Plain film radiography routine and specialized techniques and projection. In Resnick D, Niwayama G, eds. Diagnosis of bone and joint disorders, 2d ed. Philadelphia: WB Saunders, 1988.

8. Grae DL. Lateral ankle ligament injuries. Clin Orthop 1989;103:153.

9. Sauser DD, Nelson RC, Laurine MH, et al. Acute injuries of the lateral ligaments of the ankle: comparison of stress radiography and arthrography. Radiology 1983;148:653.

10. Rubin G, Witten M. The talar tilt ankle and the fibular collateral ligaments: a method for the determination of talar tilt. J Bone Joint Surg 1960;42A:311.

11. Chrisman OD, Snook CA. A reconstruction of lateral ligament tears of the ankle: an experimental study and clinical evaluation of seven patients treated by a new modification of the Elmslie procedure. J Bone Joint Surg 1969;51A:904.

12. Gould N, Seligson D, Glassman J. Early and late repair of lateral ligaments of the ankle. Foot Ankle 1980;1:84.

13. Laurin CA, Ouellet R, St. Jacques R. Talar and subtalar tilt: an experimental investigation. Can J Surg 1968;11:270.

14. Resnick D. Conventional tomography. In Resnick D, Niwayama G, eds. Diagnosis of bone and joint disorders, 2d ed. Philadelphia: WB Saunders, 1988.

15. Arner O, Ekergner K, Hulting B, Lindholm A. Arthrography of the talocruciate joint: anatomic, radiographic and clinical aspects. Acta Chir Scand 1957;113:253.

16. Smith GR, Wirguist RA, Allan NK, Northrop CH. Subtle transchondral fractures of the talar dome: a radiological perspective. Radiology 1977;124:667.

17. Haller J, Resnick D, Sartoris D, Mitchell M, et al. Arthrography, tomography and bursography of the ankle and foot. Clin Podiatr Med Surg 1988;5:893.

18. Ala-Ketola L, Purarer J, Roivisto L, Punpoa M. Arthrography in the diagnosis of ligament injuries and classification of ankle injuries. Radiology 1977;125:63.

19. Holder LE. Clinical radionuclide bone imaging. Radiology 1990;176:593.

20. Matin P. Basic principles of nuclear medicine techniques for detection and evaluation of trauma and sports medicine injuries. Sem Nuc Med 1988;18:90.

21. Rupani HP, Holder LE, Espinola DA, Engin SI. Three-phase radionuclide bone imaging in sports medicine. Radiology 1985;156:187.

22. McDougall IR, Keeling CA. Complications of fractures and their healing. Healing 1980;18:113.

23. Gupta NC, Prezio JA. Radionuclide imaging in osteomyelitis. Sem Nuc Med 1988;18:287.

24. Fornage BD, Rifkin MD. Ultrasound examination of the hand and foot. Radiol Clin North Am 1988;16:109.

25. Smith RW, Staple TW. Computerized tomography scanning technique for the hindfoot. Clin Orthop 1983;177:34.

26. Solomon MA, Gilula LA, Oloff LM, et al. CT scanning of the foot and ankle. Part 1, Normal anatomy. AJR 1986;146:1192.

27. Solomon MA, Gilula LA, Oloff LM, et al. CT scanning of the foot and ankle. Part 2, Clinical applications and review of the literature. AJR 1986;146:1204.

28. Rosenberg S, Feldna F, Singon RD. Intraarticular calcaneal fractures—computed tomographic analysis. Skeletal Radiol 1987;16:105.

29. Daffner RH. Ankle trauma. Radiol Clin North Am 1990;28:395.

30. Manwaring BL, Daffner RH, Reimer BL. Pylon fractures of the ankle: a distinct clinical and radiologic entity. Radiology 1988;168:215.

31. Feldman F, Singon RD, Rosenberg FS, et al. Distal triplanar fractures: diagnosis with CT. Radiology 1987;164:429.

32. Sarro RC, Carter BL, Barkoff MS, et al. Computed tomography in tarsal coalition. J Comput Assist Tomogr 1987;8:1155.

33. Ferkel RD, Flannigan BD, Elkins BS. Magnetic resonance imaging of the foot and ankle: correlation of normal anatomy with pathologic conditions. Foot Ankle 1991;11:289.

34. Mink JH, Deutsch AL. MRI of the musculoskeletal system. New York: Raven Press, 1990.

35. Paulov H. Imaging of the foot and ankle. Radiol Clin North Am 1990;28:991.

36. Beltran S, Herner LJ, Burk JM, et al. Femoral head avascular necrosis: MR imaging with clinical pathologic correlation. Radiology 1980;188:215.

37. Modic MT, Pflanz W, Feiglin DNI, et al. Magnetic resonance imaging of musculoskeletal infections. Radiol Clin North Am 1986;24:247.

38. Beltran J, McGhee RB, Shaffer PB, et al. Experimental infection of the musculoskeletal system: evaluation with MR imaging and Tc-99m MPP and Ga-67 scintigraphy. Radiology 1988;167:167.

Arthroscopic Surgery: The Foot and Ankle,
by Richard D. Ferkel.
Lippincott-Raven Publishers, Philadelphia © 1996.

3

Instrumentation

Richard D. Ferkel

*A*rthroscopy of the ankle evolved from the principles of knee arthroscopy, and initially the instrumentation used for the knee was applied to the ankle. As expertise and experience with ankle arthroscopy increased, it became apparent that special, smaller instruments were necessary to visualize the ankle and foot joint entirely and operate through a smaller space. In addition, because of the architecture of the ankle and foot joint, the diminished working area, and the tightness of the joints, some form of distraction became necessary. Since 1990, instrumentation for the ankle and foot has significantly improved as a "small-joint" system has evolved. The dynamic nature of arthroscopy necessitates constant improvements that will continue to allow this field to grow.

IRRIGATION

Different fluids can be used for arthroscopic irrigation during ankle and foot arthroscopy. Lactated Ringer's is the most commonly used fluid because it is physiologically compatible with articular cartilage and is rapidly reabsorbed if extravasated from the joint.[1] Glycine and normal saline can also be used, and an experimental fluid, Synovisol (Baxter), can be used with or without electrosurgery and has the appropriate pH and osmolality for the intraarticular structures[2,3] (Table 3-1).

Gravity

Inflow can be accomplished by gravity or by the use of an arthroscopic pumping device. Gravity inflow is usually adequate when the fluid is introduced through a separate cannula, but may be inadequate if the fluid is introduced through the arthroscope sheath because the flow volume and rate may not be high enough to keep up with the evacuation provided by suction instruments. Using gravity inflow through a dedicated inflow can-

TABLE 3-1.
ARTHROSCOPY SOLUTIONS

	APPROXIMATE PH	APPROXIMATE MOSM/L	COMPATIBILITY WITH ELECTROSURGERY	TISSUE TOXICITY
Synovisol	5.0	282	Nonconductive	Minimal
Ringer's lactate	6.5	273	Conductive	Moderate
0.9% saline	5.5	308	Conductive	Moderate
Glycine	6.0	200	Nonconductive	Minimal
Water	6.8	2	Nonconductive	Severe

(Esch JC, Baker CL Jr. Arthroscopic surgery: the shoulder and elbow. Philadelphia: JB Lippincott, 1993:38.)

nula with a 3-mm inner diameter (ID) at a bag height of 3 feet above the joint, a flow rate of 750 cc/minute is produced (Fig. 3-1A). In contrast, when using the same cannula and gravity height as above, but with a 2.7-mm arthroscope in the cannula, the flow rate is reduced to 75 cc/minute (see Fig. 3-1B). Using a wider cannula (3.7-mm ID) with the same 2.7-mm arthroscope produces a much higher rate of 500 cc/minute. For comparison, a dedicated 4.5-mm inflow cannula with no scope yields 924 cc/minute; a 4-mm arthroscope with a standard 4.5-mm diagnostic (high-flow) cannula yields 110 cc/minute. A 4-mm arthroscope with a 4.5-mm operative cannula and irrigation extender yields 67 cc/minute.

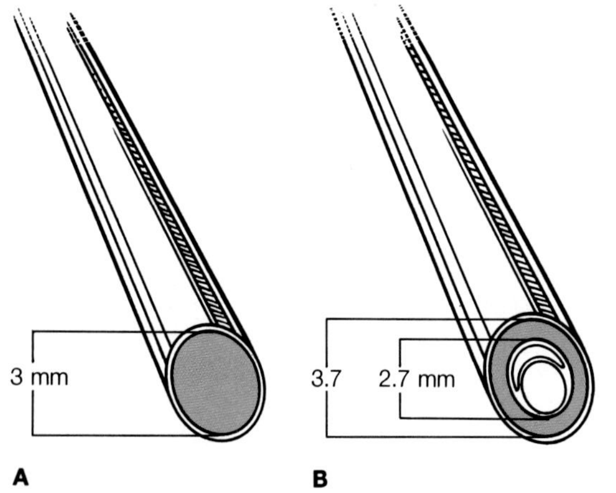

Arthroscopy Pumps

Several types of arthroscopy fluid management systems are available. They operate through the use of a pumping device or gas to pressurize an irrigating fluid into the joint. All systems have regulating devices to prevent over- or underdistention, but each works by a different mechanism (Fig. 3-2).

The operating surgeon must exercise extreme caution when using an infusion pump device during arthroscopy. The disadvantages of these systems include frequent breakdown, the need for specialized equipment and tubing, and the need for a team familiar with the operation of the device. Particularly in the foot and ankle, extravasation of fluid could lead to a compartment problem with subsequent disastrous results (Fig. 3-3).

ARTHROSCOPES

Over the last 20 years, the optical qualities of arthroscopes have improved significantly. The Hopkins rod-lens system continues to provide the best picture quality. Initially the 4-mm knee arthroscope was used in the ankle, but in some cases it was too large in diameter and had too long a lever arm and too large a sheath to allow complete visualization in the ankle without increased risk of articular cartilage scuffing. Moreover, the 4-mm arthroscope may be

FIGURE 3-1.
Inflow rates. (**A**) Using a cannula with a 3-mm interior diameter, at a bag height of 3 feet above the joint, a flow rate of 750 ml/minute is produced. (**B**) Using a cannula with a 3.7-mm interior diameter, with a 2.7-mm scope inside, yields a flow of 500 ml/minute at the same bag height.

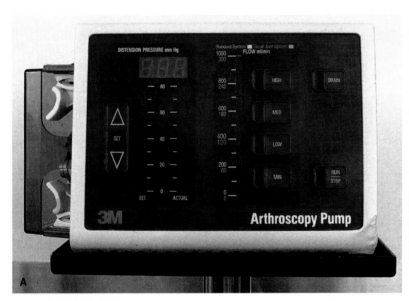
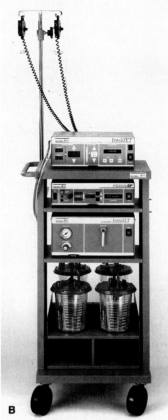

FIGURE 3-2.
Arthroscopic pumps. (**A**) The 3M arthroscopic pump (3M Health Care, St. Paul) requires a separate sensor for use in the ankle. (**B**) The Dyonics pump (Smith and Nephew Dyonics, Inc., Andover, MA) allows inflow through the arthroscopic sheath and is connected to the suction system.

too large to visualize the small spaces along the gutters of the ankle and to look into the subtalar and forefoot joints. A short 4-mm scope was developed to accommodate the more superficial ankle joint without losing the picture clarity of the larger arthroscope.

Construction and Manipulation

More recently, the Hopkins rod-lens arthroscope has been produced in 2.3-mm, 2.7-mm, and 1.9-mm diameters (Fig. 3-4). These smaller arthroscopes are available in short versions, having the advantages of a shorter lever arm, excellent picture quality, easy maneuverability, and interchangeable cannulae. The

shaft of an arthroscope must be only 67 mm long for use in ankle and foot arthroscopy. However, as the arthroscopes have become smaller and shorter, they have become correspondingly more fragile. Today the picture quality of the smaller arthroscopes is equivalent to that of the larger versions.

Field of View

There are two dimensions to the field of view[4] (Fig. 3-5). The *apparent* field of view is the diameter seen at the ocular end of the arthroscope and enhanced by magnification through the video coupler device. The closeness of the arthroscope to the object influences the surgeon's perception of the field of view.

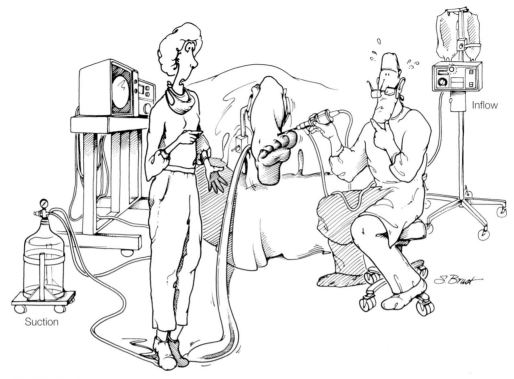

Inflow

Suction

FIGURE 3-3.
When an arthroscopic pump device is used in ankle arthroscopy, extreme caution is needed to prevent extravasation of fluid, which can lead to compartment problems.

The *actual* field of view is a measured angle of view the arthroscope produces. This angle varies from 89 for the standard 4-mm arthroscope to 100° to 115° for a wide-angle 4-mm arthroscope. In contrast, the 2.7-mm wide-angle arthroscope has a field of view of 75° to 90°. The term "wide-angle scope" refers to the actual angular field of view rather than the apparent field of view.

Inclination of View

The inclination of view is the angle of projection at the objective end of the arthroscope (Fig. 3-6). The 30° view, the most practical and the most commonly used, permits excellent visualization within the ankle and foot, particularly when a wide-angle lens is used. The 70° small-joint arthroscope allows the surgeon to see around corners but requires some experience because it is used less commonly. It is particularly

helpful in seeing over the medial and lateral domes of the talus, looking into the gutters, and evaluating certain osteochondral lesions of the talus (Fig. 3-7).

Clarity

Most current arthroscopes have a zero-to-infinity working distance and provide a clear image whether the tissue is close to the lens of the arthroscope or further away. A focusing ring permits fine adjustment to the picture quality. Once the focus is set, rarely are adjustments necessary.

Arthroscopic Movement

A careful diagnostic examination is a composite of multiple images obtained by moving the arthroscope in different positions and using the arthroscope's rotation ability and angle of inclination.

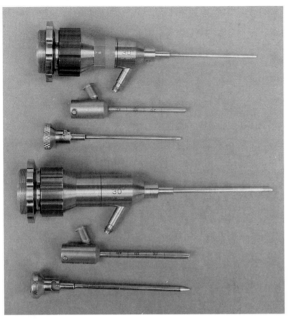

FIGURE 3-4.
Small-joint arthroscopes with interchangeable cannulae are helpful in ankle and foot arthroscopy. A 1.9-mm 30° oblique arthroscope is pictured on top, a 2.7-mm 30° oblique arthroscope below.

Pistoning

The forward and backward movement of the arthroscope is called "pistoning." Pistoning allows the surgeon to move closer or further away to visualize one particular area or to obtain a panorama of a larger field.

Angulation

Angulation is a sweeping motion that moves the arthroscope in a horizontal or vertical plane. This movement can scratch the fragile articular surfaces and must be performed gently.

Rotation

Rotation is the most valuable movement in arthroscopy. Using a 30° instead of a 0° arthroscope permits a wider view of the ankle and foot joints. Rotation of the 30° arthroscope's field of view enhances arthroscopic viewing by creating overlapping circular images. With the 70° arthroscope, a central blind spot is present (see Fig. 3-7).

Cannulae

The arthroscope is introduced into the joint by means of a cannula or sheath, which should be 1 to 2 mm shorter than the arthroscope when fully engaged. The tip of the cannula is angled in a manner to accommodate the angle of the scope lens. The proximal end of the sheath should have a quick and secure connecting mechanism to accept a trochar or arthroscope. This allows easy insertion and removal of the arthroscope from the sheath during surgery. Sheaths are available with and without side ports for fluid flow (Fig. 3-8). The amount of fluid that can

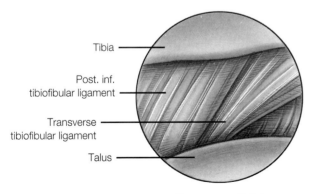
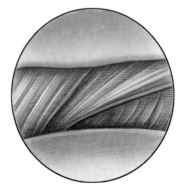

Tibia

Post. inf. tibiofibular ligament

Transverse tibiofibular ligament

Talus

Same apparent size, smaller actual view

Same apparent size, larger actual view

FIGURE 3-5.
The apparent field of view is determined by the closeness of the arthroscope to the object. The close-up (*left*) shows a smaller actual view than the more distant view (*right*).

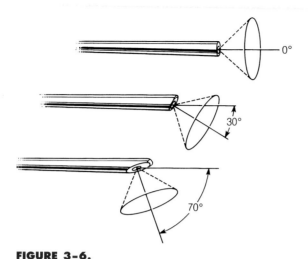

FIGURE 3-6.

The angle of inclination is 0°, 30°, or 70° relative to the arthroscope axis. The angular field-of-view cone is oriented along the axis of the angle of inclination. (Esch JC, Baker CL Jr. Arthroscopic surgery: the shoulder and elbow. Philadelphia: JB Lippincott, 1993:38.)

be introduced through the sheath depends on the size of the sheath and the pressure applied to the fluid (see Fig. 3-1).

The arthroscopic sheaths should be interchangeable so that the arthroscope and instruments can be easily placed through any of the portals desired without repeated instrumentation and subsequent soft-tissue trauma. Switching sticks that are smaller in diameter than the cannulae used should also be available, and are particularly useful if the cannula comes out of the joint inadvertently or if the surgeon needs to switch from a cannula with a side port to one without. For systems without interchangeable cannulae, plastic disposable cannulae can be used to allow exchanges of instruments through a given portal.

LIGHT SOURCES/LIGHT GUIDES

An adequate light source is just as critical to the procedure as the arthroscope. Various types of lamps have been used, including incandescent, quartz, halogen, tungsten, and xenon. The differences between lamps are the light temperature, the lumen output, and operational conditions. Currently, most light sources are metal halide or halogen; however, xenon sources, because of their similarity to sunlight, color temperature, longevity of use, and the quick-start cycle when turned off and then on again, have become very popular for use in the operating room.

To transmit the light from the light source to the distal end of the arthroscope, a light guide is interfaced between the light source and the arthroscope. Light guides or cords consist of either fiber-optic bundles or a liquid medium for light transmission. Fiber-optic guides are normally very flexible and easy to manipulate in the sterile field, but damage to individual fibers can create inadequate light transmission. Liquid light guides can transmit greater amounts of light without degradation, but are less flexible, are difficult to manipulate, and can be fragile in the sterilization process.

DISTRACTION DEVICES

Visualization of the ankle, subtalar joint, and forefoot areas can be significantly improved by the use of a distraction device. The distractor is used to increase the space between the tibia and the talus. Without distraction, certain areas of the ankle, such as the central tibial plafond and talar dome, the posterior talofibular ligament, and the calcaneofibular ligament, are poorly seen. Distraction methods can be noninvasive or invasive.

Noninvasive

Noninvasive techniques include manual distraction and gravity distraction, which are "uncontrolled" methods. Although these methods require no specific equipment, they are often inadequate for complete visualization and operative arthroscopy. Other noninvasive methods, such as the modified clove-hitch knot around the ankle, can be termed "semicontrolled"[5] (see Figs. 1-3 and 3-9). This method is inexpensive but may be inadequate for good distraction; also, the degree of force and the duration of distraction are hard to monitor. The third type of noninvasive distraction, termed "controlled," involves the use of prefabricated straps that hook around the

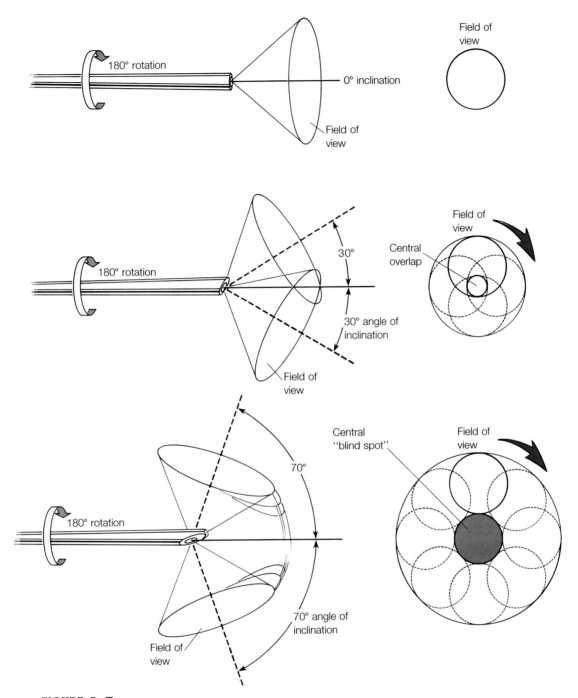

FIGURE 3-7.
Rotating the arthroscope's field of view enhances arthroscopic viewing by creating overlapping circular images with a 30° arthroscope (*center*). With a 0° arthroscope (*top*), the field of view is unchanged with rotation. With a 70° arthroscope (*bottom*), rotation occurs around a central blind spot.

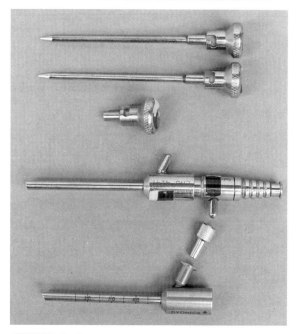

FIGURE 3-8.
Arthroscopic cannulae are available with and without side ports, inflow adapters, and side port plugs.

front of the foot and the back of the heel and are attached to an outrigger device in which a distraction force is generated (Fig. 3-10). A fracture table can also perform this type of distraction. Other devices are available that allow this type of distraction while the patient's knee is bent at 90°. Some of these devices permit the amount of pressure and force to be monitored and maintained mechanically.

Invasive

Invasive distractors use pins in the tibia and talus or calcaneus to provide mechanical distraction. A "controlled" system usually has a strain gauge to measure the amount of force and permit some degree of freedom within the ankle joint (Fig. 3-11*A*). The disadvantages of these systems include the need to insert pins and the risk of damage to the neurovascular structures, infection, and fracture. However, they allow large amounts of distraction force to be applied across the joint in a controlled manner. More recently, a "multimode" Distraction System (Acufex) has been de-

veloped to allow both invasive and noninvasive distraction to be applied through the same device.[6] This apparatus allows the surgeon to start with a noninvasive technique and progress to invasive techniques only if adequate distraction and visualization are not obtained (see Fig. 3-11*B*).

In the great toe and lesser toes, noninvasive distraction is performed in a semicontrolled manner using a toe trap attached to a rope-and-pulley

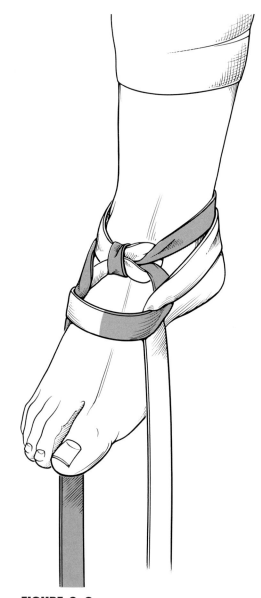

FIGURE 3-9.
Noninvasive distraction loop.

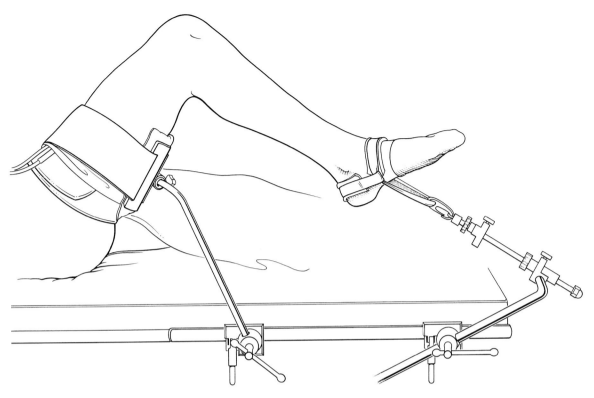

FIGURE 3–10.

Standard setup for noninvasive distraction in the supine position. Note the thigh support surrounding the tourniquet with flexion of the hip and knee. A commercial strap provides good padding over the dorsum and the posterior aspects of the ankle, and is attached to a distraction device that joins the table sterilely.

system. This is discussed further in Chapter 13. Some type of distraction is required in most arthroscopy cases of the foot and ankle.

Contraindications to the use of noninvasive distraction include impaired circulatory status, diabetes, certain generalized medical conditions, and ankle edema or fragile skin conditions. Invasive skeletal distraction is contraindicated with localized or generalized infection, osteopenia, open physis, ligamentous laxity, and active reflex sympathetic dystrophy, and in high-performance athletes who must return to their sport quickly.

VIDEO STANDARDS AND FORMATS

Standards

National Television Systems Committee (NTSC), Phase Alternating Line (PAL), and Sequential Coleur à Memoire (SECAM) are television standards used around the world to broadcast signals from one point to another. NTSC is the industry standard in the United States, Canada, several countries in the Far East, and most of Central and South America. PAL is the standard in Great Britain and is found throughout most of Europe, Africa, and Asia. SECAM is slowly losing system support but is still used remotely in France and a few European countries.

Formats

Formats are the manner in which electronic signals produced by a camera carry their color and brightness information to an accessory device for display or manipulation. Composite, RGB, and Y-C (S-VHS) are terms describing various video formats.

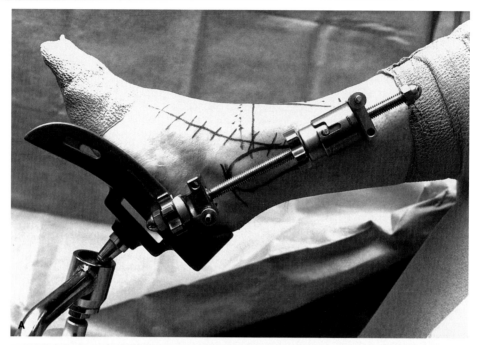

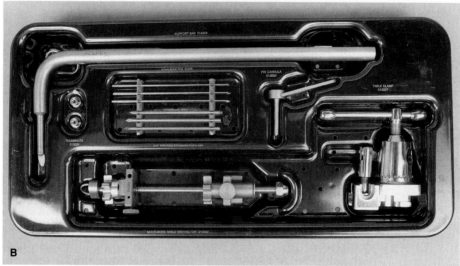

FIGURE 3–11.
(**A**) Invasive distraction device applied to the lateral aspect of the distal tibia and calcaneus, with a strain gauge to monitor distraction force. (**B**) The multimode distraction unit comes in a sterilization tray. It can be used with invasive or noninvasive distraction.

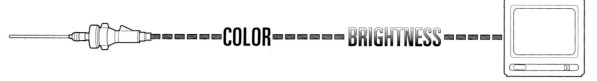

FIGURE 3-12.

Composite format, in which the color and brightness information is combined into one signal. (Graphics by J. Daugherty.)

Composite

With the composite format, color and brightness information is combined into one signal (Fig. 3-12). The primary advantage to the Composite format is consistency throughout all the different standard systems. Thus, almost all equipment, even if it is capable of Y-C (S-VHS) or RGB formats, also has a Composite format available for video compatibility.

Composite video, however, has several problems. Its band width allows only a limited amount of information to be transmitted for use. This is especially noticeable in standard videocassette recorders, as the Composite video signal has limited recording resolution capability. Several problems are created by combining color and brightness information into one signal. Because color and brightness are processed by the camera separately, an encoding function is required to combine these signals into one signal, thus adding extraneous electronic noise into the signal (signal-to-noise).[7] Combining these two signals results in cross-talk interference between the two, again increasing the electronic noise. Both of these factors lead to decreased signal-to-noise ratios. Another factor that limits the Composite signal is the "chroma" flicker, which results from this same encoding process and may be seen during the color bar screen as "chroma crawl" between the color spectrums.

Y-C (S-VHS)

In the Y-C or S-VHS format, the color and brightness information is separated into different electronic signals for transmission (Fig. 3-13). Y-C is the next most commonly available system in the United States. "Y" stands for the luminance or brightness signal, "C" for the chroma or color signal. The term "Super VHS" refers to the taping or recording systems that made this format more popular. With this format, video information is carried on two different signals (Y and C), eliminating the cross-talk between the two and improving the total signal-to-noise ratio. By separating the brightness signal and expanding its ability to carry more information, higher contrast can be obtained, meaning a sharper picture for both viewing and recording. For medical video, Y-C offers higher-resolution recording for better videotapes, excellent resolution for color prints, and a clear, bright image for viewing during surgery.

RGB

RGB is the third most commonly used video format. The term "RGB" refers to the separate transmission of the red (R), green (G), blue (B), and synchronization (S) electronic signals. A special cable is used between the camera and the monitor to conduct all these signals at the same time (Fig. 3-14).

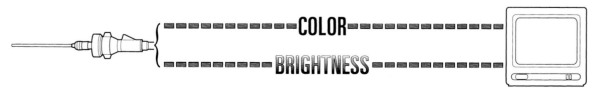

FIGURE 3-13.

Super VHS (Y-C) format, in which the color and brightness information is transmitted separately on different electronic signals. (Graphics by J. Daugherty.)

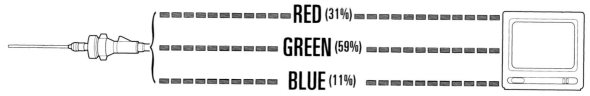

FIGURE 3-14.
RGB format, in which red, green, and blue are transmitted separately. Brightness is generated as a percentage of these colors. (Graphics by J. Daugherty. Modified from Whelan JM, Jackson DW. Video arthroscopy. Arthroscopy 1992;8:311.)

Some claim that the RGB hookup and process is superior to the other formats, and this may be true if the camera has three sensors, one for each color, and each sensor is used at its full resolution. However, there are some disadvantages to RGB. Separating a composite video signal from a single-sensor camera into RGB may actually degrade the picture due to the decrease in signal-to-noise ratio through the added electronics necessary to perform this function. Another potential disadvantage to RGB is that the color on the monitor cannot be adjusted because the RGB format renders the hue or tint knob inoperable. Therefore, if the camera-to-monitor signal is not properly balanced, alignment between the two systems is lost and there is no way to adjust it. However, for surgical facilities where constant manipulation of color adjustment creates unsatisfactory viewing, nonadjustment of the system eliminates this problem in the operating room.

Preferred Method

We currently use S-VHS for all our surgical recording, both overhead and intraarticular. An S-VHS editing system is then used to edit the tapes for presentations, patient use, and documentation.

System Resolution

Resolution is a universal term of measurement identifying the capability of an imaging system to make clear and distinguishable one object from another. Resolution is measured in lines, both vertically and horizontally. Horizontal resolution is generally used as a standard of comparison. The quality of a video camera's charged coupled device (CCD) determines the number of lines of resolution the camera can produce. The greater the number of horizontal lines, the better the image detail. The other major components of the video systems—monitor, printer, and recorder—reconvert the electronic signals created by the camera into a visual image. Each of these components has its own resolving capability; therefore, system resolution refers to the resulting resolution when these components are connected.

The "weak link theory" states that no integrated system is any stronger than its weakest link. For example, a system including a camera with 300 lines of resolution connected to a monitor with 600 lines of resolution will result in a system resolution of only 300 lines. This would be true even if the camera and monitor numbers were reversed. The results are even worse when hard-copy printers or videotape recorders are used in the video system. Therefore, the viewing image will be no better than the quality produced by the poorest-performing component of that video system (Fig. 3-15).

VIDEO CAMERAS AND COUPLERS

Video cameras have evolved just like other ankle arthroscopic instrumentation. Initially, large, heavy tube cameras were used because of the picture quality and resolution. More recently, lightweight, small CCD chip cameras have captured the market. These chip cameras are lighter in weight and smaller in size, and give a very clear picture, particularly the new three-chip cameras. In addition, many of the new small chip cameras have features such as RGB and Y-C and give improved picture quality and resolution (450 to 700 lines of resolution). Normally

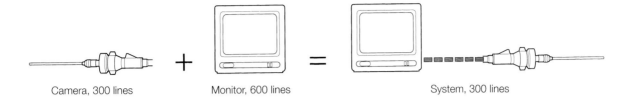

Camera, 300 lines + Monitor, 600 lines = System, 300 lines

Camera, 300 lines + Recorder, 420 lines = System, 300 lines

FIGURE 3-15.
Weak link theory. System resolution is limited by its weakest link, which in this example is a camera with 300 lines of resolution. (Graphics by J. Daugherty.)

these cameras provide automatic gain control or automatic electronic shutters to assist in low-light situations; white balance control, which sets the color spectrum of the camera; and a color bar, enabling the setup of the other components in the viewing system. Most cameras currently used in the operating room are single-chip, but three-chip cameras are becoming more popular.

The video camera must have a scope and coupling device to view the internal image. Currently 0° to 70° arthroscopes are available. These scopes range from about 1 mm to 50 mm in diameter, with working lengths of 50 to 320 mm.

There are two ways the arthroscope can be joined to the camera. The conventional arthroscope has an eyepiece that attaches to a coupler, which is linked to the chip camera (Fig. 3-16). Condensation can occur between the arthroscope and the coupler, or the coupler and the camera, thus obscuring visualization. Therefore, each of these areas must be carefully cleaned before surgery. The image size can be controlled by the magnification power of the coupler. It is important to achieve the correct image-quality balance between the size of the image on the monitor and the brightness. (Image quality is also affected by the quality of the video monitor, which will be discussed next.) The

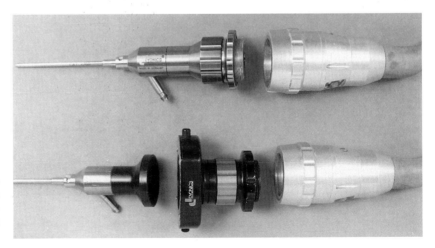

FIGURE 3-16.
The videoscope attaches directly into the camera head (*top*). In a conventional arthroscope, the eyepiece attaches to the coupler, which attaches to the camera head.

advantage of the system is that only the arthroscope must be sterile; a sterile camera bag can be placed over the coupler, camera, and camera cord.

A second way in which the arthroscope can be attached to the camera is by a "video arthroscope" (see Fig. 3-16). With this system, the arthroscope screws directly into the camera head without an intervening coupler. The advantages of this system include a shorter lever arm with a lighter arthroscope/camera combination, less possibility of moisture or condensation (fogging), and fewer potential problems when soaking the camera and arthroscope between cases. The disadvantage is that it is more difficult to switch to the 70° arthroscope: the inside of the connection is not sterile, so when the arthroscope is removed from the camera, it must be wrapped in a sterile towel or container so that contamination does not occur. When available, the most convenient method for the surgeon is to have two separate cameras attached to the 30° and 70° arthroscopes to avoid having to switch the camera back and forth and also to prevent contamination. A disadvantage is that the videoscope system must be soaked for sterilization if several cases are done in the same day, and soaking may diminish the life of the videoscope.

The degree of magnification and the size of the picture on the video monitor are affected by both the lens system and the coupler. Larger couplers produce larger screen images with a conventional arthroscope. The videoscope image can be magnified by using a different lens with the same-sized arthroscope. Some surgeons prefer a larger monitor image while operating, others a smaller image. The picture quality and brightness are better with less magnification (Fig. 3-17).

VIDEO MONITORS

The third critical component to an excellent video image is a video monitor. If the arthroscope and camera are of outstanding quality but the monitor is not, the picture seen by the surgeon will be less than desired. Current video monitors are available with up to 750 lines of resolution. The greater number of pixels produces sharper lines of curvature and greater resolution of margins within the image. The best pictures are obtained with a camera and video monitor system with RGB capability, so that the red, green, and blue can be separated.

DOCUMENTATION

Documentation is critical in ankle and foot arthroscopy, just as in other joints, and can be accomplished in various ways.

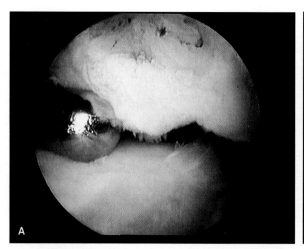
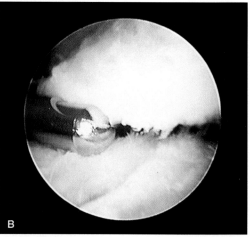

FIGURE 3-17.
Picture size and magnification are affected by coupler size. A 35-mm coupler (**A**) provides a larger picture size; a 25-mm coupler (**B**) gives somewhat better picture quality and brightness.

Video Recorders

The most common method of documentation is to record onto a videotape the image produced by the camera while watching the monitor. The entire procedure can be recorded, or "stop-and-start" editing can be accomplished by using a foot pedal, a hand-held remote control, or the remote-control buttons on the camera head. Videotape documentation is usually done on $^3/_4''$ or $^1/_2''$ tape, or on the newer $^1/_4''$ tape. In the past, $^3/_4''$ tape gave the best picture quality, but the new S-VHS recorders, combined with the appropriate monitor and camera, produce images of very similar quality. These tapes are also less expensive and provide fewer problems for storage after the tape is completed. In addition, most physicians and patients, in their offices and homes, have $^1/_2''$ videocassette recorders, making review of the tapes more convenient. In the future, $^1/_4''$ tapes may provide similar image quality, with the advantage of less storage space.

Photography

The second way to document arthroscopic surgery is by means of photographs. The best images are still produced by photographing the image directly from the arthroscope with a 35-mm film camera. However, this requires the video camera to be discon-nected from the arthroscope, and the camera to be attached to it. This also presents problems with sterility as well as picture composition. In addition, the 35-mm camera usually requires gas sterilization, thereby limiting the number of cases with which it can be used. A sterile drape can also be used to cover the camera, but this makes it more difficult to use. Some surgeons have used a photocoupler attachment to the side of the arthroscope, but to date this process has produced disappointing results. Images can also be produced by photographing a picture from the video monitor, but the picture quality is normally unsatisfactory for presentation.

Video Printing

Documentation can also be accomplished by using a video printer. The printer freezes the signal from the video camera and converts it into a digital image, which is then developed onto a special paper using thermal ink-printing techniques. The picture quality is not as good as a 35-mm direct photo from the arthroscope, but the clarity is improving each year. Most printers allow single, quad, or multiple images per print and allow the image to be modified for color, contrast, and brightness before printing.

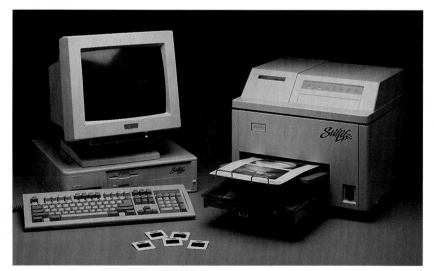

FIGURE 3-18.
A digital imaging system allows the camera signal to be processed via a computer, which transfers the image to a disk from which slides and photo-graphs can be produced.

Digital Imaging

The newer technology of digital imaging allows the camera signal to be processed through a computer, which digitizes the image and transfers it to a mobile disk such as a standard floppy disk, an optical floppy disk, CD-ROM, or a hard disk within the computer. The computer software then enhances the image to create a high-resolution image that is almost photographic in quality. With this quality of image, presentation-quality prints and slides are possible with easy interface between the surgeon and the system. This system also allows the images to be archived for patient files or for research and review. This permits great flexibility for the exchange of information with the patient, one's peers, and the referring physician (Fig. 3-18).

These systems should be easy for the surgeon and operating room staff to use and should give high-quality images for all types of presentations. These systems are sometimes expensive but are very versatile, allowing use by multiple disciplines in the operating room and for presentations and marketing purposes. These systems are the first step toward total digital imaging and the ability to process virtual reality or future telepresence, allowing the transfer of images world-wide for surgeon training or total surgical procedures via satellite. Surgeons should review their individual needs for documentation and determine which method is optimal for their practice, depending on the cost and availability of equipment.

Preferred Method

We videotape the procedure on Super VHS videotape, editing with a foot pedal or a remote-control device. The patients' names are entered onto the front of the videotape with the tape length, and when the tape is full it is stored in the office. When the patient returns for the first postoperative visit, the physician assistant and the patient review the tape together. Copies of the tape are made for the patient at this time using a second videocassette recorder hooked to the first. The tapes are logged and stored in the research area and are available for review by all surgeons. Segments of the best tapes can be used in a video presentation using a video editing system, and still pictures and slides can be shot by a camera hooked to the videocassette player.

This is quite an elaborate and expensive system and is certainly not recommended for everyone, but it shows how the system is used by one group of surgeons. The surgeon must also be aware that the tape of an arthroscopic procedure becomes part of the legal patient record and can be subpoenaed by the court.

INSTRUMENT STERILIZATION

Instruments are commonly sterilized by two methods. The first is steam sterilization, where the instruments have been wrapped. Steam sterilizers vary in design and performance characteristics, so cycle parameters vary according to the manufacturer's written instructions. Flash sterilization is steam sterilization and should be done only for emergency situations; again, time parameters vary according to the manufacturer's guidelines. The second method, gas sterilization using ethylene oxide, is the preferred method for sterilizing arthroscopes and light cables, because steam sterilization deteriorates the lens, sealants, and fiber-optic cables. The process varies according to the manufacturer and the institution. At our institution, gas sterilization is performed for 2 hours at 55° to 56°C, and aeration is done for 12 hours.

More recently, high-level disinfection with 2% activated glutaraldehyde (Metricide) for 20 minutes has been shown to be clinically safe and is currently used in many facilities, including operating rooms and surgery centers.[8,9] High-level disinfection is not sterilization, and time parameters vary according to the manufacturer's instructions. The advantage of high-level disinfection is that multiple cases can be done with the same arthroscope and camera with little delay between cases. In our surgery center and hospital, use of Metricide is common when a large number of arthroscopic cases are performed. The arthroscope is attached to the video camera and the whole unit is soaked, leaving only the tip that attaches into the camera box out of the Metricide. The arthroscope and camera unit is rinsed with sterile water after the required contact time to remove toxic and irritating residues.

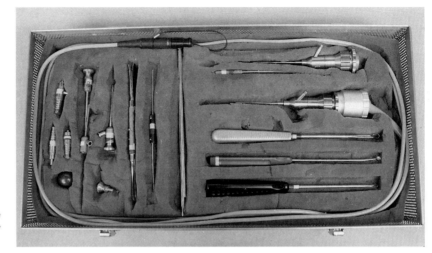

FIGURE 3-19.
Ankle arthroscopy instruments are stored in a special container for easy sterilization and organization.

ACCESSORY INSTRUMENTS

Various other instruments are needed to perform ankle and foot arthroscopy, including probes, cutting instruments, repair instruments, and retrieving instruments. Ideally, all the instruments should be kept in a large sterilization tray with compartments for the instruments (Fig. 3-19).

Spinal Needles

An 18-gauge spinal needle is commonly used to distend the joint and also to locate the anterolateral and posterolateral portals. Not only does the spinal needle allow precise positioning under direct vision of the portals, but it also gives a visual fluid backflow to verify appropriate joint penetration.

Probes

Probes come in various sizes and shapes. In the ankle, the probe should be about 1.5 mm in diameter to reach the small recesses of the gutters and to lift up under loose articular cartilage. An angled tip is particularly desirable in the ankle over the dome-shaped talus and flat tibia. The surgeon should have probes of several different sizes, at least one of which can be used through the interchangeable cannula. Although one of the least expensive of the accessory instruments, the probe is the most important to the arthroscopic surgeon (Fig. 3-20).

Dissectors

In some instances, probes may not be strong enough or large enough to free loose osteochondral fragments or ossicles from the soft tissues or surrounding

FIGURE 3-20.
Different sizes of small-joint probes allow palpation and evaluation of the internal structures of the ankle and foot.

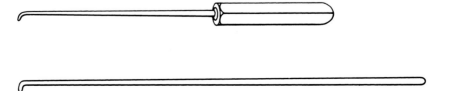

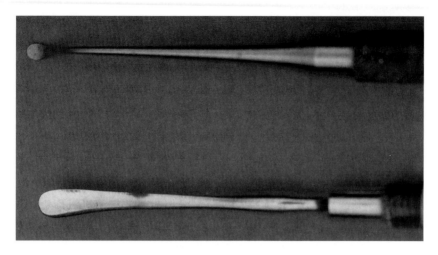

FIGURE 3-21.
Different sizes of Freer elevator tips
are useful for loosening soft-tissue and
osteochondral lesions.

bony bed. A gently curved dissector is stronger than
a probe and can accomplish these tasks more easily.
Sometimes a Freer elevator-type dissector is necessary when the bony fragments are large and
impacted, and a strong instrument is required
(Fig. 3-21).

Graspers

Another crucial instrument that should always be
available is a small grasper. The optimal grasper
should have a flat head, should be about 2.7 to 3
mm in diameter, and should be able to reach all
areas of the ankle easily. Two styles are particularly
valuable in the ankle and foot. The first is a flat-
tipped mosquito-type grasping forceps with fine
teeth, used primarily for removing small loose
bodies in soft tissue (Fig. 3-22A). The second,
a cup-shaped jaw-grasping forceps with serrated
edges, is better for larger loose bodies and soft-
tissue fragments (see Fig. 3-22B). If a large loose
body is grasped with a mosquito-type instrument,
it may spring the jaws or break the teeth. Regular
inspection of all grasping instruments is important:
pivot points or hinge pins that break inside the
joint can be difficult to retrieve. Graspers, like all
hand instruments, should be shorter for use in the
ankle and foot, allowing better tactile control and
dexterity.

The pituitary forceps is an important instrument
for not only grasping loose debris but also removing
tough fibrous material. Curved-up, curved-down,
and straight variations are available and are very

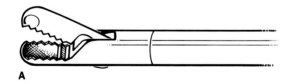

A

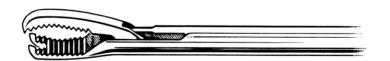

B

FIGURE 3-22.
Grasping instruments. (**A**) The grasper
is either flat or round-tipped, with fine
teeth for removing small loose bodies
and soft tissue. (Whipple TL. Arthroscopic surgery: the wrist. Philadelphia:
JB Lippincott, 1992:45.) (**B**) The pit-
bull grasper has strong serrated
edges for removing large loose bodies and soft-tissue fragments.

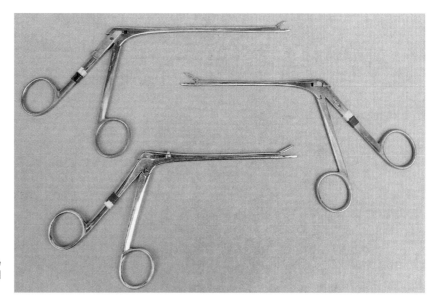

FIGURE 3-23.
Different sizes of pituitary forceps are useful for removing soft tissue and small fragments of bone.

convenient, particularly with soft-tissue lesions (Fig. 3-23).

Basket Forceps

Small-joint, short basket forceps should be available in a variety of tip designs. These include straight, angled right or left, and angled up or down. The design of these instruments should be different than those used in the knee, because scoop tips are not useful in the ankle and foot. Rather, the tip should be square or round to butt up against the synovial articular surface. The optimal size for these baskets is 2.5 to 3 mm in diameter. The instrument should be designed so that if the tip breaks, the hinge-pin mechanism remains outside the joint (Fig. 3-24).

The suction punch forceps is particularly useful

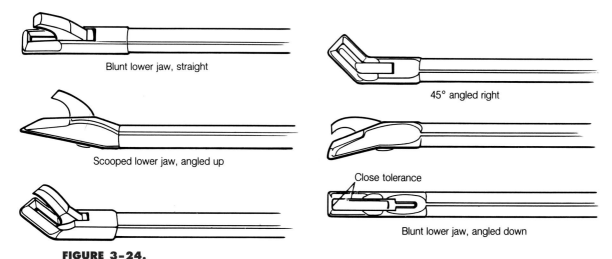

Blunt lower jaw, straight

Scooped lower jaw, angled up

45° angled right

Close tolerance

Blunt lower jaw, angled down

FIGURE 3-24.
Small-joint basket forceps with different tip designs help remove soft-tissue and chondral fragments. (Whipple TL. Arthroscopic surgery: the wrist. Philadelphia: JB Lippincott, 1992:46.)

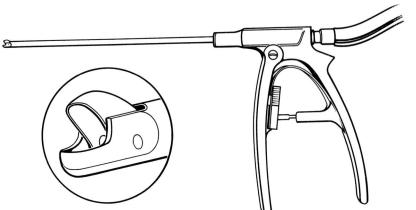

FIGURE 3-25.
The small-joint suction basket pulls the soft tissue into the teeth to facilitate cutting and tissue removal. (Whipple TL. Arthroscopic surgery: the wrist. Philadelphia: JB Lippincott, 1992:47.)

in the ankle. The blunt design permits cutting tissue close to the joint capsule and bony surface. As the tissue is cut, it is suctioned through the hollow shaft of the instrument to keep the visual field clear and ensure removal of loose debris (Fig. 3-25). Because this instrument is only 2.9 mm in diameter, it tends to clog and should be frequently cleaned with an obturator.

Knives

Different types of surgical knives are useful for excising osteochondral fragments, freeing ossicles, and removing loose articular cartilage. These blades are razor-sharp, resistant to breakage, and disposable. They are short and can be delivered through a cannula system. The blades are either straight or hooked, and are sharp on one side or both. The short 2.5-

mm banana blade is one of the most commonly used in ankle and foot arthroscopy (Fig. 3-26).

Curettes

Various small-joint curettes, either straight or curved, are available. These instruments are particularly valuable for removing osteochondral lesions, trimming articular cartilage edges, or removing articular cartilage for arthrodesis. They can be of open-ring or closed-cup design and should be rigid enough to resist bending and breakage. I prefer 3.5-mm, 4.5-mm, and 7-mm ring curettes for use in most arthroscopic situations (Fig. 3-27).

Osteotomes and Rasps

Small-joint osteotomes should be available to remove large osteophytes and to facilitate tissue elevation. Small arthroscopic rasps are useful for abrading tissue and smoothing uneven surfaces of bone.

Retrieving Instruments

Metallic rods, either hollow with suction or solid and magnetized on one end, are crucial during emergency situations. When an instrument breaks

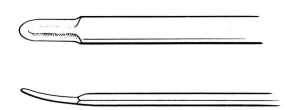

FIGURE 3-26.
Small-joint banana knife. (Whipple TL. Arthroscopic surgery: the wrist. Philadelphia: JB Lippincott, 1992:46.)

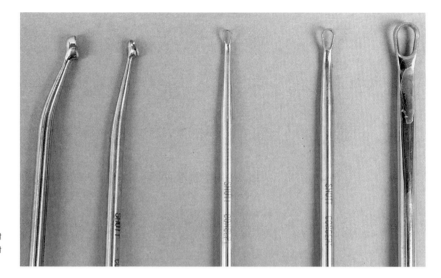

FIGURE 3-27.
Cup and ring curettes of different sizes are necessary for ankle and foot arthroscopy.

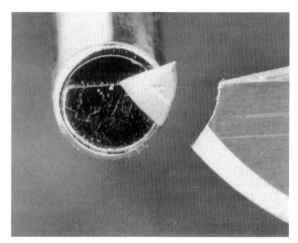

FIGURE 3-28.
A broken knife-blade fragment is held against the magnet of the Golden Retriever suction tube. (Courtesy of Instrument Makar, Okemos, Mich.) (Esch JC, Baker CL Jr. Arthroscopic surgery: the shoulder and elbow. Philadelphia: JB Lippincott, 1993:45.)

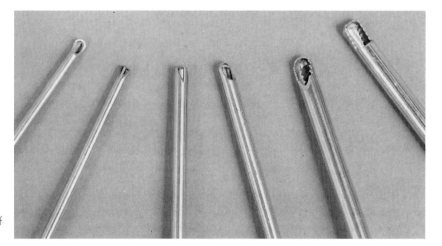

FIGURE 3-29.
Soft-tissue and cartilage resectors of different sizes and shapes.

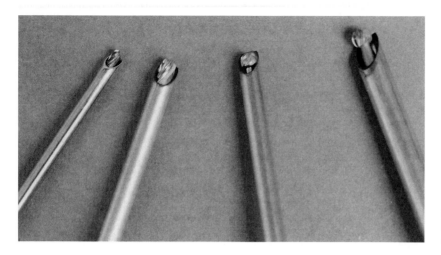

FIGURE 3-30.
Burs of different diameters are available with different-shaped tips.

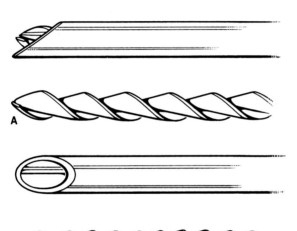

FIGURE 3-31.
(**A**) Coarse-cutting burr with deep flutes. (**B**) Fine-cutting burr with shallow flutes. (Esch JC, Baker CL Jr. Arthroscopic surgery: the shoulder and elbow. Philadelphia: JB Lippincott, 1993:47.)

and floats away, these devices should be immediately used to bring the broken piece into the anterior aspect of the ankle to facilitate removal. The combination of the magnetic tip with suction can greatly simplify the removal of a broken instrument tip, and can decrease patient morbidity and prevent exploratory arthrotomy. The Golden Retriever (Instrument Makar, Okemos, Mich.) is a very useful device for removing broken instruments (Fig. 3-28).

POWER INSTRUMENTS

It is difficult to do arthroscopy of the foot and ankle without good power instrumentation. Small-joint motorized systems are available to perform a variety of tasks quickly and efficiently. They can also excise larger volumes of tissue than conventional hand instruments and suction it quickly out of the joint.

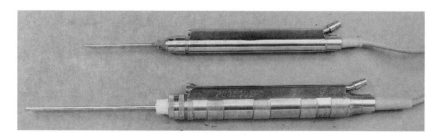

FIGURE 3-32.
Small- and large-joint motorized instruments are available for use in the ankle and foot.

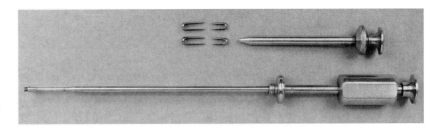

FIGURE 3–33.

Staple system for reattaching torn or loose ligaments.

These instruments come in shorter versions than those used in the knee and shoulder, and in smaller sizes (2 to 3.5 mm). Various tip designs are available, but all use a rotating blade within a fixed external sheath attached to a motor with suction. The blades can be divided into three types: full-radius resectors, cartilage cutters, and abraders. The soft-tissue and cartilage resectors run at speeds of about 2200 rpm; abraders function better between 3500 and 5000 rpm. All blades are disposable, single-use items, ensuring a sharp tip. In tight spaces, smaller 2-mm and 2.9-mm tips are used; where more space is available, the larger 3.5-mm and 4-mm tips are used (Figs. 3-29 and 3-30).

A power burr is useful for abrading or excising hard bone fragments and removing devitalized cartilage. Coarser cuts for rough large-volume work are made by burrs with fewer and deeper flutes; fine polishing work is best performed by burrs with shallower flutes and less severe angles of approach to the bone surface (Fig. 3-31). The faster the rotation of an abrader, the more aggressive the instrument. Abraders, like shavers, operate in a similar manner. If suction is applied to the handle, tissue is brought into the opening at the end of the shaver or burr. Burrs tend to clog more easily because of the amount and size of the debris being removed.

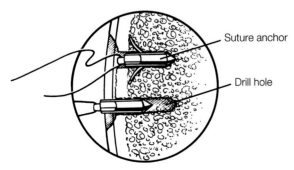

Suture anchor

Drill hole

FIGURE 3–34.

Suture anchors allow reattachment of soft tissue into the bone.

The handpiece and length of the shaver or burr tip should be appropriate for the area being treated. Various power instruments are available, and the surgeon's preference determines which one is used (Fig. 3-32).

The primary problem with all power instruments is coordination between the amount of suction and the amount of inflow. This is particularly critical in arthroscopy of the ankle and foot, where the volume of fluid in the joint is relatively small. If inflow is through the arthroscope with gravity drainage, most power instruments will quickly evacuate the joint, causing capsular tissue to collapse into the field of view. A separate portal is particularly useful to avoid this problem. In addition, the suction should be calibrated properly to match the type of shaver system used.

TABLE 3–2.

INSTRUMENTS FOR ANKLE AND FOOT ARTHROSCOPY

1. CHP camera with adapter to light source
2. Compatible light source
3. Small- and large-joint shaver systems
4. TV monitor
5. Ankle and thigh holder
6. Power reamer with Jacobs chuck and key
7. Ankle distractor, both invasive and soft tissue
8. 3/16″ threaded "trochar-tipped" Steinmann pins
9. 4.0-mm 30° standard scope and 2.7-mm 30° short scope with corresponding cannulae
10. #11 scalpel and mosquito clamp
11. 22-g by 1/2″ needle with 18-g spinal needle
12. 10-cc syringe with IV extension tubing
13. Two 50-cc syringes
14. Small ring curettes and pituitary rongeurs
15. Minidriver with K-wire attachment and K-wires
16. Miniprobes, graspers, and bites including 2.7-mm grasper, suction basket
17. Drill guide
18. 3.5-, 2.9-, and 2.0-mm shavers and burrs
19. Shoulder holder and toe trap for toe arthroscopy
20. 2.7-mm 70° arthroscope (optional)

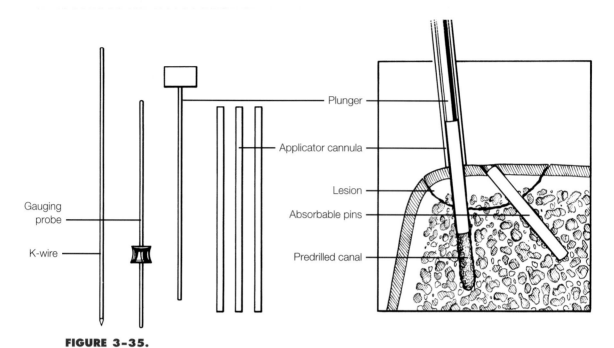

FIGURE 3–35.
Biodegradable pins are inserted by predrilling the hole and inserting the appropriate-length pin into the channel.

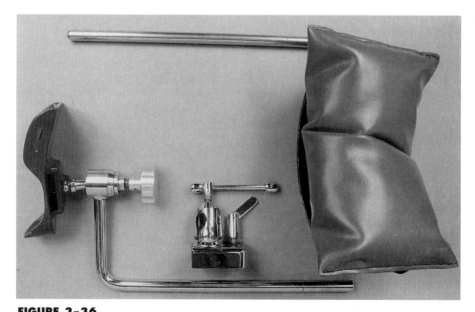

FIGURE 3–36.
A nonsterile thigh support (*right*) secures the thigh while the ankle holder attaches sterilely to the table with a clamp device.

REPAIR INSTRUMENTATION

Several systems are available for repairing ligamentous injuries about the ankle. One system uses 5.5-mm and 6.7-mm staples with a driver, impactor, and obturator system to tighten the lax anterior talofibular ligament (Fig. 3-33). A second system uses a suture anchor system inserted into the talus to tighten the ligaments, using nonabsorbable suture (Fig. 3-34). These techniques are further discussed in Chapter 10.

Biodegradable pins can be used to reattach osteochondral lesions to the talus or tibia. Several systems are available that use absorbable glycolic acid material fashioned into pins that can be inserted with appropriate instrumentation (Fig. 3-35).

OTHER INSTRUMENTS

Thigh and Ankle Holder

When arthroscopy is performed in the supine position, the thigh can be stabilized with a thigh support or a support under the popliteal fossa, as used in gynecologic procedures. These supports are placed nonsterilely and are adjusted to position the leg and foot appropriately. Some surgeons prefer to use an ankle holder to facilitate positioning of the ankle (Fig. 3-36). The ankle holder can be autoclaved and holds the foot in the appropriate position. It is particularly useful with invasive distraction. With some of the newer noninvasive techniques, the ankle holder is replaced by a strap that wraps around the ankle and foot (see Fig. 3-10).

Aiming Devices

Many jigs have been developed for arthroscopic anterior cruciate ligament reconstruction in the knee. Using the technology and principles of these devices, a small-joint Micro Vector device (Dyonics Inc., Andover, MA) has been created for adequate placement of guide wires, screws, or cannulated reamers during arthroscopic ankle and subtalar surgery (Fig. 3-37). This technique is discussed in Chapter 8.

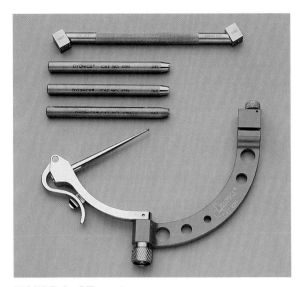

FIGURE 3-37.
A small-joint aiming device can facilitate the accurate placement of guide wires, screws, or cannulated reamers.

CAUTIONS

All instruments can fatigue and break. It is the surgeon's responsibility to check the instruments regularly. Worn or damaged instruments should be replaced to avoid intraoperative breakage. In addition, regular training sessions are critical to educate personnel responsible for cleaning, packaging, sterilizing, and storing these instruments. I use a special foam-padded surgical tray to hold all the instruments, including the arthroscopes, in precut holes so that the entire system is always in one place and readily available at all times. The instruments I use are listed in Table 3-2.

REFERENCES

1. Reagan BR, McInerny VK, Treadwell BV, et al. Irrigating fluids for arthroscopy. J Bone Joint Surg 1983;65A:629.
2. Marshall GJ, Kirchen ME, Sweeney JR, Snyder SJ. Synovisol as an irrigant for electrosurgery of joints. Arthroscopy 1988;4:187.

3. Reagan B, Zarins B, Mankin HJ. Low-conductivity irrigating solutions for arthroscopy. Arthroscopy 1991;7:105.
4. Johnson LL. Arthroscopic surgery: principles and practice. St. Louis: CV Mosby, 1986:182.
5. Yates CK, Grana WA. A single-distraction technique for ankle arthroscopy. Arthroscopy 1983; 4:103.
6. Guhl JE, Stone JW. Multimode distraction system. In Guhl JF, ed. Foot and ankle arthroscopy. Thorofare, NJ: Slack, 1983:69.
7. Whelan JM, Jackson DW. Video arthroscopy: review and state of the art. Arthroscopy 1992;8:311.
8. Crow S, Metcalf RW, Beck WC, Birnbaum D. Disinfection or sterilization? Four views on arthroscopes. AORN J 1983;37:854.
9. Johnson LL, Shneider DA, Austin MD, et al. Two percent glutaraldehyde: a disinfectant in arthroscopy and arthroscopic surgery. J Bone Joint Surg 1982;64A:237.
10. Esch JC, Baker CL Jr. Arthroscopic surgery: the shoulder and elbow. Philadelphia: JB Lippincott, 1993:38.

Arthroscopic Surgery: The Foot and Ankle,
by Richard D. Ferkel.
Lippincott-Raven Publishers, Philadelphia © 1996.

4

Operating Room Environment and the Surgical Team

Richard D. Ferkel

Arthroscopy of the ankle and foot is a technically demanding procedure that requires meticulous attention to detail, specialized instrumentation, experience, assistance, and most importantly a team effort for success. If any of these components are weak or inadequate, the result of the procedure may be compromised to the detriment of the patient.

OPERATING ROOM

The operating room—the arena in which the surgery is accomplished—must be large enough to accommodate all personnel as well as the arthroscopy cart and, when necessary, fluoroscopy. It should have the necessary equipment for general, regional, or local anesthesia, and suction should be calibrated appropriately for the type of motorized instruments used. The arthroscopy cart should be mobile to allow the procedure to be transferred to another room if needed. The arthroscopy cart should hold the video monitor, video camera, power pack, light source, video recorder, and video printer if one is used (Fig. 4-1).

PATIENT PREPARATION AND POSITION

Ankle arthroscopy can be performed in three different positions: in the supine position using a thigh and ankle holder; in the lateral decubitus position using a bean bag; and using a leg holder with the foot of the table bent at 90°.

I prefer the supine position using general or regional anesthesia. Local anesthesia is not recommended except for diagnostic purposes. If general anesthesia is used, the patient should be paralyzed to allow easier distraction and visualization. After appropriate anesthesia is administered, a suitable

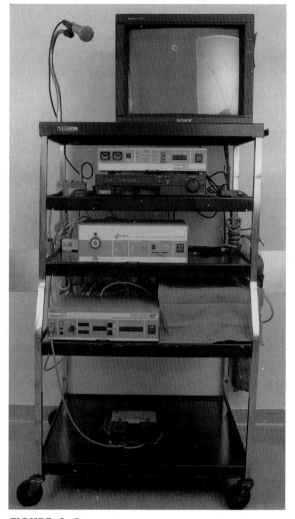

FIGURE 4-1.
The arthroscopy cart holds the monitor and power sources for the video camera, VCR, motorized shaver, and other photographic devices as needed.

antibiotic is given intravenously. A tourniquet is then applied to the upper thigh before preparing and draping the leg. A thigh support is used to secure the thigh in about 45° of hip flexion. Foam pads are placed under the thigh to prevent injury to the hamstrings and sciatic nerve. The patient is then rolled slightly until the knee and ankle are straight on the table. A bolster is attached proximal to the thigh support to prevent external rotation of the hip (Fig. 4-2). The operated extremity is then prepared and draped. A sterile clamp is attached to the table

over the drapes, and the sterile foot holder is used for invasive distraction before applying the tibial and calcaneal pins. When noninvasive distraction is used, a metal bar is inserted through the distractor and attached to a sterile clamp (Fig. 4-3). With this setup, the surgeon can sit or stand during the surgery, and both the anterior and posterior portions of the ankle are easily accessible without further manipulation of the patient's extremity.

EXTERNAL ANATOMIC LANDMARKS

The dorsalis pedis pulse should be carefully palpated and its position marked. Likewise, the saphenous vein and the anterior tibial and peroneal tertius tendons are outlined over the surface of the ankle.

Marking the superficial peroneal nerve branches is particularly important: this is the structure most at risk for injury when the anterolateral portal is created. This identification is facilitated by holding the foot in plantarflexion and inversion. The nerve can usually be palpated anterior and distal to the lateral malleolus. The joint line is identified and marked anteriorly by palpation in flexion and extension of the ankle (Fig. 4-4).

DISTRACTION

Without distraction, it is difficult to place a rigid arthroscope over a curved structure, such as the dome of the talus, without scuffing the cartilage or breaking the instrument. With distraction, the arthroscope can easily be manipulated posteriorly without damage to the tissues or equipment (Fig. 4-5). Various joint-distraction techniques have been described to improve visualization and ease of access for operative instrumentation.[1-3] Both noninvasive soft-tissue distraction setups and invasive mechanical distractors may be used. With improved noninvasive instrumentation, adequate visualization is usually possible without invasive techniques in 90% to 95% of cases.

Noninvasive

The patient's generalized ligamentous laxity should be assessed preoperatively. The anteromedial portal is established and the arthroscope inserted. A diagnostic

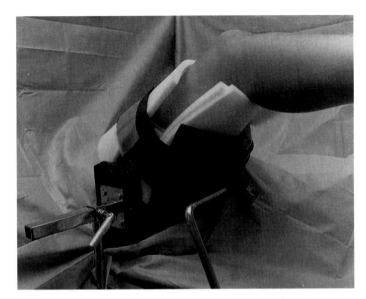

FIGURE 4-2.

The patient is secured on a thigh holder that is carefully padded, both anteriorly and posteriorly. To prevent external rotation of the thigh at the hip, a side bolster is placed over the area of the greater trochanter with extra padding.

examination can be accomplished and an assessment made as to whether the soft-tissue distraction technique used is adequate to perform both a complete diagnostic examination and surgery. The soft-tissue distraction device should be used with caution. It should grip around the inferior aspect of the ankle and foot, as well as along the dorsal surface of the midfoot. However, care must be taken to ensure the device does not exert excessive pressure over the anterior tibial neurovascular bundle, and periodic relaxation of the device helps prevent complications (Fig. 4-6).

Invasive

If noninvasive distraction does not provide adequate visualization, the invasive distractor is indicated. Invasive distraction can be applied medially, laterally, or on both sides.

Lateral

The technique for lateral invasive distraction has been described by Guhl.

1. Two threaded trochar-tipped Steinmann pins

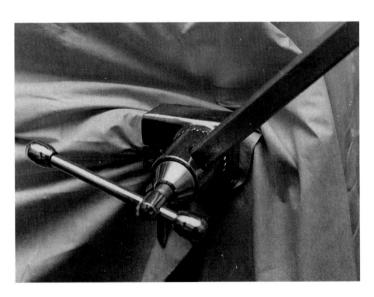

FIGURE 4-3.

A sterile clamp is attached to the table over the drapes; a sterile foot holder or multimode distractor can be inserted into this clamp.

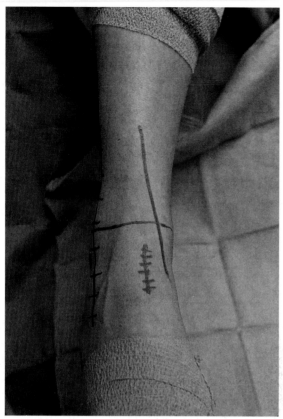

FIGURE 4–4.
Before making an incision, the nerves, vessels, tendons, and bony anatomy are marked.

(4.5″ long, ³/₁₆″ in diameter) are used. Both pins are drilled laterally to medially. The tibial pin should be placed 2.5″ to 3″ (6.5 to 7.5 cm) above the joint line. The calcaneal pin should be placed 1″ (2.5 cm) anterior and 1″ (2.5 cm) superior to the posterior inferior calcaneal margin at a 20° angle from the coronal plane toward the head (Fig. 4-7).

2. A stab incision is made in the skin 6.5 to 7.5 cm above the tibiotalar joint and a thumb-breadth below the anterior tibial crest. A small mosquito clamp is used to tunnel subcutaneously above the anterior tibial tendon to the bone.

3. A soft-tissue trochar with attached cannula is used to tunnel through the subcutaneous tissue anterior to the tibialis anterior tendon (Fig. 4-8*A*).

4. A Steinmann pin is then drilled across the lateral cortex to, but not through, the medial cortex to avoid a stress riser (see Fig. 4-8*B*).

5. The distal calcaneal pin is placed so as to avoid the peroneal tendons and the subtalar joint.

6. The skin stab incision in the calcaneus is performed using a technique similar to that used for the tibial pin placement. However, a 20° caudal inclination is used to direct the pins (Fig. 4-9).

7. The pins are drilled through the lateral cortex up to, but not through, the medial cortex. Care should be taken during placement of the tibial pin to avoid violating the tibialis anterior during insertion.

8. Once a nick is made in the skin, a cannula should be used to protect the soft tissues around the pin while drilling. Both pins should be unicortical and should not penetrate the medial cortex.

9. The joint is slowly distracted about 4 to 5 mm. Additional distraction is applied as the capsular tissues relax. Distraction should not exceed 7 or 8 mm, which usually corresponds to a reading of 50 pounds on the distractor.

10. Care should be taken to minimize bending of the pins. Distraction should be limited to 50 pounds of force for no more than 60 minutes. Periodic relaxation of the distraction device allows it to be used for a greater length of time without neurovascular injury (Fig. 4-10).

Distraction should be applied slowly because ligaments stretch more easily at slow speeds than at fast ones. Initially the joint will be distracted 4 to 5 mm; then, as the joint stretches, it will increase to 7 to 8 mm beyond normal. This should provide enough space for any type of operative procedure.

Medial

Medial-based tibiotalar distraction has been advocated by Morgan and others because pin placement in the tibia and talus allows dorsiflexion of the foot while maintaining parallel separation of the joint surfaces, rather than lateral talar tilting. In addition,

(text continues on page 79)

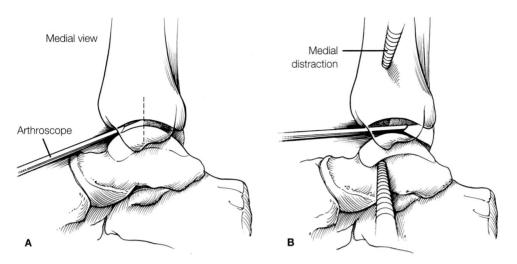

FIGURE 4–5.
Distraction of the ankle. (**A**) Without distraction, the posterior half of the tibiotalar joint is poorly seen. (**B**) With distraction, the arthroscope can be maneuvered from the anterior to the posterior portions of the joint and a complete examination of the ankle can be done.

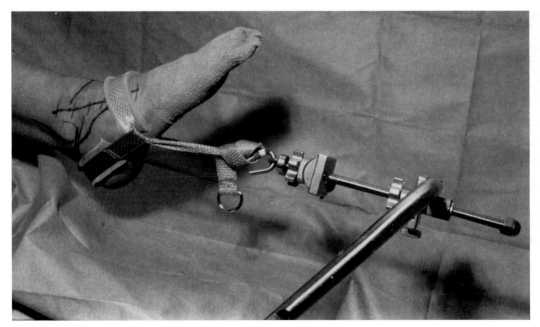

FIGURE 4–6.
Setup for soft-tissue distraction. The strap is positioned on the patient so to avoid injury to the anterior neurovascular structures and also to allow access to the ankle and subtalar portals, as needed.

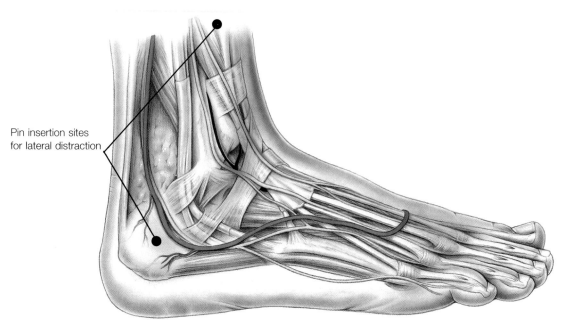

Pin insertion sites
for lateral distraction

FIGURE 4-7.
Lateral invasive distraction uses a tibial pin 2.5 to 3 inches above the joint line and a calcaneal pin 1 inch anterior
and 1 inch superior to the posterior inferior calcaneal margin.

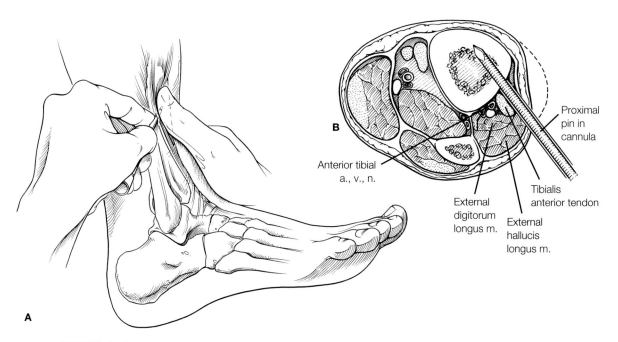

Proximal
pin in
cannula

Anterior tibial
a., v., n.

Tibialis
anterior tendon

External
digitorum
longus m.

External
hallucis
longus m.

FIGURE 4-8.
Insertion of lateral tibial pin. (**A**) Lateral view. A soft-tissue trochar is used to tunnel through the subcutaneous tissue
anterior to the tibialis anterior tendon. This trochar is placed one thumb-breadth below the anterior tibial crest to
prevent a fracture of the tibia. (**B**) Cross section. A Steinmann pin is drilled across the lateral cortex to, but not through,
the medial cortex to avoid a stress riser.

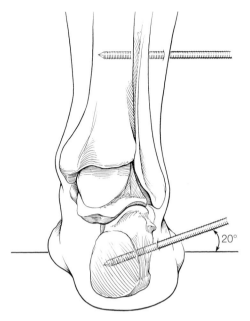

FIGURE 4-9.

Posterior view. The calcaneal pin is inserted at a 20° caudal inclination. As the ankle is distracted, the proximal and distal pins become nearly parallel.

they argue that having the distraction on the medial side allows easier instrumentation of the anterior and posterior portals.

This technique is performed by placing the proximal pin in the medial bare area of the tibia, about 1.5″ above the joint line, unicortically parallel to the joint. The distal pin is placed from medial to lateral into the body of the talus, starting from a skin incision placed just inferior and slightly anterior to the palpable tip of the medial malleolus. Recently it has been recommended that the pin be directed 10° both anterior and superior to avoid the subtalar joints and neurovascular structures.[4] The medial entry point allows plantarflexion and dorsiflexion of the talus during the procedure because the pin lies near the central rotation axis of the talar dome. The medial pin should never be placed behind the medial malleolus because of potential injury to neurovascular structures, nor should the pin be placed near the subtalar joint (Fig. 4-11).

Preferred Method

I prefer to use a soft-tissue distractor to aid arthroscopic visualization. If at the time of surgery it is evident that adequate distraction cannot be obtained

through noninvasive methods, then an invasive distraction device is applied on the lateral side of the ankle and foot.

OPERATING ROOM PERSONNEL

To perform arthroscopy of the ankle and foot successfully, each member of the surgical team must understand his or her responsibilities, and all must work together to accomplish the goal of a successful procedure (Fig. 4-12). The scrub nurse and circulating nurse help prepare the room for surgery and open all the equipment to be used. I also use an orthopedic physician assistant to help in surgery. The physician assistant is directly responsible for placing the patient's name on the videotape and ensuring that all the video equipment is working and

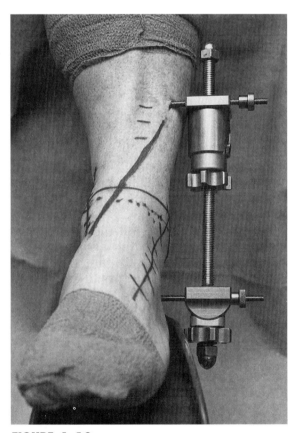

FIGURE 4-10.

Anterior/posterior view of an invasive distraction device with the pin positioned in the tibia and calcaneus on the lateral side.

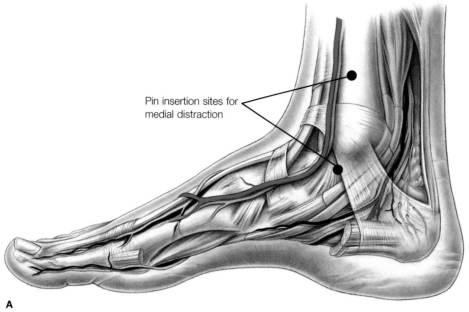

Pin insertion sites for
medial distraction

A

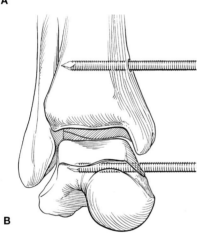

B

FIGURE 4-11.
Medial pin insertion. (**A**) Medial pins are inserted along the distal tibia and talus.
The pin should be directed 10° both anterior and superior to avoid the ankle
and subtalar joints and the neurovascular structures. (**B**) Anterior view. In the
coronal plane, the pins are inserted close to the lateral cortex of the tibia and
talus, but not through them.

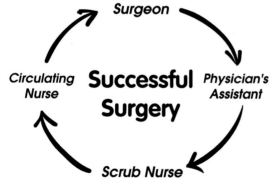

FIGURE 4-12.
The surgical team must work together to accomplish the goal of a
successful procedure.

that all instrumentation has been opened for the
procedure. The surgeon and the physician assistant
then secure the patient on the thigh holder and pad
all areas after appropriate anesthesia has been
administered.

The circulating nurse prepares the leg, plugs all
the equipment into the video cart, and sets up irrigation and suction. It is the circulating nurse's responsibility to monitor the irrigation carefully so the fluid
does not run out, and to keep the suction canisters
empty and the suction functioning. The use of the
Levelert (Dyonics Inc., Andover, MA) is helpful to
warn the nurse that the irrigating solution is running
low while he or she is monitoring other areas of the

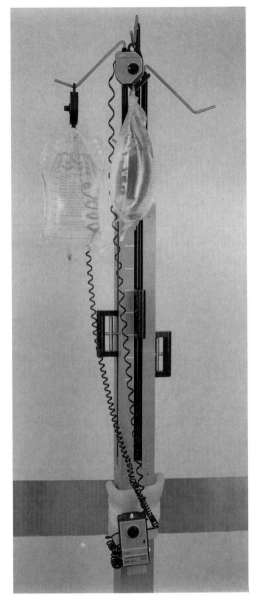

FIGURE 4-13.
The Levelert has an alarm to alert the nurse that the fluid bag is running low.

room (Fig. 4-13). In addition, the circulating nurse must be familiar with the video equipment in case there is a problem while the rest of the operating room personnel are scrubbed.

The anesthesiologist carefully monitors the patient and maintains muscle paralysis so that adequate distraction is obtained. In addition, the anesthesiolo-

gist notifies the surgeon every 15 minutes of the length of the tourniquet time. The assistant helps with the organization of the equipment during the procedure as well as with distraction and holding of instrumentation. The scrub nurse must know what procedure will be performed and organizes the appropriate equipment.

OPERATING ROOM SETUP

The operating room is set up to allow maximum space for surgery and the use of overhead lights, and provides room for nonsterile and sterile personnel to move freely. The operating room should be equipped with a full supply of disposable motorized tools, additional sterile light cords, sterile arthroscopes, and cameras, in case of equipment malfunction (Fig. 4-14). A backup arthroscopic set must be available in case of emergencies and equipment problems. With appropriate care of the

TABLE 4-1.
SURGICAL TEAM RESPONSIBILITIES

Anesthesiologist	• Administer appropriate general anesthesia with muscle paralysis or regional anesthesia
	• Monitor carefully the patient's vital signs
	• Maintain careful vigilance of the tourniquet time and tourniquet function
Physician assistant	• Prepare the arthroscopy cart and check that all video and arthroscopic equipment is working properly
	• Maintain surgical tape and note the patient's name before and after each case
	• Assist in patient positioning
	• Check with the scrub nurse that all needed equipment is sterile and on the field
	• Assist with surgery, including holding arthroscope and steadying surgical instruments
	• Assist with wound closure and application of dressings
Scrub nurse	• Facilitate the execution of the surgical procedure
Circulating nurse	• Must be familiar with objectives and techniques of the surgical procedure

(Whipple TL. Arthroscopic surgery: the wrist. Philadelphia: JB Lippincott, 1992.)

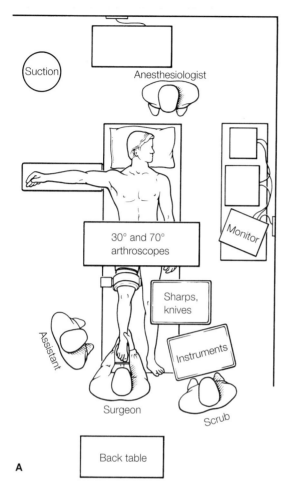

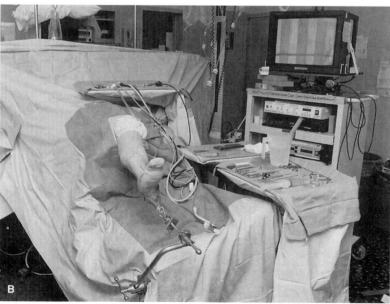

FIGURE 4-14.

Operative setup. (**A**) Overhead view showing the typical arrangement of the anesthesiologist, surgeon, assistant, scrub nurse, and various surgical stands and tables, as well as the video equipment. (**B**) Actual operative setup.

equipment, proper attention to detail, and understanding of individual responsibilities by all personnel, the procedure should proceed expeditiously and smoothly. Table 4-1 summarizes the responsibilities of the anesthesiologist, physician assistant, scrub nurse, and circulating nurse.

After the patient is positioned correctly, his or her leg is prepared and draped. Draping is done in the following order: an impermeable split sheet is applied around the lower leg to just above the knee; a heavier split sheet is then applied over the first sheet; and an extremity sheet is applied for a third layer of draping.

Equipment Location

Three Mayo stands are used for surgery. The first is only for sharp instrumentation. The second is for the most commonly used surgical instruments, and the third goes over the leg to hold the 30° and 70° arthroscopes, camera, and large and small joint shavers (see Fig. 4-14).

Procedure

The surgeon usually performs the procedure either standing or using a combination of standing and sitting on a roller stool. The sitting position is used to make the posterior portal and also to visualize the ankle through the posterior portal while the surgeon operates from the anterior compartment.

REFERENCES

1. Yates CK, Grana WA. A single distraction technique for ankle arthroscopy. Arthroscopy 1983;4:103.
2. Guhl JF, Stone JW. Multi-mode distraction system. In Guhl JF, ed. Foot and ankle arthroscopy. Thorofare, NJ: Slack, 1983:69.
3. Guhl JF. New concepts: distraction in ankle arthroscopy. Arthroscopy 1988;4:160.
4. Skie MC, Ebraheim NA, Hannum SQ, Podeszwa DA. Anatomic considerations for the placement of distraction pins in the talus. Foot Ankle 1994;15:221.

BIBLIOGRAPHY

Peters VJ, Ferkel RD. Arthroscopic surgery of the ankle. Orthop Nurs 1989;8(5):12.

Arthroscopic Surgery: The Foot and Ankle,
by Richard D. Ferkel.
Lippincott-Raven Publishers, Philadelphia © 1996.

5

Correlative Surgical Anatomy

Richard D. Ferkel and Richard A. Weiss

EVOLUTION

Some 24 million years ago, during the Miocene era, the tree-dwelling primates began to evolve into more terrestrially adapted species. The descent from the trees by the Miocene apes represents a critical period in the evolution of human locomotion. The shift to an upright position and bipedalism required a dramatic restructuring of pelvic, lower limb, and foot morphology. The human foot differs from that of other primates in three fundamental ways:

1. The human foot has both transverse and longitudinal arches.
2. The human foot is a rigid structure, with strong ligamentous support.
3. The human foot does not function as a grasping organ.

Because the foot brings humans into immediate and direct physical contact with their environment, it must withstand great stress, constant exposure, and the weight of the entire body. During the course of evolution, the human foot has developed into a superbly designed and exquisitely functional appendage.[1]

EMBRYOLOGY

The limb buds, consisting of mesoderm covered by ectoderm, first appear during the fourth week of embryonic development. The mesoderm gives rise to the future bones, muscles, tendons, and ligaments; the ectoderm goes on to form skin, nails, hair, and the sweat and sebaceous glands. The nerves and vascular elements grow into the limb buds from the trunk. The development of the lower limb parallels but lags slightly behind that of the upper limb. Structures appear in a proximal-to-distal sequence, from the thigh toward the foot. The future hallux, the preaxial or tibial border, and the postaxial or fibular border of the leg-foot axis are distinguishable shortly after the fifth week of embryonic life. Next the metatarsal condensations and future digits appear. By the end of the eighth week, as the embryonic phase ends and the fetal phase begins, the feet are fully formed, with the soles facing each other and the entire lower extremity in marked external rotation. This is the so-called "praying" position, where the feet remain until the seventh prenatal month. There is no angulation yet between the foot and the leg, and the ankle is in an equinus position.

During the ensuing fetal period, the leg-foot axis undergoes important rotational changes. There is progressive internal rotation of the thigh and leg, with subsequent dorsiflexion and pronation of the foot, bringing it close to the adult neutral position. The rotational changes during this critical period are due largely to the growth and interaction of the talus and calcaneus. Congenital foot disorders such as vertical talus and talipes equinovarus are thought to be related to abnormalities in talocalcaneal development during this phase of gestation.[2]

SKIN AND SUBCUTANEOUS FASCIA

The skin of the foot and ankle is similar in basic organization to skin elsewhere in the body. It consists of a layer of dense connective tissue, the dermis, covered by an outer layer of stratified squamous epithelium, known as the epidermis. The dermis is arranged in two layers: a deep or reticular layer, and a superficial or papillary layer. The deeper reticular layer is responsible for the strength and toughness of the skin. It is also within this layer that sweat glands, sebaceous glands, smooth muscle, and hair follicles are found. The skin on the sole of the foot has no hair follicles and lacks sebaceous glands.

The arrangement of connective tissue bundles in the retinacular layer gives rise to various patterns of cleavage or tension lines within the skin, known as Langer's lines. An appreciation of the pattern of cleavage lines is important to the surgeon because incisions made along Langer's lines are apt to heal with a fine, linear scar, whereas incisions that cross the cleavage lines are more likely to result in unsightly, irregular scars. On the medial aspect of the leg and across the anteromedial aspect of the ankle and dorsum of the big toe, Langer's lines run parallel to the long axis of the foot. On the rest of the dorsal surface of the foot, the lines of cleavage are arranged

obliquely at a 45° angle to the long axis, curving around the tip of the lateral malleolus. On the plantar aspect, the lines are arranged longitudinally with a gentle curvature, convex to the fibular side, and form a U-shaped pattern along the border of the heel (Fig. 5-1).

The skin on the plantar aspect of the foot is tightly bound to the underlying fascia by strong fibrous septa that limit movement between the two. The septa divide the subcutaneous fat into small chambers that act as protective shock absorbers in areas of increased pressure. Typically, the subcutaneous chambers are enlarged under the metatarsal heads and calcaneus. The skin on the anterior aspect of

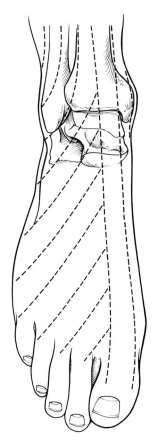

FIGURE 5–1.

Cleavage lines on the dorsal skin of the foot. On the dorsomedial aspect, the cleavage lines are parallel to the medial border of the foot. On the remaining surface, the lines are oblique, making about a 45° angle with the long axis of the foot. (Direction of cleavage lines adapted from Cox HT. The cleavage lines of the skin. Br J Surg 1941;29:234.)

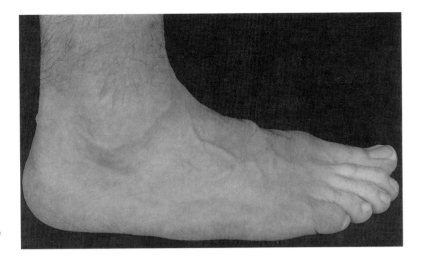

FIGURE 5-2.
Topical lateral ankle anatomy. Note the
position of the lateral malleolus.

the ankle and dorsum of the foot is thin and only
loosely connected to the underlying fascia. The skin
in this area is supple and easily moved over the
underlying structures.

LANDMARKS

Several bony landmarks and soft-tissue structures are
easily palpated on the ankle and provide constant
orientation during arthroscopic surgery. The lateral
and medial malleoli are readily identifiable bony
landmarks. The lateral malleolus lies 1 cm distal and
2 cm posterior to the medial malleolus (Figs. 5-2,
5-3). Passive dorsiflexion facilitates palpation of the

anterior joint line, which lies on a line drawn 2 cm
proximal to the tip of the lateral malleolus and 1
cm proximal to the tip of the medial malleolus
(Fig. 5-4).

The posterior articular margin of the tibia is positioned about 5 cm distal to the anterior joint line,
but is not palpable because it is located deep to a
thick layer of fibroadipose tissue between the Achilles and flexor tendons (Fig. 5-5). Posterolaterally,
however, between the lateral aspect of the Achilles
tendon and the peroneal tendons, only a thin layer
of fibrous tissue lies between the skin and the posterior joint capsule. The bony landmarks to be palpated on the medial aspect of the foot are the sustentaculum tali, located 2.5 cm below the tip of the

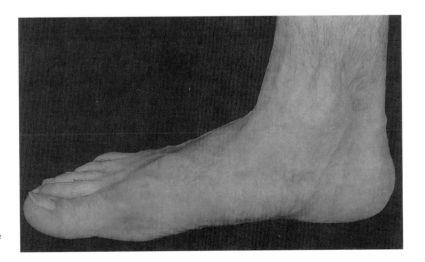

FIGURE 5-3.
Topical medial ankle anatomy. Note the
position of the medial malleolus.

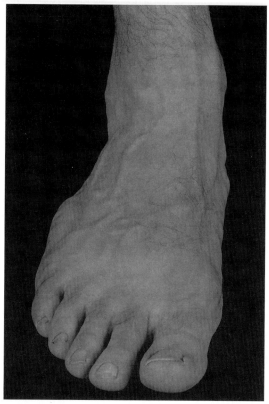

FIGURE 5-4.
Topical anterior ankle anatomy.

the midpoint of the bimalleolar axis to the proximal end of the first intermetatarsal space (see Fig. 5-6). On the lateral aspect of the ankle, the peroneal tendons pass immediately behind the lateral malleolus as they cross the ankle joint (Fig. 5-7). On the medial aspect of the ankle, a soft-tissue depression is palpable between the posterior aspect of the medial malleolus and the Achilles tendon. Within this depression lie the tendons of the tibialis posterior, flexor digitorum longus, and flexor hallucis longus, as well as the posterior tibial artery and tibial nerve (Fig. 5-8). Pulsation in the posterior tibial artery is palpable behind the medial malleolus, 2.5 cm anterior to the medial border of the Achilles tendon.

Subcutaneous Layer

Three sensory nerve systems and accompanying superficial veins can be found in the subcutaneous layer of the ankle: the superficial peroneal, saphenous, and

medial malleolus; the navicular tuberosity; and the medial aspect of the talar head, found at the midpoint of a line drawn between the medial malleolus and the navicular tuberosity. On the lateral border of the foot, the flared tuberosity at the base of the fifth metatarsal is easily found; one fingerbreadth proximal to the tuberosity is the calcaneocuboid articulation. The sinus tarsi can be felt by applying finger pressure to the soft-tissue depression just anterior to the lateral malleolus. If the foot is then inverted, the lateral aspect of the talar dome can be felt by deep palpation of the sinus.

Tendon landmarks of the foot and ankle are also easy to identify and palpate. On the anterior aspect of the ankle, the digital extensor tendons and anterior tibialis tendon can be felt. They run parallel to each other and under the extensor retinacula (Fig. 5-6). Pulsation of the dorsalis pedis artery can be felt between the tendons of the extensor hallucis longus and extensor digitorum longus on a line drawn from

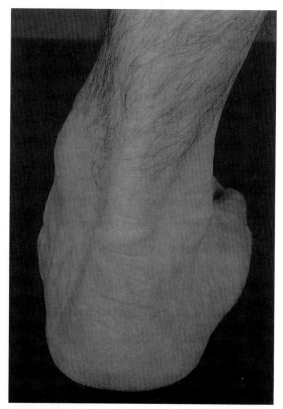

FIGURE 5-5.
Topical posterior ankle anatomy.

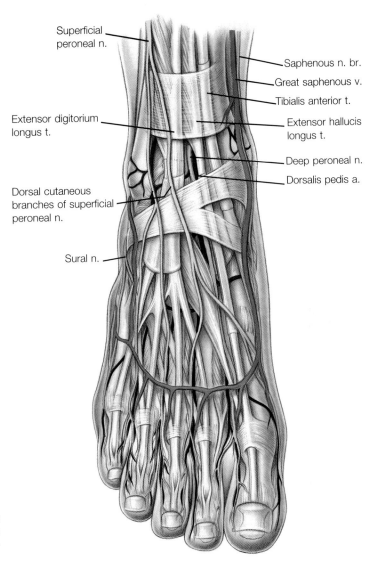

FIGURE 5-6.
Dorsal anatomy of the ankle and foot. Note the
position of the deep peroneal nerve and dorsalis
pedis artery and branches of the superficial peroneal nerve.

sural. The cutaneous nerves and superficial veins of
the ankle are important structures to identify and
protect when establishing portals for arthroscopy.

Superficial Peroneal Nerve

The superficial peroneal nerve is found subcutaneously and often can be palpated as a thin, tense
cord along the lower leg and ankle with inversion
and plantarflexion of the foot (Fig. 5-9). It arises
from the common peroneal nerve and passes down
the leg between the peroneus longus muscle and

the fibula. The nerve then becomes more superficial, descending the leg between the peroneal
group of muscles and the extensor digitorum longus, piercing the crural fascia about 6.5 cm above
the tip of the lateral malleolus. At this point it
divides into its terminal branches, the intermediate
and medial dorsal cutaneous nerves (Fig. 5-10).
The intermediate dorsal cutaneous nerve passes
over the inferior extensor retinaculum, crosses the
common extensor tendons of the fourth and fifth
digits, and then runs in the direction of the third
metatarsal space before dividing into dorsal digital

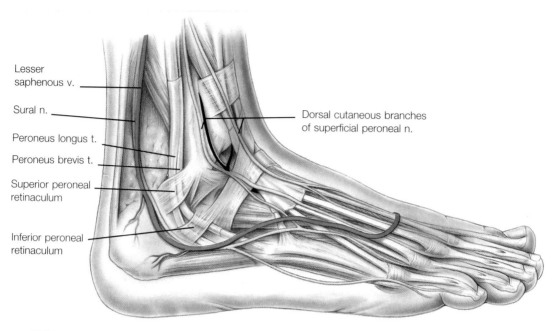

FIGURE 5-7.

Lateral anatomy of the ankle and foot. The internervous plane lies between the superficial peroneal nerve and the sural nerve, along the posterior fibula and peroneal tendons, and extends along toward the base of the fourth metatarsal.

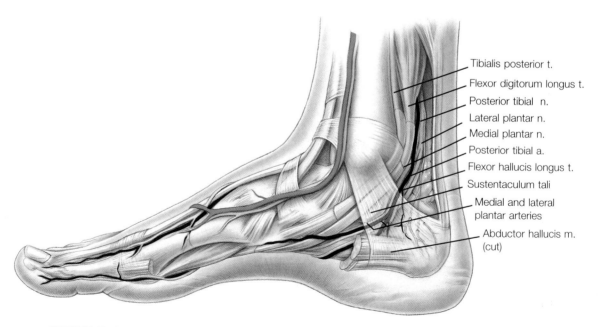

FIGURE 5-8.

Medial anatomy of the ankle and foot. The posterior tibial nerve lies between the flexor digitorum longus and the flexor hallucis longus, divides into the medial and lateral plantar nerves, and gives off calcaneal branches.

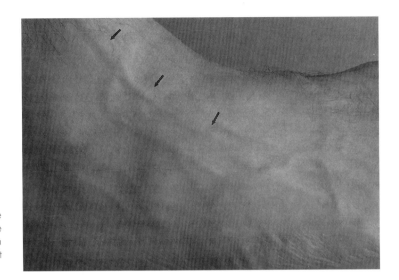

FIGURE 5-9.
The superficial peroneal nerve (*arrows*) can be identified by plantarflexing and inverting the foot. Usually only one of the two branches can be identified subcutaneously. (Head is to the left and toes are to the right.)

branches. The medial terminal branch of the superficial peroneal nerve, the medial dorsal cutaneous nerve, passes over the anterior aspect of the ankle overlying the common extensor tendons. It runs parallel to the extensor hallucis longus tendon and divides distal to the inferior extensor retinaculum into three dorsal digital branches. The terminal cutaneous branches of the superficial nerve lie in close proximity to the dorsal venous plexus of the anterior aspect of the ankle.

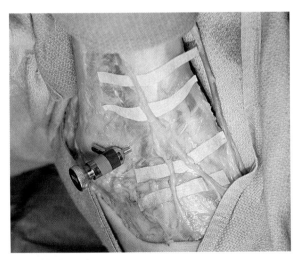

FIGURE 5-10.
Anatomic dissection of the superficial peroneal nerve and its branches. Note the proximity of the anterolateral portal to the superficial peroneal nerve.

This classic description of the course of the superficial peroneal nerve[2–4] has recently been expanded to include four anatomic variations[5] (Fig. 5-11). In a cadaveric study of 85 legs, the nerve was noted to lie solely in the lateral compartment in only 62 (73%) of the specimens, piercing the crural fascia 3 to 18 cm proximal to the lateral malleolus. The other descriptions included passage through the fascia from the anterior compartment in 12 specimens (14%), branches in both anterior and lateral compartments in 10 specimens (12%) before dividing, and one case of the nerve descending on the superficial surface of the peroneus longus fascia and then dividing, never running deep to the muscle. It is important to be aware of these variations because injury to the superficial peroneal nerve is the most common complication of ankle arthroscopy (see Chap. 15).

Sural Nerve

Posterolaterally, the sural nerve and short saphenous venous plexus lie in the subcutaneous tissue just posterior to the peroneal tendons behind the lateral malleolus (Figs. 5-12 through 5-14). The sural nerve passes 1.5 cm below the tip of the lateral malleolus and lies anterior to the short saphenous vein. The sural nerve divides into its lateral and medial terminal branches at the base of the fifth metatarsal. The short saphenous vein receives tributaries from

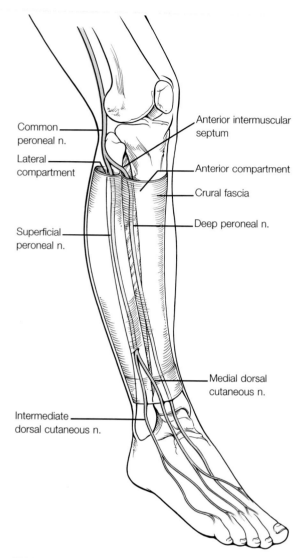

FIGURE 5-11.
The superficial peroneal nerve pierces the crural fascia and gives off two branches to supply sensation to the dorsal aspect of the ankle and foot.

The saphenous nerve supplies the skin of the anteromedial aspect of the leg. It is distributed distally to the medial side of the foot and may reach as far as the first metatarsophalangeal joint.

Deep Fascial Layer

The deep fascial layer contains the flexor and extensor tendons of the foot and ankle, as well as the two deep neurovascular bundles. The anterior compartment of the leg (Fig. 5-15) contains the tibialis anterior muscle, the extensor hallucis and extensor digitorum longus muscles, and their blood supply (the anterior tibial vessels) and innervation (the deep peroneal nerve).

The tibialis anterior is the largest muscle in the anterior compartment of the leg. It functions in foot inversion and ankle dorsiflexion and helps maintain the longitudinal arch. It arises from the inferior surface of the lateral condyle and the proximal two thirds of the lateral surface of the body of the tibia, from the interosseous membrane, from the deep surface of the crural fascia, and from the intermuscular septum between it and the extensor digitorum longus. The muscle fibers give way to a strong tendon in the distal third of the leg. The tendon passes downward on the anterior crest of the tibia, passing through the most medial compartment of the extensor retinaculum. It is inserted into the medial and plantar surface of the first cuneiform bone and into the base of the first metatarsal. In the upper part of the leg, the tibialis anterior covers the anterior tibial vessels and the deep peroneal nerve.

The extensor hallucis longus muscle is located between the tibialis anterior and the extensor digitorum longus. It arises from the anterior surface of the fibula and from the interosseous membrane. The muscle fibers give way to a tendon that occupies its own fibrous compartment in the inferior extensor retinaculum. The tendon crosses the anterior tibial vessels from lateral to medial at the ankle and inserts into the dorsum at the base of the distal phalanx of the great toe.

The extensor digitorum arises from the lateral tibial condyle, the anterior surface of the fibula, and the interosseous membrane. Between it and the tibialis anterior lie the proximal portions of the anterior tibial vessels and deep peroneal nerve. The extensor digitorum tendon passes under the extensor retinaculum with the peroneus tertius and divides into four

the lateral calcaneal veins and from the dorsalis pedis vein as it reaches the lateral aspect of the foot.

Saphenous Nerve

The saphenous nerve passes over the anterior aspect of the medial malleolus and is found posteromedial to the great saphenous vein. Both the nerve and vein cross over the anteromedial joint capsule.

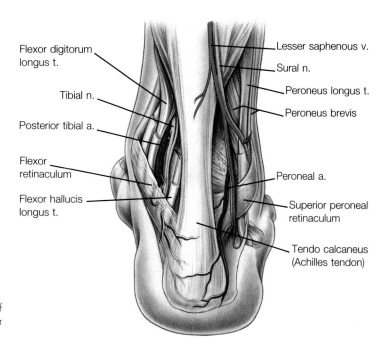

Flexor digitorum
longus t.

Tibial n.

Posterior tibial a.

Flexor
retinaculum

Flexor hallucis
longus t.

Lesser saphenous v.

Sural n.

Peroneus longus t.

Peroneus brevis

Peroneal a.

Superior peroneal
retinaculum

Tendo calcaneus
(Achilles tendon)

FIGURE 5-12.
Posterior view of the hindfoot. Note the relation of
the Achilles tendon to the posterior neurovascular
bundle and sural nerve.

slips, which reach the middle and distal phalanges of the four lesser toes.

The anterior tibial artery is one of the terminal branches of the popliteal artery. The artery and its two venae comitantes pass through the aperture at the proximal border of the interosseous membrane to lie on the anterior surface of that membrane, gradually descending toward the tibia. Close to the level of the ankle joint, the artery passes anterior to the joint and lies more superficial, where it becomes the dorsalis pedis artery.

The deep peroneal nerve arises from the division of the common peroneal nerve between the fibula and the peroneus longus. The deep peroneal nerve reaches the anterior intermuscular septum and joins the anterior tibial artery in the proximal third of the leg. The nerve lies just lateral to the artery as the two structures descend on the interosseous membrane, anterior to the artery at the middle of the leg, and then returns to its lateral position in the distal third of the leg. Multiple muscular branches of the deep peroneal nerve supply the anterior compartment musculature, as well as an articular branch to the ankle joint. The nerve then terminates in lateral and medial branches on the dorsum of the foot.

On the medial aspect of the ankle, the tarsal tunnel carries, from front to back, the posterior tibial

tendon, the flexor digitorum longus tendon, the posterior tibial artery and venae comitantes, the tibial nerve, and the flexor hallucis longus tendon (see Fig. 5-8). The posterior tibial artery exits the tarsal tunnel and divides into medial and lateral plantar vessels. The lateral plantar artery is the larger of the two vessels and provides the major contribution to the deep plantar arterial arch. The tibial nerve divides into medial and lateral plantar nerves as it exits the tarsal tunnel. The lateral plantar nerve supplies most of the intrinsic muscles of the foot.

On the lateral aspect of the ankle, the peroneals function as the primary everters of the foot, as well as assisting in plantarflexion. The brevis grooves the lateral malleolus and lies close to the bone, curving distally to its insertion on the tuberosity of the fifth metatarsal. The peroneus longus lies just posterior to the brevis, and runs in a groove on the plantar surface of the foot to insert onto the first metatarsal and medial cuneiform.

Ligaments

Tibiofibular Syndesmosis

The tibiofibular syndesmosis is formed by the rough, convex surface of the medial aspect of the distal end of the fibula and a corresponding concavity on the lateral aspect of the tibia. Distal to the syndesmosis, the tibia and fibula are smooth and covered by articular cartilage, which is continuous with that of the ankle joint. The ligaments that make up the syndesmosis are the anterior and posterior inferior tibiofibular ligaments, the transverse tibiofibular ligament, and the interosseous membrane.

ANTERIOR INFERIOR TIBIOFIBULAR LIGAMENT

The anterior inferior tibiofibular ligament is a flat band of fibers extending obliquely from inferiorly on the anterior border of the lateral malleolus, upward and medially to the anterolateral tubercle of the tibia (Fig. 5-16). It is divided into two or three bands, or it may be multifascicular.[6] The fibers increase in length from above downward, and during plantarflexion contact the lateral ridge of the trochlear surface of the talus (from cadaver analysis, 20% of the ligament is seen intraarticularly via the arthroscope).

POSTERIOR INFERIOR TIBIOFIBULAR LIGAMENT

The posterior inferior tibiofibular ligament is quadrilateral in shape and smaller than its anterior counterpart. Its fibers originate from the posterior border of the lateral malleolus and extend upward

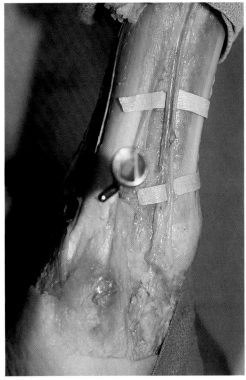

FIGURE 5-13.
Posterior view of an anatomic specimen. The sural nerve and lesser saphenous vein are identified. The posterolateral portal must be placed close to the Achilles tendon to avoid these structures.

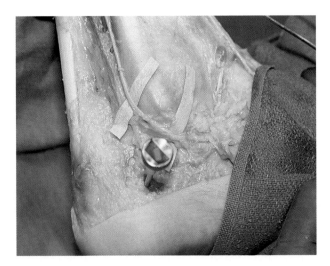

FIGURE 5-14.
Lateral view of the anatomic specimen, demonstrating the course of the sural nerve. Note the proximity of the nerve to the calcaneal distraction pin.

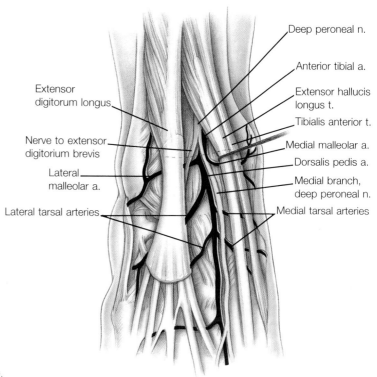

Deep peroneal n.

Anterior tibial a.

Extensor
digitorum longus

Extensor hallucis
longus t.

Tibialis anterior t.

Nerve to extensor
digitorium brevis

Medial malleolar a.

Dorsalis pedis a.

Lateral
malleolar a.

Medial branch,
deep peroneal n.

Lateral tarsal arteries

Medial tarsal arteries

FIGURE 5–15.
Anterior view. Deep fascial layer of the dorsal ankle.

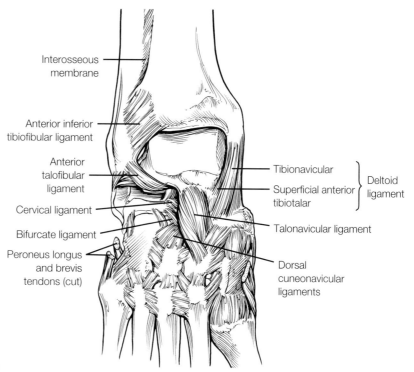

Interosseous
membrane

Anterior inferior
tibiofibular ligament

Anterior
talofibular
ligament

Tibionavicular

Deltoid
ligament

Superficial anterior
tibiotalar

Cervical ligament

Bifurcate ligament

Talonavicular ligament

Peroneus longus
and brevis
tendons (cut)

Dorsal
cuneonavicular
ligaments

FIGURE 5–16.
Anterior ligaments of the ankle and foot.

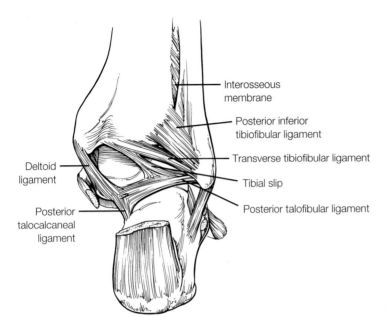

Interosseous membrane

Posterior inferior tibiofibular ligament

Transverse tibiofibular ligament

Tibial slip

Posterior talofibular ligament

Deltoid ligament

Posterior talocalcaneal ligament

FIGURE 5-17.
Posterior ankle ligaments.

and medially onto the posterolateral tibial tubercle (Fig. 5-17).

TRANSVERSE TIBIOFIBULAR LIGAMENT

The transverse tibiofibular ligament lies deep and inferior to the posterior tibiofibular ligament and is sometimes called the deep component of the posterior inferior tibiofibular ligament. This strong, thick band of yellowish fibers originates from the posterior fibular tubercle and the upper segment of the digital fossa, and inserts on the posterior aspect of the tibial articular surface, reaching the medial border of the medial malleolus. The transverse ligament projects below the posterior tibial margin and constitutes a true posterior labrum, deepening the tibial articulating surface of the talus. The transverse ligament fills the posterior aspect of the medial surface of the lateral malleolus and comes in contact with the articular cartilage of the posterolateral talar surface.[6] During plantarflexion, the transverse tibiofibular ligament is tightly squeezed between the posterior tibial

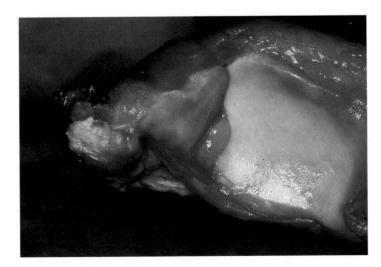

FIGURE 5-18.
Synovial fringe seen in the recess between the tibia and fibula. This tissue is usually located posteriorly, adjacent to the posterior inferior tibiofibular ligament.

margin and the posterior talofibular ligament. During dorsiflexion, however, a synovial-lined cul-de-sac and the so-called tibial slip become apparent (see below). The transverse ligament has a synovial covering that may hypertrophy and cause painful hindfoot impingement (see Fig. 5-17).

INTEROSSEOUS MEMBRANE

The interosseous membrane consists of numerous short fibrous bands running from the medial aspect of the distal fibular shaft to the lateral surface of the distal tibia. The fibers form a vault over the underlying tibiofibular synovial recess. This recess, which is about 1 cm high, contains a reddish synovial fringe that can be seen arthroscopically as it descends into the ankle joint between the fibula and the lateral talar surface as the ankle is brought into plantarflexion (Fig. 5-18).

Ankle Joint

The articular capsule of the talocrural or ankle joint is attached to the margins of the articular surfaces of the tibia and malleoli proximally and to the talus distally (Fig. 5-19). The capsule is thin anteriorly and posteriorly but is stabilized medially and laterally by strong collateral ligaments.

DELTOID LIGAMENT

The thick deltoid or medial collateral ligament consists of two sets of fibers, superficial and deep. The superficial fibers are broad and triangular, and fan out as an extraarticular sheet from the medial malleolus to the navicular, talus, spring ligament, and calcaneus (Fig. 5-20).

The most anterior of the superficial fibers form the tibionavicular portion of the ligament, inserting onto the navicular tuberosity, and the anterior tibiotalar fascicle, inserting onto the dorsum of the talar neck. Immediately posterior to this, the tibioligamentous fascicle inserts onto the superior border of the calcaneonavicular ligament. The tibiocalcaneal ligament, the strongest component of the superficial deltoid, originates from the medial aspect of the anterior colliculus, descending almost perpendicularly to be inserted onto the sustentaculum tali of the calcaneus. The superficial posterior tibiotalar ligament inserts onto the posteromedial talar tubercle, medial to the groove for the flexor hallucis longus tendon. The deep layer of the deltoid ligament

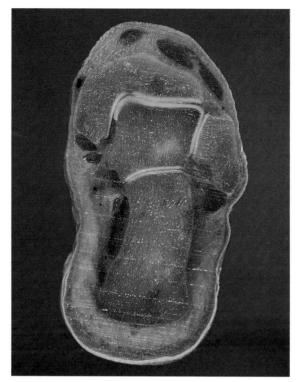

FIGURE 5–19.
Coronal section demonstrating the articular surfaces of the ankle and subtalar region, with the associated muscles and ligaments. (Courtesy of Professor Berend Hillen, University of Utrecht, The Netherlands.)

consists of a small anterior component, the anterior talotibial ligament, and a strong posterior talotibial ligament. The anterior talotibial ligament runs obliquely inferiorly and anteriorly to its attachment on the medial surface of the neck of the talus. It varies in size and may be very small or absent. The posterior talotibial ligament, the strongest component of the entire medial complex, is conical, with its base superior and apex posteroinferior. It runs obliquely inferiorly and posteriorly to insert on the medial surface of the talus as far as the posteromedial talar tubercle (see Fig. 15-19). The deep portion of the deltoid ligament is intraarticular and covered only by synovium.

Lateral Ligaments

The lateral collateral ligamentous complex consists of three distinct structures: the anterior talofibular ligament, the calcaneofibular ligament, and the posterior talofibular ligament (Fig. 5-21).

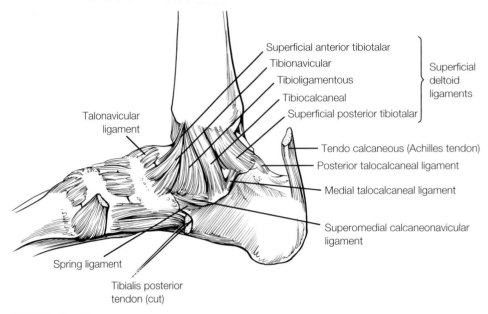

FIGURE 5-20.
Medial ligaments of the hindfoot. The fibers of the deltoid ligament provide stability to the medial aspect of the ankle.

ANTERIOR TALOFIBULAR LIGAMENT

The anterior talofibular ligament arises from the anterior border of the lateral malleolus and passes obliquely forward and somewhat medially to insert onto the talus just anterior to the lateral articular facet. It is a flat, relatively strong ligament, often separated into two distinct bands. The anterior talofibular ligament is closely related to the capsule of the talofibular joint, and be-

comes taut in plantarflexion as it braces the body of the talus (see Fig. 5-21).

CALCANEOFIBULAR LIGAMENT

The calcaneofibular ligament, a strong, cordlike ligament, is the largest of the three collateral ligaments. It originates from the lower segment of the anterior border of the lateral malleolus and courses inferiorly

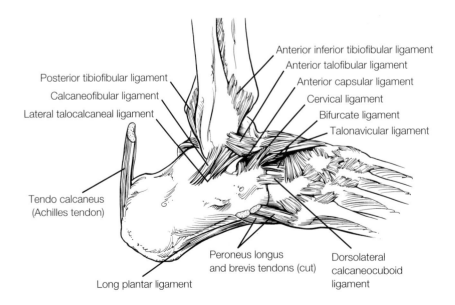

FIGURE 5-21.
Lateral ligaments of the ankle.

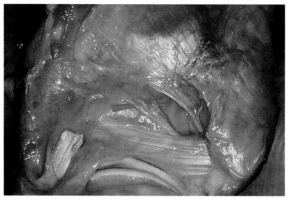

FIGURE 5-22.
The tibial slip (*marker*) runs from the posterior talofibular ligament and inserts on the posterior tibial margin, blending with the fibers of the transverse tibiofibular ligament.

and slightly posteriorly to its insertion onto a small tubercle at the upper part of the lateral surface of the calcaneus. The ligament is crossed superficially by the peroneal tendons and their sheaths, which may leave an imprint on the ligament (see Fig. 5-21).

POSTERIOR TALOFIBULAR LIGAMENT

The posterior talofibular ligament arises from the depression at the medial and posterior aspect of the lateral malleolus and runs almost horizontally to its insertion onto a prominent tubercle on the posterior surface of the talus, immediately lateral to the groove for the tendon of the flexor hallucis longus. The posterior talofibular ligament is the strongest and most deeply seated of the lateral ligaments (see Fig. 5-17). It is intracapsular but extrasynovial.

During dorsiflexion, the posterior talofibular ligament moves distally to expose a synovial-lined cul-de-sac. The floor of this recess occasionally demonstrates a thin band known as the "tibial slip." The tibial slip extends from the superior border of the posterior talofibular ligament and runs medially and upward. It inserts on the posterior tibial margin, blending with fibers of the transverse tibiofibular ligament, and its insertion may reach the posterior surface of the medial malleolus[6] (see Figs. 5-17, 5-22). Paturet called this structure the "posterior intermalleolar ligament."[7]

Synovial Folds

Synovial folds, or plicae, are membranes that invest the deep surfaces of the ligaments. The folds contain helical vascular networks that aid in turnover of the synovium. They also allow the synovium to glide on the overlying capsule or articular cartilage and are normal components of the chondrosynovial junction in all movable joints. The ankle joint normally contains plicae at the anterior and posterior tibiotalar junctions, the inferior tibiofibular syndesmosis, and the medial and lateral talomalleolar spaces. Trauma, adhesions, or chronic impingement may cause the synovial folds to hypertrophy, resulting in pain (see Figs. 5-18, 5-23).

Portals

The selection of portal locations is immediately related to the many anatomic structures on both the anterior and posterior aspects of the ankle. There are eleven possible arthroscopic approaches to the ankle. Portal locations can be grouped into anterior, posterior, and transmalleolar. Table 5-1 lists the key anatomic structures; this subject is discussed in detail in Chapter 6.

CROSS-SECTIONAL ANATOMY

A knowledge of regional cross-sectional anatomy is necessary to do ankle arthroscopy, especially when placing distraction pins (Fig. 5-24).

Distal Tibia

The tibial distraction pin is placed about 2.5 cm proximal to the ankle joint (see Fig. 5-24*A*). At this level, the anterior tibial crest presents a prominent subcutaneous border. The flat tendon of the tibialis anterior muscle lies on the anterior tibial crest. Adjacent and just lateral to the tibialis anterior tendon is the tendon of the extensor hallucis longus muscle. Between the two tendons and at a slightly deeper level, directly on the tibial surface, are the anteriortibial vessels and the deep peroneal nerve. Posteromedially, the posterior tibial vessels and the tibial nerve lie deep to the soleus muscle, between the flexor hallucis longus and the flexor digitorum longus muscles.

(*text continues on page 102*)

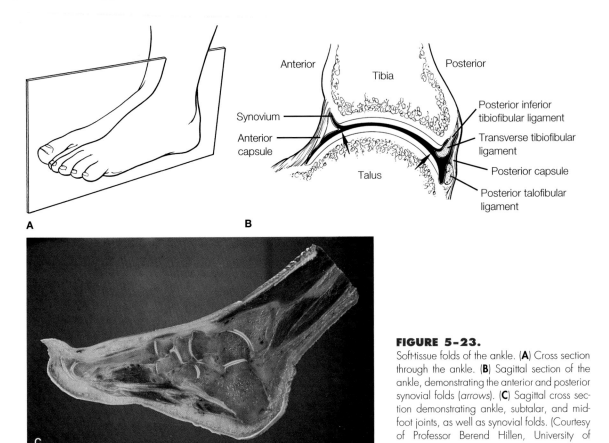

FIGURE 5-23.
Soft-tissue folds of the ankle. (**A**) Cross section through the ankle. (**B**) Sagittal section of the ankle, demonstrating the anterior and posterior synovial folds (*arrows*). (**C**) Sagittal cross section demonstrating ankle, subtalar, and midfoot joints, as well as synovial folds. (Courtesy of Professor Berend Hillen, University of Utrecht, The Netherlands.)

TABLE 5-1.
PORTALS AND THE NEAREST ANATOMY AT RISK

PORTAL	TENDONS	NERVES	VESSELS
Anterior approaches			
Anterolateral	Extensor digitorum, peroneus tertius	Superficial peroneal	
Anteromedial	Anterior tibialis	Saphenous	Greater saphenous vein
Anterocentral	Extensors	Deep peroneal	Dorsalis pedis artery
Posterior approaches			
Posterolateral	Peroneal	Sural	Small saphenous vein
Posteromedial	Posterior tibial, flexor digitorum, flexor hallucis	Tibial	Posterior tibial artery
Transachilles	Achilles		
Transmalleolar			
Medial	None	Saphenous	Saphenous
Lateral	Extensor	Superficial peroneal, deep peroneal	Anterior, tibial

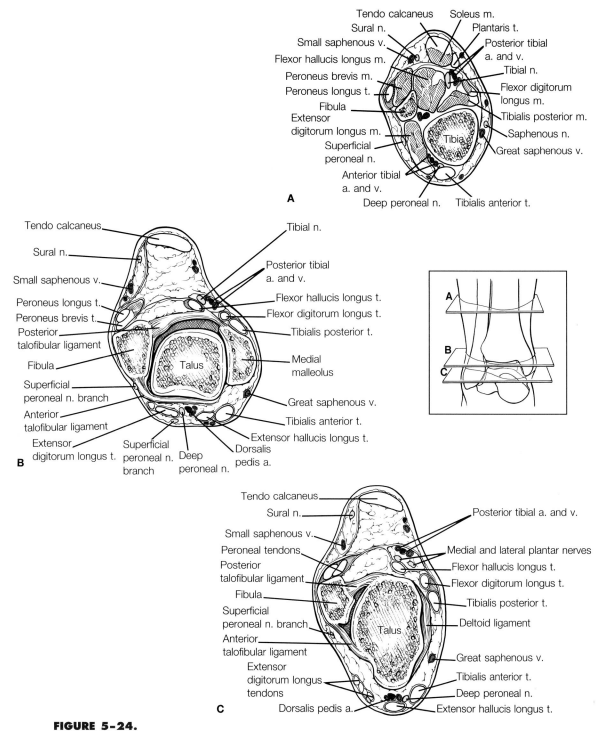

FIGURE 5-24.

(**A**) Cross-sectional anatomy of the distal tibia about 2.5 cm proximal to the ankle joint. (**B**) Cross-sectional anatomy at the level of the ankle joint. (**C**) Cross-sectional anatomy through the talus.

Ankle Joint

At the level of the ankle joint, the anterior neurovascular bundle is crossed from the lateral to the medial side by the tendon of the extensor hallucis longus (see Fig. 5-24*B*). The anterior tibial vessels and the deep peroneal nerve, therefore, lie between the extensor hallucis longus tendon and the first tendon of the extensor digitorum longus. The order of the structures that pass anterior to the ankle joint from the medial to the lateral side is the tibialis anterior tendon, extensor hallucis longus tendon, anterior tibial artery and venae comitantes, deep peroneal nerve, extensor digitorum longus tendon, and peroneus tertius tendon. Figure 5-24*B* shows the relatively superficial position of these structures. The tendons are readily palpable, as is the pulsation of the anterior tibial artery.

The posterior tibial neurovascular bundle is located behind the posteromedial aspect of the tibia, between the flexor digitorum longus and flexor hallucis longus tendons.

Talus

The central axis of rotation of the talar dome lies just distal and slightly anterior to the tip of the medial malleolus (see Fig. 5-24*C*). When placing distraction pins, it is imperative to stay anterior to the medial malleolus and superior to the sustentaculum tali to prevent injury to the long flexor tendons, the posterior tibial tendon, and the posteromedial neurovascular bundle.

REFERENCES

1. Jaffe WL, Gannon PJ, Laitman JT. Paleontology, embryology and anatomy of the foot. In Jahss MH, ed. Disorders of the foot and ankle. Philadelphia: WB Saunders, 1991:3.
2. Saraffian SK. Development of the foot and ankle. In Saraffian SK. Anatomy of the foot and ankle. Philadelphia: JB Lippincott, 1983:1.
3. Goss CM, ed. Gray's anatomy, 29th American ed. Philadelphia: Lea & Febiger, 1973:1000.
4. Holinshead WH. Anatomy for surgeons, 2d ed., vol 3. New York: Harper & Row, 1969:822.
5. Adkison DP, Bosse MJ, Gaccione DR, Gabriel KR. Anatomic variations in the course of the superficial peroneal nerve. J Bone Joint Surg 1991; 73A:112.
6. Saraffian SK. Anatomy of the foot and ankle: descriptive, topographical and functional, 2d ed. Philadelphia: JB Lippincott, 1993.
7. Paturet G. Traite d'anatomie humaine, vol. 2. Paris: Masson, 1951:704.

Arthroscopic Surgery: The Foot and Ankle,
by Richard D. Ferkel.
Lippincott-Raven Publishers, Philadelphia © 1996.

6

Diagnostic Arthroscopic Examination

Richard D. Ferkel

Arthroscopy of the ankle and foot is a useful diagnostic modality to evaluate pathology and determine appropriate treatment. However, it must not be used as a substitute for careful history, physical examination, and diagnostic testing. Its primary advantages over the other methods of evaluation are that it provides direct "eyeball" visualization of the internal structures of the ankle and foot, and allows these structures to be evaluated dynamically. When used with the proper indications, it is virtually 100% accurate in diagnosing intraarticular disorders of the ankle and foot.

PORTALS

Portals provide an entry to visualize the structures of the ankle and foot. In this section we will emphasize portals and diagnostic examination of the ankle; Chapters 12 and 13 discuss these principles in the hindfoot and forefoot.

Proper portal placement is critical to performing good diagnostic and therapeutic arthroscopy. If the portals are positioned improperly, visualization can be impaired, making diagnosis and treatment more difficult. A thorough knowledge of ankle anatomy is necessary to avoid complications.

Anterior Portals

Three primary anterior portals are used in arthroscopy of the ankle: anteromedial, anterolateral, and anterocentral (Fig. 6-1). The anteromedial portal is placed just medial to the anterior tibial tendon at the joint line. Care must be taken not to injure the saphenous vein and nerve traversing the ankle joint along the anterior edge of the medial malleolus. Just medial to the anterior tibial tendon at this site is a premalleolar depression or "soft spot" that often bulges in the presence of an effusion. The anterolateral portal is placed just lateral to the tendon of the peroneus tertius at or slightly

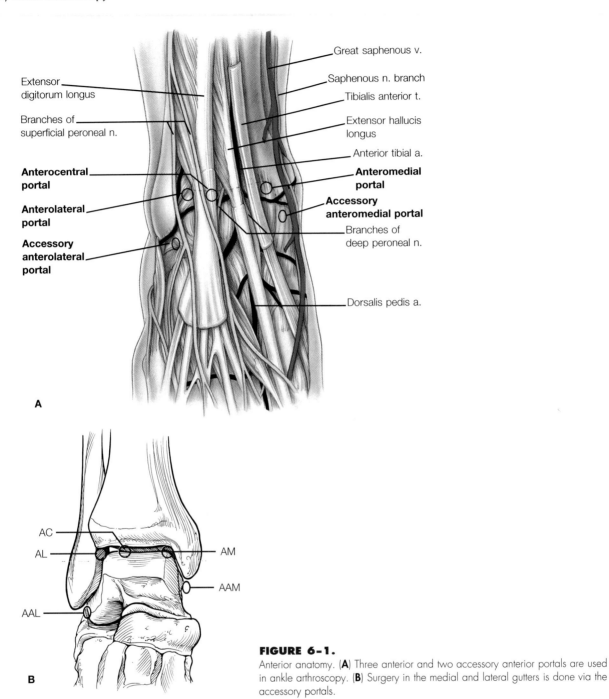

FIGURE 6-1.
Anterior anatomy. (**A**) Three anterior and two accessory anterior portals are used in ankle arthroscopy. (**B**) Surgery in the medial and lateral gutters is done via the accessory portals.

proximal to the joint line. The superficial peroneal nerve divides 6.5 cm proximal to the tip of the fibula into the intermediate dorsal and medial dorsal cutaneous branches.[1] The intermediate dorsal cutaneous nerve passes over the inferior extensor retinaculum, crosses the common extensor tendons of the fourth and fifth digits, and runs in the direction of the third metatarsal space before dividing into the dorsal digital branches. The medial terminal branch of the superficial peroneal nerve, the medial dorsal cutaneous nerve, passes over the anterior aspect of the ankle overlying the common extensor tendons.

It runs parallel to the extensor hallucis longus and divides distal to the inferior extensor retinaculum into the three dorsal digital branches. These nerve branches must be avoided during portal placement (see Fig. 5-11 in Chapter 5). Between these portals, an anterior central portal may be established between the tendons of the extensor digitorum communis. Placing the portal between the tendons helps to avoid injury to the neurovascular structures, including the dorsalis pedis artery and the deep branch of the peroneal nerve. The dorsalis pedis artery and the deep branch of the peroneal nerve lie deep in the interval between the extensor hallucis longus and the medial border of the extensor digitorum communis tendons. The medial branches of the superficial peroneal nerve must also be avoided when using this portal. In the past, use of this portal has been advocated to allow greater ease of passage of instruments and the arthroscope from the anterior and posterior compartment because of the different degree of concave curvature of the dome of the talus in the medial/lateral or coronal plane. However, in my experience, use of this portal has never been necessary in more than 600 ankle arthroscopies, and its use is strongly discouraged due to the increased potential for complications.

Accessory Anterior Portals

The accessory anterior portals are used in addition to the usual anteromedial and anterolateral portals. They can be useful while working in the tight spaces of the medial and lateral gutters for instrumentation or excision of soft tissue or bony lesions. Two accessory anterior portals are most commonly used, the anterolateral and the anteromedial (see Fig. 6-1). The accessory anteromedial portal is established 0.5 to 1 cm inferior and 1 cm anterior to the anterior border of the medial malleolus. It is especially useful in facilitating the evaluation of the medial gutter and deltoid ligament, particularly for the removal of ossicles inherent to the deep portion of the deltoid ligament while visualizing from the anteromedial portal.

The accessory anterolateral portal is established 1 cm anterior to and at or just below the tip of the anterior border of the lateral malleolus, in the area of the anterior talofibular ligament. When visualizing

ossicles from the anterolateral portal, an instrument can be inserted through the accessory anterolateral portal to facilitate removal as well as probing of the anterior talofibular ligament, the posterior talofibular ligament, and surrounding bony architecture.

Posterior Portals

Posterior portals are routinely used in ankle arthroscopy and may be established posteromedial, posterolateral, or directly through the Achilles tendon (trans-Achilles; Fig. 6-2).

The posterolateral portal, the most commonly used and the safest, is located directly adjacent to the lateral edge of the Achilles tendon, about 1.2 to 2.5 cm above the tip of the fibula; the exact level depends on the type of distraction used. This portal is usually at or slightly below the joint line. Branches of the sural nerve and the small saphenous vein must be avoided with the posterolateral approach.

The trans-Achilles portal is established at the same level as the posterolateral, but through the center of the Achilles tendon. It was originally designed to allow a two-portal instrumentation technique in the posterior aspect of the ankle, as well as to avoid injury to neurovascular structures lateral to the Achilles tendon. However, in my experience, this portal does not allow easy mobility of the arthroscope and instruments and may lead to increased morbidity in the Achilles tendon region. It has been abandoned for these reasons.

The posteromedial portal is made just medial to the Achilles tendon at the joint line. The posterior tibial artery and the tibial nerve must be avoided, and the tendons of the flexor hallucis longus and flexor digitorum longus must also be protected. The calcaneal nerve and its branches may separate from the tibial nerve proximal to the ankle joint and traverse in an interval between the tibial nerve and the medial border of the Achilles tendon. Because of the potential for serious complications, the posteromedial portal is contraindicated in all but the most extreme situations.

Accessory Posterior Portals

The accessory posterolateral portal is made at the same level as or slightly higher than the posterolateral portal. It is established 1 to 1.5 cm lateral to the

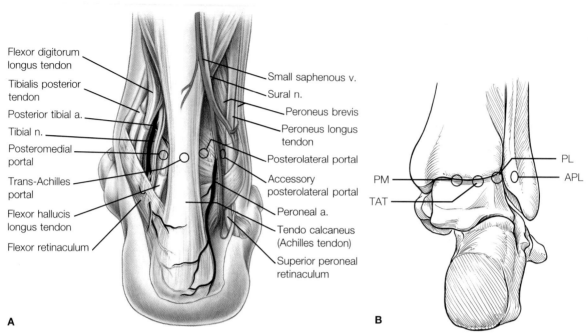

A **B**

FIGURE 6-2.

Posterior anatomy. (**A**) There are three posterior portals and one accessory posterior portal in the ankle. Usually only the posterolateral portal is used. (**B**) Note the relations of the posterior portals to the bony anatomy.

posterolateral portal, and extreme caution must be exercised to avoid injury to the neurovascular structures (see Fig. 6-2). It is particularly useful for the removal of posterior loose bodies when posterior visualization is necessary, and for the debridement and drilling of very posterior osteochondral lesions of the talus.

Transmalleolar and Transtalar Portals

Transmalleolar portals may be used for various operative techniques to gain better access to osteochondral lesions of the talar dome. It is more frequently used on the medial side than on the lateral side because lateral talar dome lesions are located more anterior than those on the medial side, and the lateral malleolus is farther posterior than the medial malleolus. It is particularly useful for drilling Kirschner wires under arthroscopic control through the tibia or fibula into the talar dome using a small-joint drill guide. Bone grafting of certain osteochondral lesions of the medial dome of the talus has also been done

through this portal (see Chap. 8 for a more detailed discussion of this subject).

Transtalar portals can be used to drill or bone-graft osteochondral lesions of the talus, especially medial lesions. The lateral transtalar portal is made

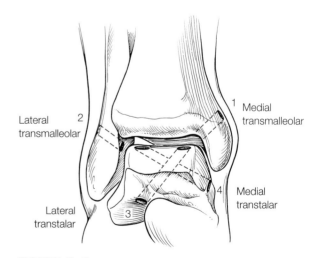

FIGURE 6-3.

Anterior view. The transmalleolar and transtalar portals of the ankle.

at the lateral talar process and is discussed further in Chapter 8 (Fig. 6-3).

SURGICAL TECHNIQUE (PREFERRED METHOD)

After the patient is brought to the operating room and appropriate anesthesia is administered, the patient is secured in the supine position with a thigh holder as detailed in Chapter 4. If general anesthesia is used, the patient should be paralyzed to allow maximum ankle distraction. The extremity is then prepared and draped and all tendinous, bony, and neurovascular structures are carefully marked. Before starting the procedure, the ankle and foot, including the toes, should be plantarflexed and inverted so that the superficial peroneal nerve and its branches can be identified, if possible (Fig. 6-4).

The anteromedial portal is always established first because it is easier to access, has less risk of injuring neurovascular structures, and is most reproducible.

Ten to 15 cc of sterile lactated Ringer's solution is infused in the ankle joint with an 18-gauge needle angled in a posterolateral direction. Joint distention is verified by outpouching of the anterolateral capsular wall. A #11 scalpel is used to make a vertical skin incision with one hand while palpating the anterior tibial tendon with the other (Fig. 6-5). Dissection using a mosquito clamp is then carried out through the subcutaneous tissue and capsule, and a blunt trochar with the attached arthroscopic cannula is carefully placed into the ankle joint. Additional lactated Ringer's solution is infused into the joint via a syringe through the arthroscopic side port, and the joint is visualized from the anteromedial portal.

An 18-gauge spinal needle is inserted in the ankle joint to locate under direct vision the position for the anterolateral portal. The location of this portal varies depending on the location of the primary pathology in the ankle, so it should not be established first. Similar techniques are used to incise the skin, taking extreme caution to avoid injuring branches of the superficial peroneal nerve as the mosquito clamp bluntly dissects down onto the capsule. This is followed by insertion of an inflow cannula into the ankle joint. At this juncture, an

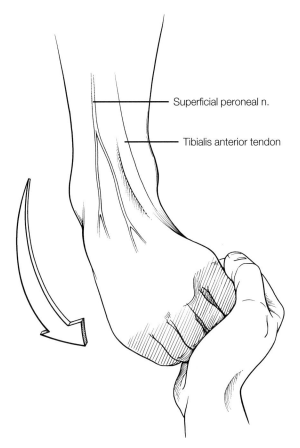

FIGURE 6-4.
The superficial peroneal nerve is checked preoperatively by plantarflexion and inversion of the ankle and foot.

assessment can be made as to whether a soft-tissue, noninvasive or invasive distraction technique will be necessary.

The posterolateral portal is always established, not only to facilitate inflow but also to permit visualization of the posterior structures. This is accomplished by distracting the joint and gently maneuvering the arthroscope under the medial notch of Harty until the posterior capsule and posterior ligaments are visualized. With good inflow from the anterolateral portal distending the capsule, an 18-gauge spinal needle is introduced through the posterolateral portal just medial to the transverse tibiofibular ligament (Fig. 6-6A,B).

The exact site of puncture through the capsule varies depending on whether the pathology is more lateral or more medial. For typical posteromedial osteo-

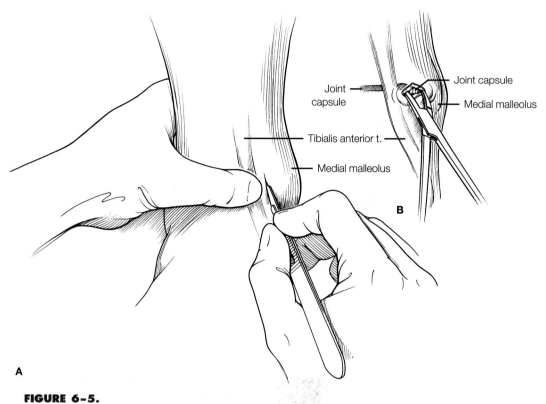

Joint capsule

Joint capsule

Medial malleolus

Tibialis anterior t.

Medial malleolus

B

A

FIGURE 6–5.

Establishing the anteromedial portal. (**A**) An incision is made medial to the anterior tibial tendon while palpating the tendon with the thumb. (**B**) Blunt dissection is performed with a clamp through the skin to the capsule.

chondral lesions of the talus, the puncture through the capsule should be in the soft spot interval between the transverse tibiofibular ligament and the extraarticular flexor hallucis longus tendon. For more central or posterolateral lesions, the portal should be established closer to the transverse tibiofibular ligament or in the interval between the transverse tibiofibular ligament and the posterior inferior tibiofibular ligament. This puncture should be angled toward the pathology to permit easier visualization. Once again, the key to establishing the posterior portal is good joint distention with constant distraction.

The posterior cannula is then inserted with care to avoid injury to the branches of the sural nerve and the short saphenous vein (see Fig. 6-6C). The posterolateral portal is initially used as a primary inflow portal, and it may be subsequently used for visualization or instrumentation by means of an interchangeable system of cannulae.

ARTHROSCOPIC ANATOMY

Normal Ankle

The intraarticular anatomy of the ankle as seen during arthroscopic examination has been described extensively.[2] The ankle joint can be divided into anterior and posterior cavities, each of which can then be subdivided further into three compartments for methodical inspection of the joint.[3]

I have developed a 21-point systematic examination of the anterior, central, and posterior ankle joint to increase the accuracy and reproducibility of the arthroscopic examination.[4,5] Use of this system allows the surgeon to document the findings in a reproducible fashion and to diagnose accurately any potential intraarticular pathology. In addition, it guarantees that all areas of the ankle joint are carefully inspected, and provides a videotape record that is complete and can be reviewed

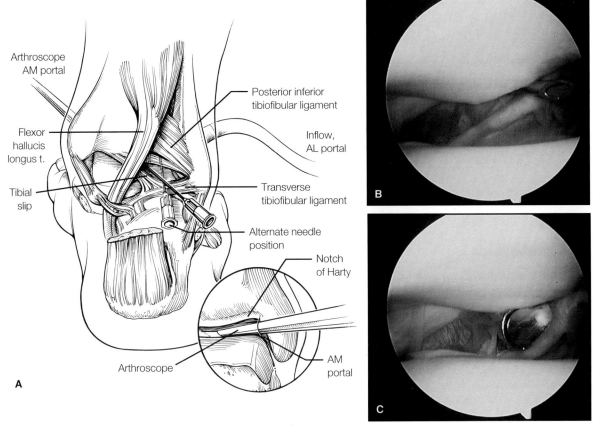

FIGURE 6-6.

Establishing the posterolateral portal. (**A**) Posterior view. Inflow is placed through the anterolateral (AL) portal and the arthroscope is inserted through the anteromedial (AM) portal. (Inset) Anterior view. The arthroscope is then maneuvered through the notch of Harty to visualize the posterior structures. A spinal needle is then inserted to determine the appropriate direction for the posterolateral portal. (**B**) Arthroscopic view from the anterolateral portal, demonstrating the spinal needle penetrating the joint capsule medial to the transverse tibiofibular ligament. (**C**) After the spinal needle determines the appropriate direction, the interchangeable cannula is inserted through the posterolateral portal under direct vision, medial to the transverse tibiofibular ligament.

in the future for both patient care and clinical studies of ankle arthroscopy patients.

Anterior Ankle Examination

The arthroscopic examination is always done initially through the anteromedial portal, then through the anterolateral and posterolateral portals (Fig. 6-7).

The first structure visualized during the anterior examination is the deep portion of the deltoid ligament as it arises from the tip of the medial malleolus and its fibers run vertically down to the medial trochlear surface of the talus (Area 1A). This is an area where ossicles may be hidden, and it should be carefully evaluated for pathology. Also noted is the articular surface of the tip of the medial malleolus as it corresponds and articulates with the medial talar dome and the posterior recess and posterior ligaments (1B). Area 1 is visualized more completely with the 70° scope.

Area 2, the medial gutter, includes the area from the deltoid ligament to below the medial dome of the talus (2A). Areas of articular damage here should be carefully noted, particularly in patients with medial malleolar pain.

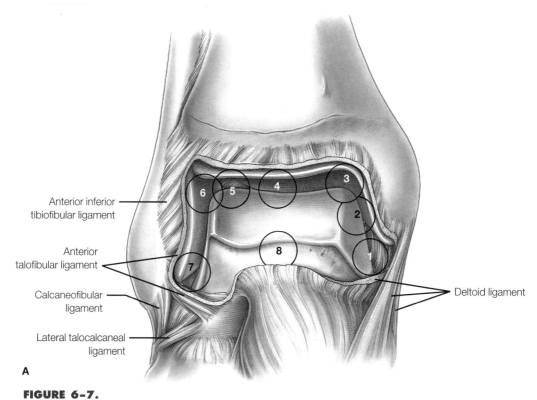

FIGURE 6-7.

Eight-point anterior examination (viewed from the anteromedial portal). (**A**) The anterior ankle is examined starting at the tip of the medial malleolus and making a circle within the ankle joint. (**B**) Arthroscopic views are demonstrated at positions 1, 3, 4, 6, and 7.

Area 3, the medial talar dome, is where the tibial plafond and the medial malleolus meet at the medial bend. The tibia articulates with the medial dome of the talus and is termed the medial corner of the ankle (3A). In this region, the anterior articular margin of the tibia deviates from its more horizontal configuration centrally and laterally to a more convex configuration in the coronal plane. At this medial articular notch (notch of Harty), the arthroscope may be maneuvered most easily into the central and posterior aspects of the joint without scuffing the articular surfaces (3B).

Area 4 is the medial talus articulation with the tibial plafond (4A). In this area, the distal portion of the tibial lip directs slightly anteriorly in the sagittal plane. This portion of the talus articulates within a depression in the talar surface called the sagittal groove. This groove lies between the medial and lateral shoulders of the talus, and projects from anterior to posterior. The anterior tibial lip has hyaline cartilage that extends from the undersurface of the tibial plafond

around the anterior corner superiorly (4B). At the area between the anterior tibial lip and the capsular reflection is a periosteum-covered subchondral bone, the synovial recess. Although the recess is more prominent in this area, it extends from medial all the way to the lateral portion of the ankle. This is where tibial osteophytes develop and synovium and capsule become adherent at the margins of the osteophyte. Some authors argue that the anterocentral portal permits better visualization than the anteromedial and anterolateral because of the sagittal groove in the talus. However, the anterior tibial lip provides an overhang that appears to make arthroscopic visualization from this portal more difficult; this is another reason why the anterocentral portal is not recommended.

The fifth and sixth areas of the anterior ankle examination are the lateral talus and the talofibular articulation (5A). This area is called the trifurcation, as it includes the distal lateral tibial plafond, the lateral talar dome, and the fibula, and is bounded by the

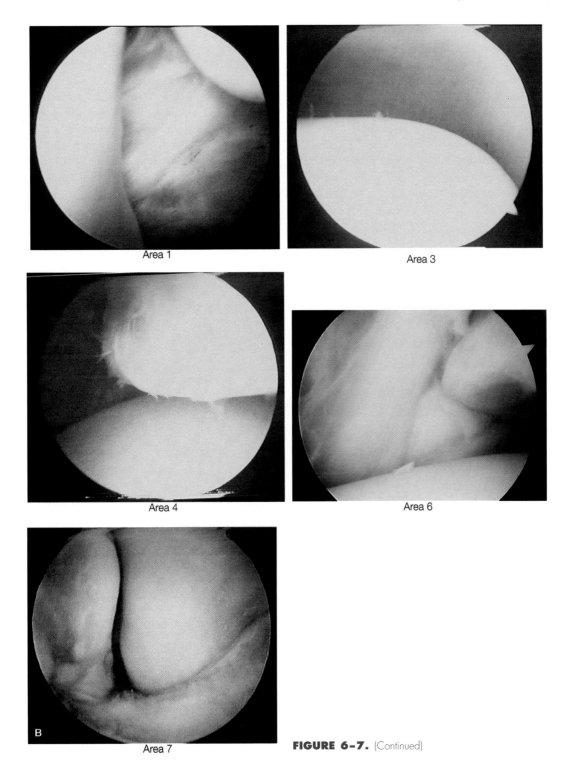

FIGURE 6-7. (Continued)

anterior inferior tibiofibular ligament superiorly. This relation is a key one in the ankle, as this is often the site of soft-tissue and bony pathology. The syndesmotic or anterior inferior tibiofibular ligament runs at about a 45° angle from the lateral portion of the distal tibia to the fibula, just below the level of the lateral talus (6A). From our dissections, it appears to be about 20% intraarticular and the rest extraarticular. Both Bassett and I have noted on occasion a

separate fascicle to the anterior inferior tibiofibular ligament that may impinge against the talus.[6] Behind this thick strong ligament is a synovial recess, as well as the tibiofibular articulation (6B). Although normal synovial tissue exists in this region, it is often the site of synovitis, particularly after inversion ankle sprains. The anterolateral talar dome is also the site of osteochondral lesions of the talus, and access is usually easy in this region.

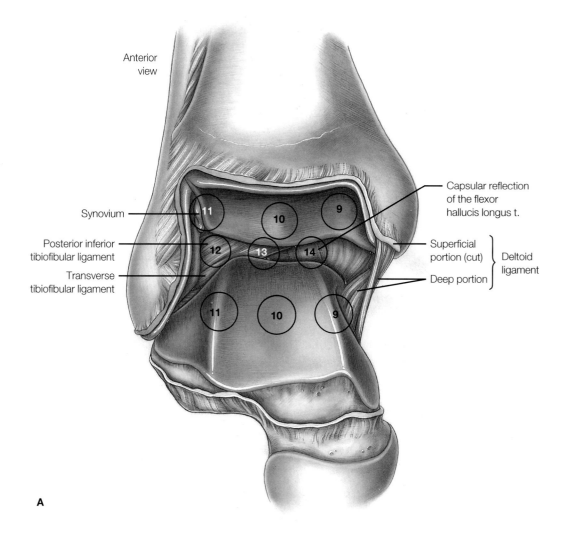

A

FIGURE 6-8.

Six-point central examination (viewed from the anteromedial portal). (**A**) The central examination is performed by maneuvering the arthroscope into the center of the ankle and examining the tibiotalar articulation. The arthroscope is then placed more posteriorly to examine the posterior capsular structures. (**B**) Arthroscopic views of points 11, 12, 13, and 14. (**C** and **D**) Arthroscopic views of point 13.

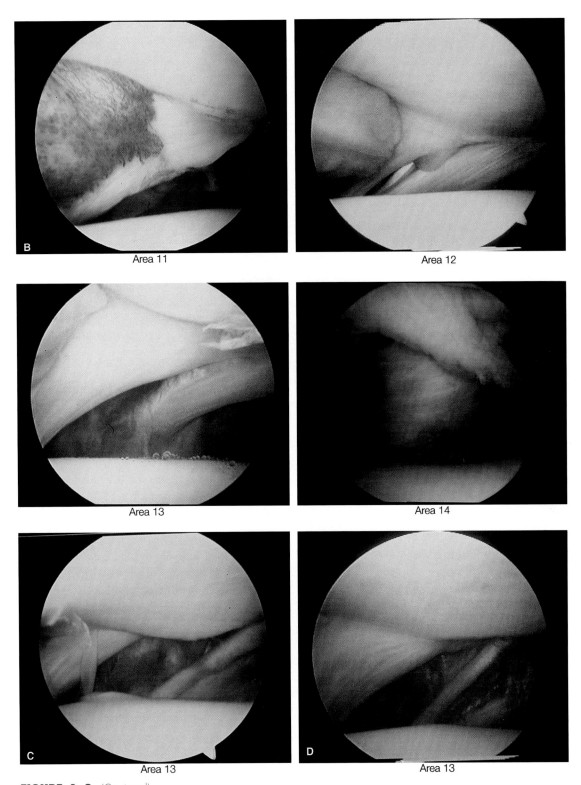

Area 11

Area 12

Area 13

Area 14

Area 13

Area 13

FIGURE 6-8. (Continued)

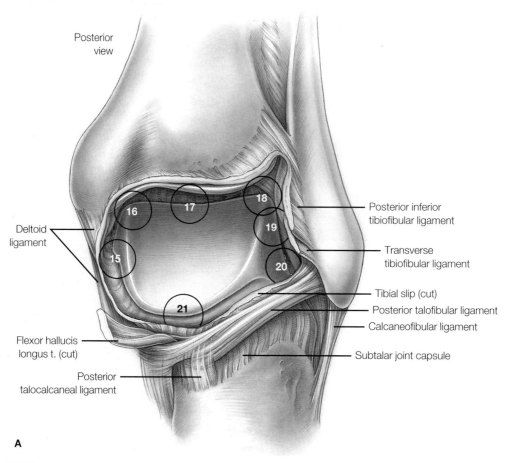

Posterior
view

Deltoid
ligament

15

16

17

18

19

20

21

Posterior inferior
tibiofibular ligament

Transverse
tibiofibular ligament

Tibial slip (cut)

Posterior talofibular ligament

Calcaneofibular ligament

Subtalar joint capsule

Flexor hallucis
longus t. (cut)

Posterior
talocalcaneal ligament

A

FIGURE 6-9.

Seven-point posterior examination (viewed from the posterolateral portal). (**A**) The posterior examination is initiated along the posterior medial malleolar–talar articulation and is carried clockwise to end in the posterior recess. (**B**) Arthroscopic views of points 15, 16, 18, and 20.

The seventh area anteriorly is the lateral gutter, a space between the medial border of the fibular articulation and the lateral border of the talar articulation (7A). It extends from below the anterior inferior tibiofibular ligament to the anterior talofibular ligament. This is often the site of chondromalacia, as well as ossicles at the tip of the fibula within the ligament substance. The anterior talofibular ligament represents a capsular reflection running from the tip of the fibula to the inferior lateral portion of the talus. Soft-tissue impingement often occurs within this space, which includes the soft-tissue envelope of the capsule. The 70° arthroscope allows increased visualization of the lateral gutter (7B).

The final area to be examined anteriorly is the anterior gutter (8), which represents the capsular reflection

anteriorly of the ankle as it inserts along the talar neck. There is a normal bare area proximal to the capsular insertion, similar to the area on the central portion of the distal tibia (8A). A synovial recess can also be found at the anterior inferior aspect of the talar dome. In this area anterior talar osteophytes may articulate or butt against osteophytes of the anterior tibial lip. However, if the osteophytes are more distal along the capsular reflection, extreme care must be taken to avoid injury to the neurovascular structures immediately above.

Central Ankle Examination

After the anterior ankle has been carefully examined, the arthroscope is maneuvered through the medial tibial notch so that the central portion of the tibiota-

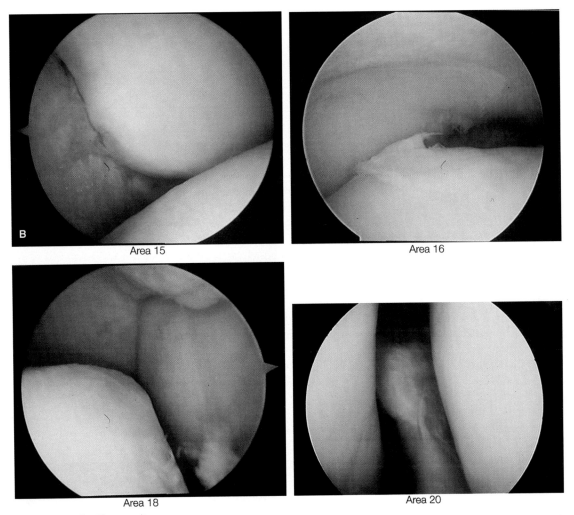

Area 15

Area 16

Area 18

Area 20

FIGURE 6-9. (Continued)

lar articulation can be evaluated (Fig. 6-8). The normal convexity of the distal tibia allows maneuvering of the arthroscope in this region.

Area 9 is the medial dome of the talus, with the tibial plafond as it blends into the medial malleolar region (9A). This is an area where osteochondral lesions of the talus often begin. Throughout the central portion of the examination, assessment and grading of chondromalacia of the articular surface should be done.

Area 10 is the central portion of the tibia and talus. Sometimes central osteochondral lesions of the tibia or talus develop, particularly cystic lesions within the distal tibia (10A).

Area 11 involves the articulation of the lateral talar dome with the distal tibia and fibula and the

syndesmotic articulation (11A). This area often has synovitis or synovial nodules that may compress against the articulation and generate pain (11B).

Posterior Ankle Examination

With the arthroscope in the central portion of the ankle and with adequate distraction, several posterior structures are visualized. With the arthroscope laterally, the posterior inferior tibiofibular ligament is well visualized as it runs obliquely at about a 45° angle from the posterior tibia to the fibula (12A). This ligament is quite large and strong, and can also be the site of soft-tissue pathology (12B). Just medial and inferior to this ligament is the transverse tibio-fibular ligament (13A). Usually there is a small gap between the transverse tibiofibular ligament and the posterior inferior tibiofibular ligament (13B), but sometimes a larger separation can be seen (13C). The transverse tibiofibular ligament can also vary in size from very thick to cordlike and rarely is even a double structure (13D). Occasionally it can hypertrophy or thicken and cause soft-tissue pain. In some ankles, a soft-tissue interval or synovial recess may exist between these two ligaments; in others, the space is quite small.

Some confusion exists as to whether this ligament represents the tibial slip. After careful dissections and analysis of many anatomy texts, it appears that the transverse tibiofibular ligament should not be termed the tibial slip. Rather, the tibial slip runs from the posterior talofibular ligament to the transverse ligament, and it too can be hypertrophied with trauma (see Chap. 5).

Medial to the transverse tibiofibular ligament is the capsular reflection of the flexor hallucis longus tendon (14A). It usually cannot be seen, but sometimes a hole in the synovial covering reveals it (14B). The medial and lateral synovial recesses should also be assessed, but the posterior aspect of the talus as it curves backward is normally not easily seen from this portal.

The posterior examination continues from the posterolateral portal (Fig. 6-9). This portal is made lateral to the Achilles tendon, and generally the capsular penetration is between the transverse tibio-fibular ligament and the flexor hallucis longus. Occasionally this capsular penetration varies, depending on the site of the pathology. The posterior portion of the ankle, including this capsule, is smaller than the anterior portion. Visualization starts with area 15A, revealing the deltoid ligament and posteromedial gutter. The posterior portion of the deltoid ligament as it runs from the medial malleolus to the talus is carefully assessed, as is the entire medial gutter (15B). This recess is not as large as that seen anteriorly.

The second area of concern is the posterior medial talar dome and tibial plafond (16A). This is the most common area of osteochondral lesions of the medial dome of the talus, and often these lesions are seen better from the posterior portal than the anterior (16B).

The third area is the central talus and distal tibia (17). The sagittal groove is seen posteriorly as well,

although it is not as obvious. The distal tibial overhang is usually obscured by the transverse tibiofibular ligament (17A). This ligament, together with the posterior tibiofibular ligament, forms a firm, thick covering over the posterior tibial lip that Hamilton calls the posterior labrum of the ankle.

Areas 18 and 19 include the lateral talar dome, the posterior tibia, and the posterior talofibular articulation. These areas are more difficult to see with the capsular penetration of the posterior portal but easier to see with the capsular penetration switched between the posterior tibiofibular ligament and the transverse tibiofibular ligament (18A). Synovitis and other soft-tissue pathology can be seen in this area (18B). The posterior syndesmotic ligament runs obliquely at a 45° angle, similar to its anterior component. The posterior talofibular articulation is rarely the site of pathology (19A).

Area 20 is the lateral gutter, where the inferior portions of the fibula and talus articulate (20A). This area is more easily seen in some ankles than others because of variations in anatomy. The posterior talofibular ligament reflection can also be seen as it joins from the tip of the posterior fibula to the posterolateral dome of the talus (20B).

The final area to examine in the posterior ankle is the posterior gutter with the synovial and capsular

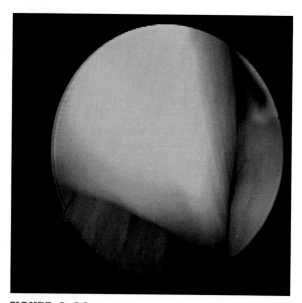

FIGURE 6-10.
The flexor hallucis longus tendon can be seen running in a sheath just posterior to the ankle capsule.

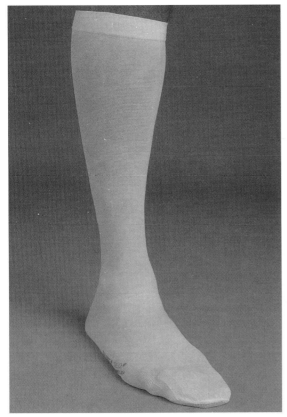

FIGURE 6–11.
Postoperatively, a compression stocking can be used on patients who do not require immobilization.

reflections (21A). It is much smaller than the anterior gutter and can be more difficult to see. It is not uncommon for loose bodies to hide in this area.

Occasionally, the surgeon can slip out of the posterior capsule just enough to look down the sheath of the flexor hallucis longus tendon as it runs in its groove on the posterior talus (Fig. 6-10). Extreme caution should be made to avoid injury to this structure.

POSTOPERATIVE MANAGEMENT

After the arthroscopic examination is completed, all wounds are closed with a 4-0 nonabsorbable nylon suture and a compression dressing is applied. The dressing is then held in place with either a short-leg TED compression stocking or a short-leg posterior splint, depending on the type of pathology encoun-

tered and the extent of the surgery (Fig. 6-11). Usually, the fluid that has extravasated about the ankle into the subcutaneous tissues is absorbed or leaks out of the portals over a short time.

A TED stocking, if used, can be removed at 48 hours and the bandages thrown away. The stocking is then reapplied and the patient can start partial weight bearing with crutches and general range of motion and strengthening. If a short-leg posterior splint has been applied, it is usually removed at 5 to 7 days. With either form of postoperative treatment, sutures are removed within a week and further ankle compression is maintained with the short-leg TED stocking. Patients are then placed in a short-leg walking boot for 1 to 2 weeks as they increase their weight bearing (Fig. 6-12).

More recently a multi-application ankle sup-

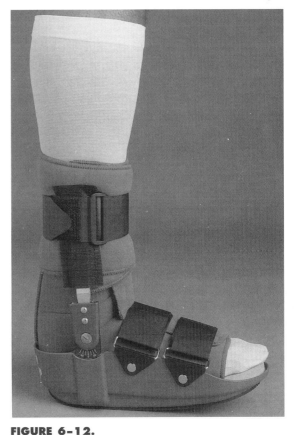

FIGURE 6–12.
One week postoperatively, the stitches are removed and a compression stocking and hinged ankle boot are applied to allow progressive weight bearing.

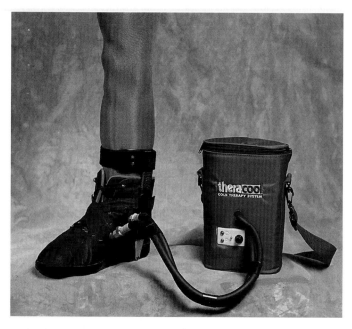

FIGURE 6-13.
The multi-application ankle support is used postoperatively to provide both air compression and ice therapy using a dual bladder system.

port has been used 1 week after surgery. This shoe has a dual bladder to provide air compression as well as cold therapy to reduce swelling, improve circulation, and facilitate a more rapid recovery from surgery. The patient uses a small hand pump to inflate or deflate the air cells, and a rehabilitation circulation container to cool the circulating water (Fig. 6-13).

Crutches are usually discarded at between 7 and 14 days, depending on the patient's discomfort. The patient usually works at home on range of motion and strengthening, but formal therapy can be initiated 2 to 3 weeks after surgery, if indicated, depending on the surgical procedure performed. Showers can be started as soon as the stitches are removed, but swimming or soaking the ankle in a bath are delayed until 14 days postoperatively.

Return to full activity, including sports, depends on the surgical procedure performed. Some caution must be exercised in returning patients too quickly to running or jumping or contact sports, particular if invasive pin distraction has been used. Rehabilitation is discussed in more detail later in Chapter 14.

REFERENCES

1. Adkison DP, Bosse MJ, Gaccione DR, Gabriel KR. Anatomic variations in the course of the superficial peroneal nerve. J Bone Joint Surg 1991;73A:112.
2. Chen YC. Arthroscopy of the ankle joint. In Watanabe M, ed. Arthroscopy of small joints. Tokyo: Igaku-Shoin, 1985:104.
3. Drez D, Guhl JF, Gollehon DL. Ankle arthroscopy: technique and indications. J Foot Surg 1981;2:138.
4. Ferkel RD. An illustrated guide to small joint arthroscopy. Andover, MA: Smith & Nephew Dyonics Inc, 1989.
5. Ferkel RD, Fischer SP. Progress in ankle arthroscopy. Clin Orthop 1989;240:210.
6. Bassett FH, Gates HS, Billys JB, et al. Talar impingement by the anteroinferior tibiofibular ligament: A cause of chronic pain in the ankle after inversion sprain. J Bone Joint Surg 1990; 72A:55.

BIBLIOGRAPHY

Feiwell LA, Frey C. Anatomic study of arthroscopic portal sites of the ankle. Foot Ankle 1993;14:142.
Guhl JF. Foot and ankle arthroscopy, 2d ed. Thorofare, NJ: Slack, 1993.
Kelikian H, Kelikian A. Disorders of the ankle. Philadelphia: WB Saunders, 1985.

Section Two

Surgical Arthroscopy

Arthroscopic Surgery: The Foot and Ankle,
by Richard D. Ferkel.
Lippincott-Raven Publishers, Philadelphia © 1996.

7

Soft-Tissue Lesions of the Ankle

Richard D. Ferkel

*S*oft-tissue lesions of the ankle present a difficult diagnostic problem. Even after careful history, physical examination, and diagnostic testing, the diagnosis may not be readily apparent. These lesions usually involve the synovium, but the capsule or ligamentous tissues may also be affected. Soft-tissue pathology accounts for about 30% to 50% of lesions seen in the ankle and subtalar joints.

In the past, acute and chronic soft-tissue complaints in the ankle have been treated primarily by nonoperative means, with a specific diagnosis often lacking. If the patient's symptoms persisted, aspiration and occasionally arthrotomy with synovial biopsy was done. Arthroscopy has allowed the entire visualization of the joint without obscuring tissue planes (unlike an arthrotomy). It allows complete diagnosis and treatment of soft-tissue problems.

ANATOMY AND HISTOLOGY

Nearly all articulations of the extremities are synovial or diarthrodial joints. Because they have a joint cavity, they are fairly movable. Anatomic features of the synovial joint are shown in Figure 7–1. The articular cartilage and the articulation are enveloped by a joint capsule and supported by ligaments. The outer stratum of the joint capsule (fibrosum) is made up of dense fibrous tissue. The inner layer (synoviale) consists of loose, highly vascular connective tissue and synovium (synovial membrane).[1] This synovial membrane is usually smooth and glistening and may exhibit infoldings (synovial folds) and slender projections, the larger ones called synovial villae. It is richly supplied with nerves, lymphatics, and blood vessels.

There are two types of membrane or synovial cells, type A and type B. Type A cells are probably the producers of hyaluronic acid of the synovial fluid.

The joint cavity contains a viscous fluid, the synovial fluid, produced by the synovial membrane. Analysis of this fluid is helpful in the differential

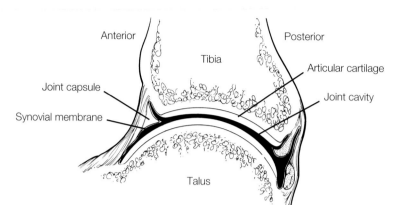

FIGURE 7-1.

Cross-sectional view of a typical synovial joint of the ankle.

diagnosis of joint swelling because it can distinguish noninflammatory, inflammatory, and septic processes.[2]

CLASSIFICATION

Numerous classifications of synovial disorders can be made. The system presented below incorporates the source of synovial irritation and will be used throughout this chapter:

1. Congenital: plicae or congenital bands within the ankle
2. Traumatic: sprains, fractures, and previous surgery
3. Rheumatic: rheumatoid arthritis, pigmented villonodular synovitis, crystal synovitis, hemophilia, and synovial chondromatosis
4. Infectious: bacterial and fungal
5. Degenerative: primary and secondary
6. Neuropathic: Charcot joint
7. Miscellaneous: ganglions, arthrofibrosis.

PATIENT EVALUATION

Patients with complaints of aching, swelling, tenderness, and other signs of joint inflammation should always be carefully evaluated to determine the specific causes of their symptoms. A detailed differential diagnosis must be considered and must include the above problems. A history of trauma or injury is more likely to cause a nonspecific type of synovitis,

either localized or generalized; however, trauma can also trigger an underlying specific pathologic process.

Patient evaluation includes a careful history, physical examination, and radiologic testing. Arthritis tests should be used throughout for rheumatoid arthritis, lupus, gout, and other rheumatologic conditions whenever suspicion is present. CT scanning is helpful for three-dimensional imaging of the ankle, especially with bony and soft-tissue lesions.[3] MRI is particularly helpful in demonstrating soft-tissue lesions about the foot and ankle: it allows the observer to distinguish blood vessels, nerves, fat, ligaments, tendons, bone marrow, muscles, and fluid clearly, as each has different signal characteristics.[4] A detailed discussion of radiologic techniques is given in Chapter 2.

CONGENITAL PLICAE

Plicae, or shelves, have been clearly demonstrated in the knee but are more difficult to find in the ankle. More commonly, congenital bands are seen as an incidental finding when examining the ankle for other types of pathology.

TRAUMA

Nonspecific Generalized Synovitis

This type of synovitis can be caused by sprains or after fractures or previous surgery. The ankle joint can respond to both indirect and direct trauma. With a traumatic episode, a generalized or localized synovitis can occur, as well as fibrous bands and adhesion formation. Patients with generalized nonspecific synovitis usually complain of pain, swelling, and soreness, and their history may involve a traumatic event, either significant or trivial. Occasionally, no inciting event can be recalled. If, after adequate and appropriate workup, the patient fails to respond to conservative treatment, ankle arthroscopy is indicated.

At surgery, chronically inflamed synovium is commonly seen and may contain hemosiderin or other fibrin debris. With synovitis, the villae produce a fibrin exudate. The formation of fibrous bands represents aggregates of the fibrin exudate. These are usually seen anteriorly, but can also be seen in the syndesmosis or posteriorly. They are associated with minimal to mild chondromalacia, depending on the duration of the symptoms (Fig. 7-2).

The most common causes of nonspecific synovitis are ankle sprains and fractures. After such injuries, the hematoma produces exudate and swelling, followed by extensive cellular response, fibrous tissue reaction, hyalinization, and ultimately chronic synovitis. Significant synovitis, adhesive band formation, and scarring and fibrosis can be seen with severe injury, and are usually associated with arthrofibrosis

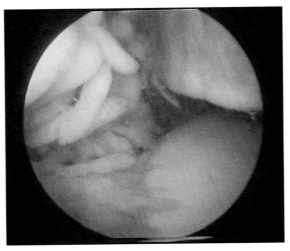

FIGURE 7-3.
Arthroscopic view of local synovitis of the anterolateral ankle joint in a 33-year-old male 15 months after minor trauma.

of the joint. This problem is discussed further in Chapter 9.

Nonspecific Localized Synovitis

A localized synovitis of the medial or lateral talomalleolar joint can develop after trauma and produces localized soreness and swelling. On physical examination, localized tenderness with minimal swelling and full range of motion is usually seen. The diagnostic workup is usually negative, although there may be some signal alteration on MRI. At arthroscopy, mild synovitis, papillary formation, and fibrosis is noted. Excision of this tissue in a localized area often produces excellent results if all conservative treatment methods have failed (Fig. 7-3).

Soft-Tissue Impingement

Ankle sprains are one of the most common injuries in sports. One inversion ankle sprain occurs per 10,000 persons per day.[5-7] In a study at West Point, 30% of cadets suffered an ankle sprain in their 4 years at the school.[8] Most commonly, these involved basketball (45%), volleyball (25%), and soccer (31%). After an ankle sprain, 10% to 50% of patients have some chronic pain.[9-11] Commonly, ankle inversion

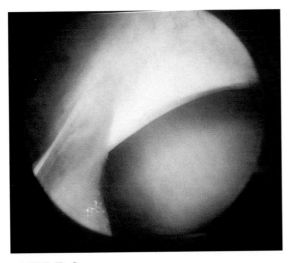

FIGURE 7-2.
Arthroscopic view of a fibrous band occluding the lateral gutter in a 43-year-old male 1 year after inversion ankle sprain. Excision of this band relieved his pain.

injuries are associated with the following sequence: torn anterior talofibular ligament, torn calcaneofibular ligament, and torn posterior talofibular ligament. During this sequence, the syndesmotic ligaments, anteriorly, posteriorly, or both, can also be injured (Fig. 7-4).

The differential diagnoses of chronic postsprain pain include osteochondral lesions of the talus, calcific ossicles beneath the medial or lateral malleolus, peroneal tears or subluxation, tarsal coalition, degenerative joint disease, nerve entrapment, occult fractures of the talus and calcaneus, subtalar dysfunction, reflex sympathetic dystrophy, and soft-tissue impingement. The primary cause of chronic pain after an ankle sprain is soft-tissue impingement. This can occur along the syndesmosis, the anterior gutter, the syndesmotic interval between the tibia and fibula, underneath the ankle, or posteriorly in the syndesmosis and posterior gutter.

Anterolateral Impingement

Anterior impingement of the ankle is the most common type of soft-tissue impingement because of the mechanism of most ankle sprains. Wolin

and colleagues in 1950 described 9 patients with persistent pain and swelling over the anterolateral aspect of the ankle several weeks to months after an inversion sprain.[12] Arthrotomy of the ankle in these patients revealed a massive hyalinized connective tissue extending into the joint from the anterior inferior portion of the talofibular ligament. They called this a ''meniscoid'' lesion because it looked like a torn meniscus in the knee. They thought that disability resulted from entrapment of this tissue between the tibia and the fibula; excision of the scar tissue relieved the symptoms in all cases.

ANATOMY

A thorough understanding of the region's anatomy is necessary. Impingement can occur at the anterior inferior tibiofibular ligament, the lateral gutter, and the anterior talofibular ligament (Fig. 7-5).

CLINICAL PRESENTATION

Because the most common mechanism of ankle injury is plantarflexion inversion, chronic lateral ankle pain is much more common than chronic medial pain following a sprain. Typically, the patient complains of vague anterior pain, usually along the

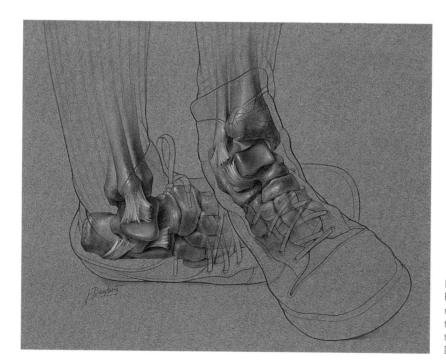

FIGURE 7-4.
Plantarflexion inversion injury of the right ankle leading to single and multiple tears of the lateral ligamentous complex. (Illustration by John Daugherty and Richard Ferkel.)

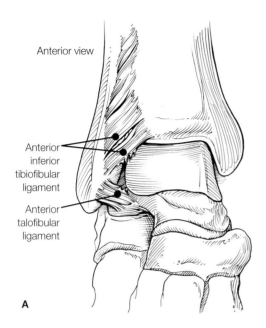

Anterior view

Anterior inferior tibiofibular ligament

Anterior talofibular ligament

A

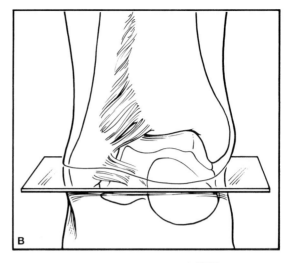

B

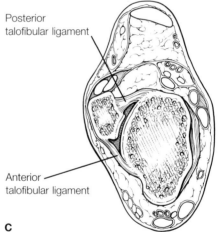

Posterior talofibular ligament

Anterior talofibular ligament

C

FIGURE 7-5.

Anterolateral ankle anatomy. (**A**) Soft-tissue impingement sites. Note the accessory fascicle of the anterior inferior tibiofibular ligament, which can impinge across the lateral talar dome. (**B**) Plane of cross section through the lateral gutter. (**C**) Cross-sectional picture of lateral gutter. This gutter is bounded by the talus medially, the tibia laterally, and the anterior and posterior ligaments.

anterior and anterolateral aspect of the ankle, sometimes involving the syndesmosis and sinus tarsi regions. Pain is usually absent at rest and present with most activities, limiting the patient's ability to participate in a given sport. Often the patient has seen several physicians and is frustrated by his or her lack of progress.

Physical examination may reveal tenderness along the syndesmosis, anterior gutter, including the anterior talofibular ligament and the calcaneofibular ligament, and many times also the posterior subtalar joint or sinus tarsi. It is important to try to differenti-

ate lateral gutter pain from subtalar pain, especially in the sinus tarsi (Fig. 7-6).

Radiologic evaluation may reveal calcification or heterotopic bone in the interosseous space, which indicates previous injury to the distal tibiofibular syndesmosis, with ossicles along the tip of the fibula and the lateral talar dome consistent with injuries of the anterior talofibular ligament. Often the x-rays are normal, as are the bone scan and CT scan. In about 30% of cases, MRI may be helpful in indicating the abnormality in the lateral gutter (Fig. 7-7; see also Fig. 2-32 in Chapter 2). Occasionally, a

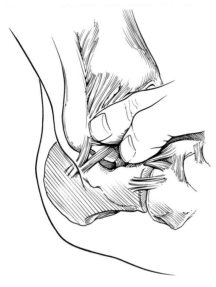

FIGURE 7-6.
Differentiating pain in the lateral gutter from subtalar pain is done by careful palpation. Selective injections can also be helpful in distinguishing the area of maximum pain.

ize the entire ankle, 2.7-mm or 4.0-mm 30° and 70° arthroscopes are used. Motorized shavers, burrs, graspers, and baskets are used to treat the associated pathology. Distraction is used to visualize the entire joint and to facilitate inflow as well as treatment.

PREFERRED METHOD

The patient is placed in a supine position with a nonsterile thigh holder, and the foot is prepared and draped. All anatomic landmarks are carefully marked out, and the ankle is distended with 10 cc saline from the anteromedial portal. The anteromedial portal is then established and a 2.7-mm short videoscope with a 2.9-mm interchangeable cannula is inserted. The probe is placed through the anterolateral portal, and inflow is through the posterolateral portal.

Usually a noninvasive distraction strap can be applied (see Chap. 3). Use of the strap allows complete inspection of the entire joint, but still permits

kinematic MRI is useful to show the impingement lesion dynamically. Stress x-rays in this group are usually negative.

ARTHROSCOPIC APPEARANCE

At arthroscopy, the medial malleolar-talar articulation and the central portion of the ankle on the anterior gutter are usually normal. Pathology is generally limited to the syndesmosis and the lateral gutter. Patients generally have a synovitis surrounding the anterior inferior tibiofibular ligament, both in front and behind, as well as synovitis of the anterior talofibular ligament. Also noted at surgery is fibrosis of the lateral gutter and chondromalacia of the talus and the fibula in some cases. In addition, a small ossicle or loose body may be hidden in the soft tissues at the tip of the fibula. Rarely, an adhesive thick scar band, previously described as a meniscoid lesion, is present, extending from the anterolateral aspect of the distal tibia to the lateral gutter (Fig. 7-8).

TREATMENT

Anterolateral impingement lesions can be approached using either the supine, lateral decubitus or the 90° flexed position for arthroscopy. To visual-

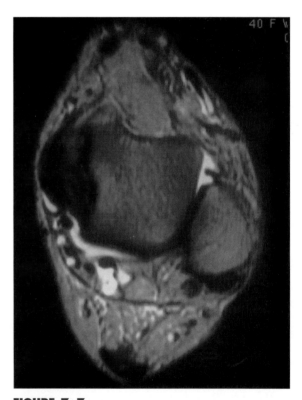

FIGURE 7-7.
Axial T2-weighted image showing fluid in the lateral gutter with torn remnant of syndesmotic ligament.

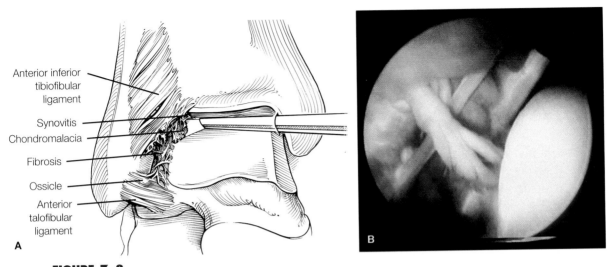

Anterior inferior
tibiofibular
ligament

Synovitis

Chondromalacia

Fibrosis

Ossicle

Anterior
talofibular
ligament

A

B

FIGURE 7-8.
Soft-tissue impingement. (**A**) Viewed through the anteromedial portal, anterolateral soft-tissue impingement with synovitis and fibrosis and chondromalacia in the anterolateral gutter. (**B**) Arthroscopic view of the anterolateral impingement lesion. Note the hemosiderin staining of the lateral gutter and associated scar bands and synovitis.

easy relaxation of distraction to allow surgery in the anterolateral portion of the ankle. The more distraction applied, the more occluded the anterolateral compartment of the ankle becomes, thereby making visualization difficult in this region. The best way to visualize the anterolateral gutter is to dorsiflex the ankle (with distraction relaxed) so the entire lateral gutter space opens up. With dorsiflexion of the ankle, the anterior capsule is relaxed and the lateral malleolus moves away from the medial malleolus. At the same time, the fibula is pulled slightly superiorly, while the fibers of the interosseous and tibiofibular ligaments tend to become more horizontal. In addition, the fibula is medially rotated with dorsiflexion (Fig. 7-9).

Although the 30° arthroscope is routinely used with anterolateral impingement, the 70° arthroscope is usually used during the surgical portion of the procedure. It allows increased visualization of the syndesmosis, anterolateral gutter, and talus, and allows better visualization along the posterior gutter from the anterior portals (Fig. 7-10).

Before beginning the surgery, visualization should be done from the anteromedial, anterolateral, and posterolateral portals. The inflow cannula is then left in the posterolateral portal to give a high-flow system. The arthroscope is reinserted in the ante-

romedial portal, and the anterolateral gutter is debrided with the 2.9-mm full-radius shaver, baskets, and graspers as necessary. Debridement usually includes removing inflamed synovium, thickened adhesive bands, osteophytes, and loose bodies (Fig. 7-11). All involved tissue is excised down to the underlying cartilage. The synovium, as well as any inflamed capsular or ligamentous tissue, is removed. Care must be taken *not* to excise the anterior talofibular ligament remnant. Inflammatory tissue may be seen not only in the lateral gutter but also in the syndesmosis in the articular space between the tibia and fibula.

POSTOPERATIVE TREATMENT

After surgery, patients are placed in a posterior splint for 1 week. They are then put in a rehabilitation shoe or a cam walker for an additional 3 weeks. Subsequently, they are given a small ankle brace to wear inside a tennis shoe and begin formal physiotherapy. Patients can return to full activity, including sports, when all the goals of rehabilitation have been achieved (see Chap. 14).

PATHOLOGIC FINDINGS

Histologic analysis was performed on all patients with soft-tissue impingement syndrome, and moderate synovial hyperplasia with subsynovial capillary

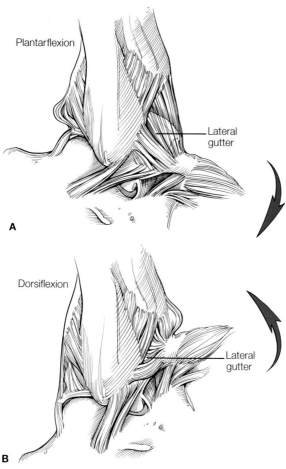

FIGURE 7-9.
The effect of flexion/extension of the ankle on the lateral gutter.
(**A**) With plantarflexion, tension is applied across the lateral gutter,
narrowing this space and making visualization difficult. (**B**) Dorsiflexion of the ankle relaxes the lateral gutter structures while the
fibula is pulled slightly superiorly, optimizing visualization of this
entire area.

inversion ankle sprain. Between 1983 and 1994, we
have treated more than 120 patients arthroscopically
for anterolateral impingement. Our initial group of
31 patients with more than 2 years of follow-up has
been reported, with 26 of 31 (84%) as excellent/
good, subjectively and objectively; 4 of 31 (13%)
fair; and 1 poor.[13] In the subsequent 89 cases, the
results have remained similar. Liu,[14] Martin,[15] and
Meislin[16] and their colleagues recently reported similar results in treating this condition.

The term "chronic post-ankle sprain pain"

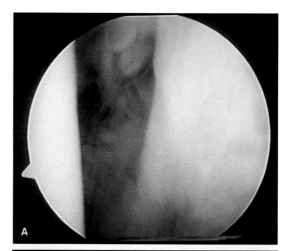

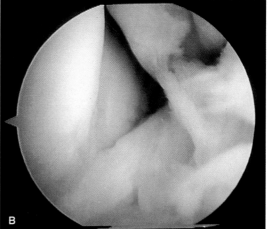

FIGURE 7-10.
Visualization of the lateral gutter of the left ankle from the anteromedial portal. (**A**) Picture obtained with a 30° arthroscope. It is
difficult to see the fibula and the anterior talofibular ligament. (**B**)
Using the 70° arthroscope to look over the lateral dome of the
talus, the articulation of the fibula with the talus and the anterior
talofibular ligament are well seen.

proliferation was seen in all cases. Also noted in
many patients were hyaline cartilage degenerative
change and fibrosis (Fig. 7-12). These findings were
consistent with the chronic inflammatory process.[13]
In general, ligamentous tissue was not seen on histologic analysis.

CLINICAL RESULTS

Arthroscopic treatment of anterolateral impingement of the ankle has proven successful, alleviating
the chronic aching pain that patients exhibit after an

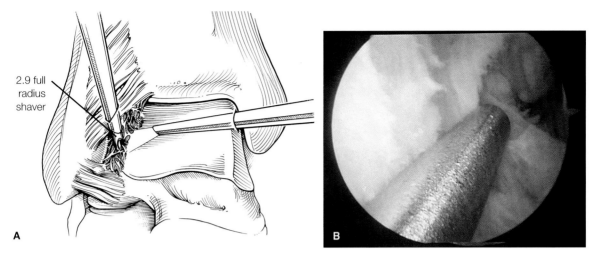

FIGURE 7-11.
Debridement of the lateral gutter. (**A**) Debridement is performed with a small-joint shaver and includes removing inflamed synovium, thickened adhesive bands, osteophytes, and loose bodies. (**B**) Arthroscopic view through the anteromedial portal. A full-radius shaver is debriding the lateral gutter while avoiding injury to the anterior talofibular ligament.

should be discarded, as the term "anterolateral impingement of the ankle" is more appropriate to describe this condition.

Syndesmotic Impingement

The inferior tibiofibular joint is intimately involved with dorsi- and plantarflexion of the ankle. The mode of action of the inferior tibiofibular joint depends on the shape of the trochlear surface of the talus. The width of the trochlear surface is smaller posteriorly (2.5 cm) than anteriorly (3.0 cm), as shown in Figure 7-13*A*. Therefore, if the medial and lateral surfaces of the talar body are to be held tightly, the intermalleolar space must vary within certain limits: it must be smallest during plantarflexion and greatest during dorsiflexion[17] (see Fig. 7-13*B,C*).

During plantarflexion of the ankle, the malleoli

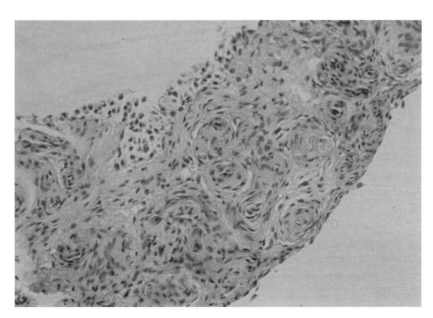

FIGURE 7-12.
Photomicrograph of the synovial biopsy specimen from an anterolateral impingement patient shows moderate synovial hyperplasia with subsynovial capillary proliferation (hematoxylin and eosin, ×100).

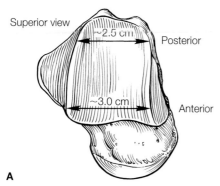

A

FIGURE 7-13.

Tibiofibular joint mechanics. (**A**) The width of the trochlear surface of the talus is smaller posteriorly than anteriorly. (**B**) During plantarflexion of the ankle, the malleoli are approximated actively as the lateral malleolus is pulled inferiorly and rotated medially. (**C**) With dorsiflexion of the ankle, the lateral malleolus moves away from the medial malleolus and is pulled slightly superiorly as the fibula is medially rotated.

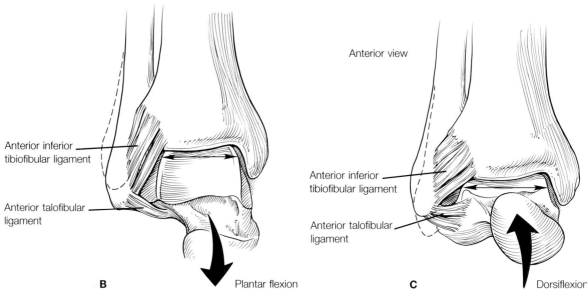

FIGURE 7-14.

Syndesmotic impingement. (**A**) Plane of cross section through the syndesmosis. (**B**) Cross-sectional view through the syndesmosis demonstrates that impingement can occur anteriorly, centrally, or posteriorly.

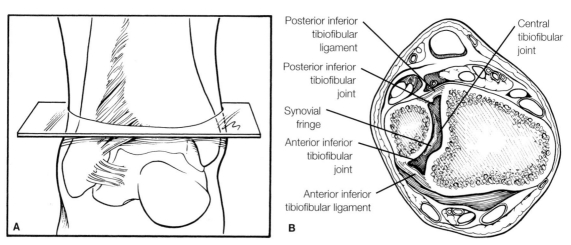

are approximated actively as the lateral malleolus is pulled inferiorly and rotated medially (see Fig. 7-13*B*). Conversely, during dorsiflexion of the ankle, the lateral malleolus moves away from the medial malleolus and is pulled slightly superiorly as the fibula is medially rotated[17] (see Fig. 7-13*C*).

Injuries to the syndesmosis are vastly underestimated and often occur with sprains and fractures that go undetected. Syndesmotic sprains have been estimated to occur in as many as 10% of all ankle injuries, and tend to be most common in collision sports such as ice hockey, football, and soccer. Syndesmotic sprains may involve any or all of the following structures: the anterior inferior tibiofibular ligament; the posterior inferior tibiofibular ligament, including its distal and deep component, the transverse ligament; and the interosseous membrane (see Figs. 7-5*A*, 7-14).

CLINICAL PRESENTATION

Although not entirely clear, the mechanism of injury appears to be primarily an external rotation injury, although hyperdorsiflexion has also been reported to lead to tears of the syndesmosis. On physical examination, these patients have exquisite tenderness along the syndesmosis and more proximally on the interosseous membrane. A positive squeeze test is usually seen with this injury, as is a positive external rotation stress test[18,19] (see Chap. 2). A positive test generates pain over the anterior and posterior tibiofibular ligament's interosseous membrane.

Bassett and associates found syndesmotic impingement occurring with a separate distal fascicle of the anterior inferior tibiofibular ligament.[20] With a tear of the anterior talofibular ligament, laxity occurs in the lateral ankle and the anterolateral talar dome extrudes anteriorly with dorsiflexion, leading to the soft-tissue impingement (Fig. 7-15).

ARTHROSCOPIC APPEARANCE

Syndesmotic impingement cannot always be differentiated from anterior or posterior impingement because in many instances the injury and subsequent impingement problem involve multiple areas. At surgery, the inflamed synovium envelops the anterior inferior tibiofibular ligament as well as the inferior articulation of the tibia and fibula (Fig. 7-16). In addition, synovial nodules are frequently seen in this area. The synovitis involves the anterior and also the posterior aspects of the syndesmotic ligament, and sometimes this ligament is torn or frayed (Fig. 7-17). Associated loose bodies, chondromalacia, and osteophytes may be noted.

PREFERRED METHOD

The ankle is evaluated with 30° and 70° 2.7-mm short arthroscopes. A full-radius 2.9-mm shaver is used to debride the anterior inferior tibiofibular ligament, and sometimes part of it is excised with either a shaver or a suction basket (Fig. 7-18). Previous cadaver studies indicate that about 20% of this ligament is visualized intraarticularly, and no instability

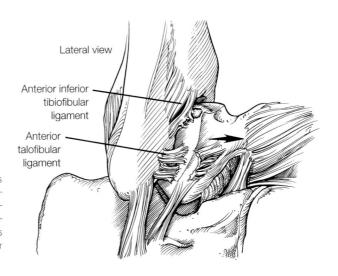

FIGURE 7-15.
With a tear of the anterior talofibular ligament, laxity occurs in the lateral ankle and the anterior talar dome extrudes anteriorly. With dorsiflexion, the distal fascicle of the anterior inferior tibiofibular ligament may impinge against the talus. (Redrawn with permission from Bassett FH, Gates HS, Billys JB, et al. Talar impingement by the anteroinferior tibiofibular ligament. J Bone Joint Surg [Am] 1990;72:55.)

Lateral view

Anterior inferior tibiofibular ligament

Anterior talofibular ligament

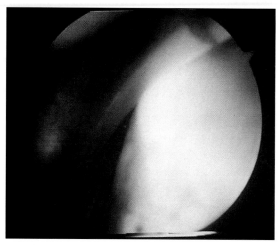

FIGURE 7-16.
Arthroscopic view of a fascicle of the anterior inferior tibiofibular ligament impinging against the lateral dome of the talus.

has been produced at the syndesmotic joint by resecting this intraarticular portion. The ligament should always be excised when there is corresponding rubbing along the lateral talus or if it is torn or frayed and obviously incompetent. Vigorous debridement of the synovitis is done, and a suction basket is particularly helpful in removing the inflamed synovium and synovial nodules in the tibiofibular interspace.

Posterior Impingement

Posterior impingement also usually occurs along the lateral side and involves the posterior tibiofibular ligament, including the transverse tibiofibular ligament and occasionally the tibial slip (see Figs. 7-19, 7-5C). This impingement can occur alone or in combination with anterolateral and syndesmosis impingement. However, usually a more generalized posterolateral impingement occurs with fibrosis, capsulitis, and synovial swelling along the posterior portions of the ankle. This type of impingement can be missed if careful anterior and posterior viewing is not done. Without some type of distraction device, it can be difficult to see some of the synovial problems of the posterolateral corner of the ankle (Fig. 7-20).

The transverse tibiofibular ligament can vary in size and shape and can become pathologic in certain

cases (see Chap. 6). Occasionally this ligament is associated with a specific tibial slip; other times it is not. When both ligaments are seen together, there is a higher chance of an impingement-type problem. Excision of this hypertrophied ligament can lead to significant pain relief. Rarely, the transverse tibiofibular ligament is torn and can lead to posterior ankle pain (Fig. 7-21).

Hamilton has also described the "meniscus of the ankle" in the posterior ankle joint of ballet dancers.[21] He has found cases of tears in this posterior ankle meniscus that would displace in the joint and become symptomatic (Fig. 7-22). In addition, he has described a labrum on the posterior lip or edge of the tibia. Although this is infrequent, when injured the tibial labrum can become hypertrophied or torn and can cause significant symptoms.

Posterior impingement lesions are treated by alternating portals, depending on the site of the pathology, using motorized and basket instruments (Fig. 7-23).

Evaluating Chronic Ankle Pain

Although the incidence of impingement of the ankle after ankle sprain is unknown, an estimate can be made. Between 1983 and 1994, about 4000 ankle sprains were treated at the Southern California Or-

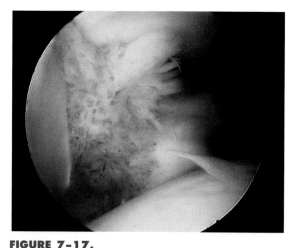

FIGURE 7-17.
Arthroscopic view of a right ankle demonstrating hemosiderin staining and inflamed synovium posterior to the anterior inferior tibiofibular ligament.

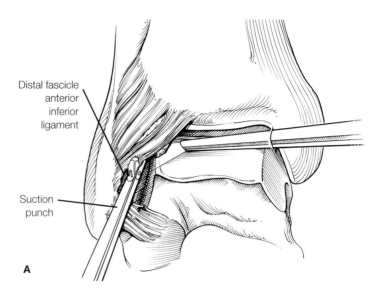

Distal fascicle
anterior
inferior
ligament

Suction
punch

A

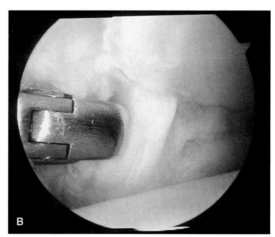

B

FIGURE 7-18.
Excision of torn syndesmotic ligament. (**A**) Visualization is done from the anteromedial portal, and a suction punch or small basket is brought into the joint through the anterolateral portal to remove the torn fascicle. (**B**) Arthroscopic view of excision of the torn syndesmotic ligament using a suction basket.

thopedic Institute. At present, about 120 patients have been operated on for this problem, for an incidence of 3%.

A proposed sequence for the development of chronic impingement of the ankle is described in Table 7-1. An algorithm is useful to help evaluate and treat chronic sprain pain patients (Table 7-2).

RHEUMATIC DISEASES

Although a discussion of rheumatic diseases and their classification is beyond the scope of this chapter, the arthroscopic surgeon must understand certain points to diagnose and treat these problems correctly.

Rheumatoid Arthritis

Rheumatoid arthritis is a chronic systemic inflammatory problem characterized by the method in which it affects the joints. Although the etiology is unknown and various causes have been postulated, no consensus exists as to its exact cause. The clinical presentation of rheumatoid arthritis is highly inconsistent, ranging from pauciarticular illness of brief duration to progressive destruction with polyarthritis and vasculitis. Its appearance in the ankle is similar to that in the knee, wrist, hip, and other areas of the body.

Although rheumatoid arthritis can affect any diarthrodial joint, it initially involves small joints of

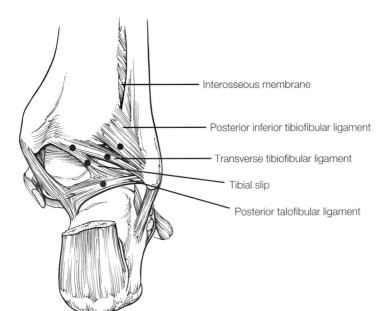

Interosseous membrane

Posterior inferior tibiofibular ligament

Transverse tibiofibular ligament

Tibial slip

Posterior talofibular ligament

FIGURE 7-19.
Posterior impingement sites. Note that the tibial slip can also be an area of soft-tissue impingement.

the hands, wrists, knees, and feet. The disease may progress to affect the elbow, shoulder, ankle, and subtalar region. The ankles and feet are affected with pain and limited motion, particularly in the ankle and subtalar region.

Surgery in the rheumatoid patient is based on correct timing, with careful assessment of the region and estimation of the patient's general condition.[22]

In the ankle, chondromalacia and synovitis may be seen, depending on the severity of the disease. In some situations, areas of articular cartilage necrosis on the tibial plafond or the talar dome may be the primary pathology.[23] If the patient fails conservative therapy, then ankle arthroscopy should be considered after a consultation with a rheumatologist. The main indications for surgery are pain, swelling, and

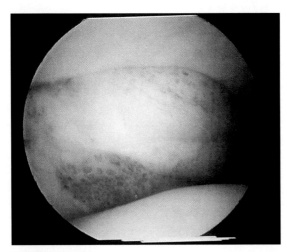

FIGURE 7-20.
Posterolateral synovial nodule in a right ankle.

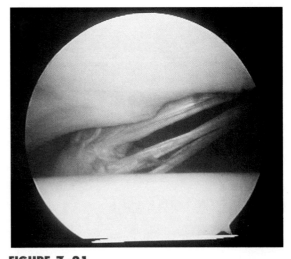

FIGURE 7-21.
Tear of the transverse tibiofibular ligament in a 30-year-old ballerina.

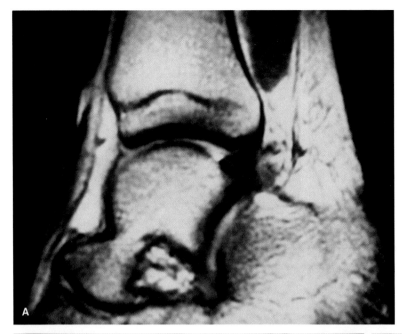

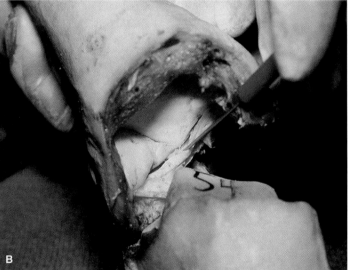

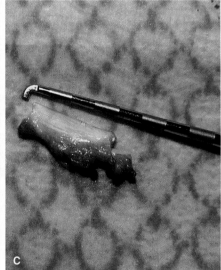

FIGURE 7-22.
Pseudomeniscus. (**A**) MRI showing posterior pseudomeniscus. (**B**) Photo showing location of lesion on the tibial slip arising from the posterior talofibular ligament. (**C**) Gross appearance of posterior pseudomeniscus after surgical excision. (**A, B,** and **C** courtesy of William Hamilton, MD.)

locking and catching sensations. Preoperatively, it is important to aspirate the ankle or subtalar region. A CT scan or MRI may be useful to look for synovitis, effusion, articular damage, and other unsuspected abnormalities. If synovitis is present, it is removed using 2.9-, 3.5-, or 4.5-mm full-radius shaver blades. The use of distraction is helpful in performing a complete synovectomy.

Pathologic examination of the synovium shows synovial hyperplasia with villae, papillary formation, and necrosis. Because of areas of surface necrosis, many synovial villae have a creamy yellowish appearance referred to as "rice bodies." Complete synovectomy is impossible: even with thorough debridement, up to 5% of the original rheumatoid granulation may remain.[24] Early synovectomy provides better overall results than later synovectomy.[25] It appears that early synovectomy may provide the

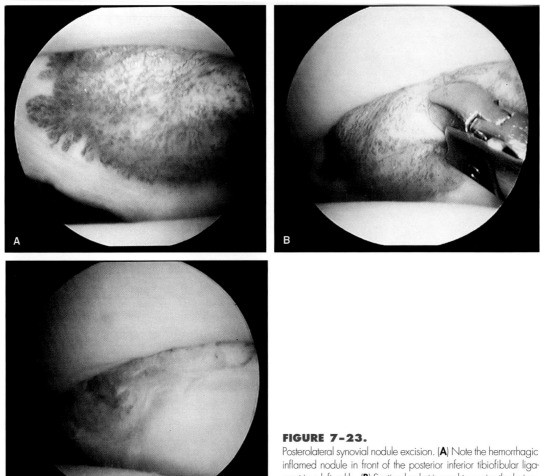

FIGURE 7-23.
Posterolateral synovial nodule excision. (**A**) Note the hemorrhagic inflamed nodule in front of the posterior inferior tibiofibular ligament in a left ankle. (**B**) Suction basket is used to excise the lesion. (**C**) Postexcision view of the articulation between the tibia and the fibula with the synovial nodule removed.

joint several years of good function. However, results are limited and are not as promising if bone and cartilage lesions are already present. Some investigators have also questioned the benefit of synovectomy in general.[26]

As the disease progresses and the rheumatoid granulations develop, joint incongruity and loss of joint space occur. If, on preoperative x-ray films, significant joint disruption has occurred, synovectomy should be avoided, as the results are generally poor and short-term in nature. Even in the best circumstances, debridement and synovectomy slow but do not prevent articular destruction, and they provide only temporary relief (Fig. 7-24). The subtalar joint is also affected by rheumatoid arthritis; arthroscopic subtalar synovectomy may provide

some pain relief, but no results have currently been reported.

Pigmented Villonodular Synovitis

Pigmented villonodular synovitis is thought by some to be a benign neoplasm in the synovium.[27] It occurs most frequently in the knee, but it can occur in the ankle. It can be seen in either a generalized or a localized (circumscribed) form. The more localized solitary lesion is more common in the ankle than the former type. On physical examination the ankle is warm, swollen, and tender, with decreased range of motion. Aspiration of the joint reveals dark, serosanguineous fluid, and x-rays are occasionally helpful

Table 7–1.
SEQUENCE OF LATERAL ANKLE PAIN

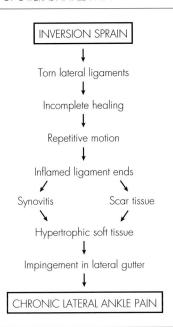

in the diagnosis. The arthrogram may show nodular masses and MRI can demonstrate swollen synovial tissue[28] (see Figs. 2-24, 2-35 in Chapter 2).

Arthroscopy is helpful to confirm the diagnosis when synovitis, papillary formation, and hemosiderin deposits are seen. In addition, brownish-red or yellow components may be visible on the surface of the lesion (Fig. 7-25). Treatment includes total synovectomy, as in rheumatoid arthritis, by means of an invasive or noninvasive distractor. Histologic examination shows deep synovial cell proliferation, increased vascularity, and fibrosis with infiltration of lymphocytes, multinucleated giant cells, iron deposition, and lipid-laden macrophages, interspersed with areas of hemorrhage.[29] With the localized form, arthroscopic excision of the lesion is usually curative. However, with the generalized form, tenosynovectomy may not give lasting results, as recurrences are more common.

Synovial Chondromatosis

Synovial chondromatosis is seldom seen in the ankle and is almost always monoarticular.[30] Diagnosis is made by limited range of motion, locking, swelling, and visualization of multiple calcifications on x-rays of the ankle. At arthroscopy, synovial chondromatosis presents with multiple foci of cartilage metaplasia within the synovium.[31] As these masses grow, they form nodules within the synovial tissue and then become excrescences. These nodules can calcify or ossify. Three phases of this process have been described by Milgram:[32]

1. Active intrasynovial phase without formation of loose bodies
2. Transitional phase, characterized by both active synovial disease and the formation of numerous (often hundreds) chondral loose bodies in the joint. In the early form there is no osseous development, so x-rays and scans are not helpful except for the arthrogram, CT scan, and MRI. In the second stage, bone formation within the synovial tissue and the formation of detached osteochondral fragments can be seen in a regular x-ray and are more representative of chronic synovial chondromatosis (Fig. 7-26*A*).
3. "Burned-out" phase, in which there is no intrasynovial activity but the joint is filled with multiple osteochondral loose bodies. On radiologic examination, both degenerative joint disease and the loose bodies are noted. On radiologic analysis, this entity may be confused with chondrocalcinosis (pseudogout).

Diagnosis is best made by arthroscopic examination and synovial biopsy. Usually at arthroscopy chronic synovitis is seen with chondral and osteochondral fragments within the synovium, along with loose bodies (see Fig. 7-26*B,C*). Later, degenerative joint disease can develop. The presence of loose bodies alone within the ankle joint does not establish a diagnosis of synovial chondromatosis. Loose bodies can also be present in such conditions as degenerative joint disease, rheumatoid arthritis, neurotrophic arthritis, osteochondritis dissecans, tuberculosis, arthritis, and osteochondral fractures. The absence of true cartilaginous metaplasia within the synovial membrane helps to exclude these other conditions.[33]

For treatment, a distraction device is used to perform synovectomy and loose body removal

Table 7-2.
MANAGEMENT OF CHRONIC ANKLE PAIN

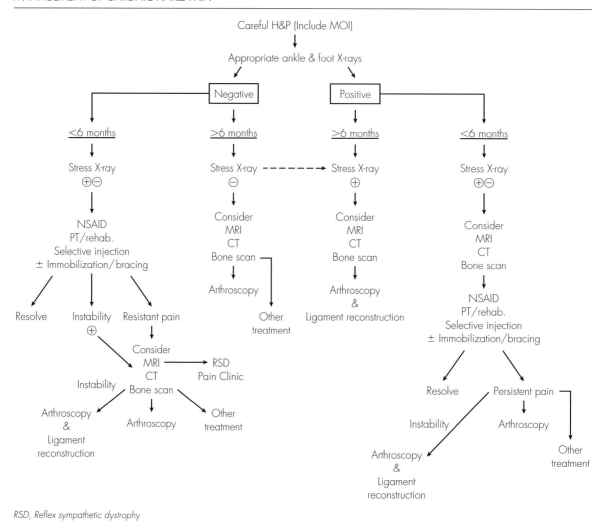

RSD, Reflex sympathetic dystrophy

with stages 1 and 2. Stage 3 debridement and loose body removal are done without synovectomy. With open surgery, about 5% of the problems recur, but no series of arthroscopic treatment has been reported. Even with recurrence, arthroscopy is recommended for repeat surgery.

An aggressive form of synovial chondromatosis has been described that tends to recur, occasionally with distal metastases. If the metastases occur, it should be considered a form of synovial chondrosarcoma.[34]

Hemophilia

The ankle is commonly affected with hemophiliac hemarthrosis, which usually occurs from trauma. Acutely the joint is swollen, red, and tender, and extensive loss of joint space occurs. On x-ray, effusion with spurs and sclerosis can be seen. Arthroscopic synovectomy can be used in chronic situations. Along with proper medical supervision, arthroscopic synovectomy may decrease the number and severity of future bleeding episodes.

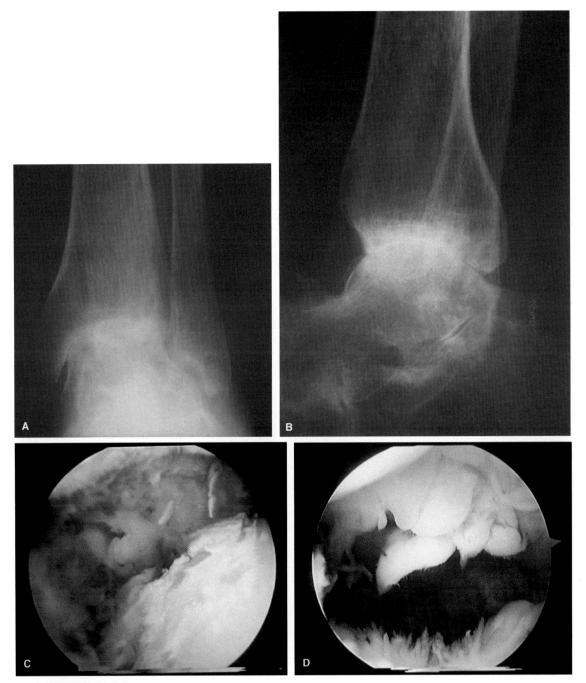

FIGURE 7-24.

Rheumatoid arthritis. (**A,B**) Preoperative anteroposterior and lateral radiographs of a 53-year-old woman with rheumatoid arthritis. Note the severe loss of joint space. (**C**) Arthroscopic view of the same patient shows loss of articular cartilage and hemorrhagic synovium. (**D**) Synovitis and degeneration of the articular cartilage in a 45-year-old man with rheumatoid arthritis.

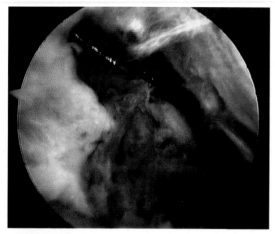

FIGURE 7-25.
Pigmented villonodular synovitis of the ankle. Note the hemosiderin deposits within the synovium.

Other Inflammatory Arthritides

Chen has described some cases of gonarthritis and Crohn disease.[35] Treatment is usually complete arthroscopic debridement. Gout, chondrocalcinosis, and seronegative spondyloarthropathies can affect the ankle and subtalar joints; arthroscopy is used for debridement and occasionally synovectomy (Fig. 7-27).

INFECTION

Acute infection of the ankle is best diagnosed and treated by arthroscopic means. Appropriate cultures, as well as debridement and synovectomy, are per-

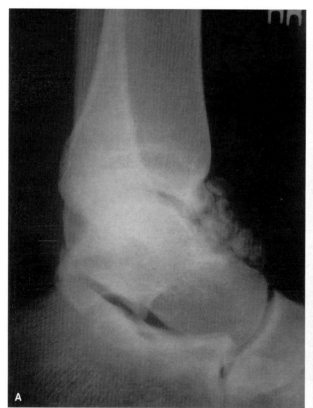

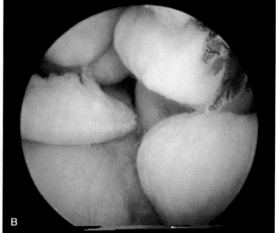

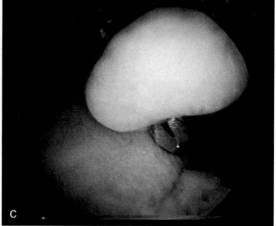

FIGURE 7-26.
Synovial chondromatosis. (**A**) Lateral ankle radiograph showing multiple loose bodies along the anterior border of the ankle, consistent with synovial chondromatosis. (**B**) At arthroscopy, many loose bodies are seen in the anterior joint. (**C**) "Pit bull" grasper is inserted to remove the loose bodies.

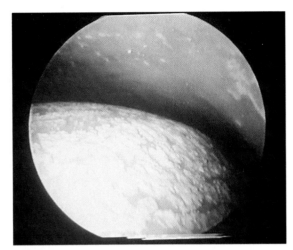

FIGURE 7-27.

Crystal deposition involving the distal tibia and talus in a 38-year-old male with a history of gout.

formed. In the chronic situation, often the etiology of the arthritic joint is unknown and can be facilitated by arthroscopic debridement and biopsy.

Coccidioidomycosis is endemic in the southwestern United States and Mexico. Transient arthralgias develop in up to one third of the patients with acute infection. The organism disseminates in an estimated 0.1% to 0.2% of the patients, and 20% of these develop bone and joint involvement. Usually the disease is monoarticular and can involve the ankle with destructive changes over the years. Arthroscopic synovial biopsy and culture facilitate the diagnosis and treatment. Synovectomy is useful only in the early stages; by the time the diagnosis is usually made, degenerative joint disease has already occurred.

Lyme disease can also involve the foot and ankle. This disease is now the most prevalent arthropod-borne infection in the United States and is endemic in the Northeast, Minnesota, California, and Oregon. The late stages of Lyme disease may cause persistent musculoskeletal symptoms that may resemble an overuse syndrome, mechanical derangement of the joint, or tendinitis. Pain can be seen in the tibiotalar, subtalar, talonavicular, and metatarsophalangeal joints. Other problems associated with Lyme disease include heel pain, plantar fasciitis, Achilles tendinitis, posterior tibial tendinitis, and dorsal foot swelling. When the diagnosis is in doubt, arthroscopic synovial biopsy and culture facilitate the diagnosis. Once diagnosed, conventional treatment with appropriate antibiotics results in clinical improvement in most cases.[36]

PREFERRED METHOD OF ANKLE SYNOVECTOMY

A localized or generalized synovectomy as indicated is part of the treatment protocol in virtually all the conditions discussed above. Although the technique used is the same as that described in Chapter 6, several technical aspects are important to emphasize.

The joint must be visualized in its entirety, using the anteromedial, anterolateral, and posterolateral portals with the patient in the supine position. Distraction is critical for complete evaluation and treatment of the joint, either with invasive or noninvasive means. The 2.7-mm or 3.5-mm full-radius blades are used for ankle synovectomy, as well as 2.7-mm 30° and 70° arthroscopes with wide-angle lenses and large-screen pictures.

The first key to successful synovectomy is a good flow system into the ankle and suction out of the ankle. This can be accomplished with the use of a separate inflow cannula, usually placed at the posterolateral portal initially. Another method is to use an arthroscopic pump, but extreme caution must be taken to avoid extravasation. The two anterior portals are used for the arthroscope and instrumentation.

The second key is the use of an interchangeable cannula system, which allows the arthroscope, basket, shaver, probes, and inflow to be easily and quickly switched without excessive instrumentation of portal sites.

The third key is to perform a careful 21-point examination of the entire ankle (see Chap. 6). Synovectomy should start anteromedially and progress anterocentrally and anterolaterally, and then to the anterior and posterior portions of the ankle joint. Instruments and the arthroscope are switched repeatedly between the anterior and posterior portals as needed.

Patients with rheumatoid arthritis have friable, thin synovium. When debriding anterodorsally or posteromedially, extreme caution must be used to avoid injuring the neurovascular structures. Generally, a blade without exposed cutting edges ("whisker") is used to prevent injury to the neurovascular structures; once visualization is improved, the full-radius blade can be used.

Synovectomy is best performed using the tourniquet, but before removing the instruments the tourniquet should be released and a drain inserted if extensive bleeding is seen. Posterior splinting and compression dressing for 5 to 7 days are particularly helpful in these patients. Early motion should be initiated as soon as soft-tissue swelling has abated and pain is controlled.

REFERENCES

1. Barnett HCH, Davies DV, MacConail RA. Synovial joints: their structure and mechanics. Springfield, IL: Charles C Thomas, 1961.

2. Rodman GP, Schumacher R. Primer on the rheumatic diseases, 8th ed. Atlanta: Arthritis Foundation, 1986:187.

3. Solomon MA, Gilula LA, Oloff LM, et al. CT scanning of the foot and ankle. I. Normal anatomy. Am J Roentgenol 1986;146:1192.

4. Ferkel RD, Flannigan B, Elkins B. MRI of the foot and ankle: normal anatomy with clinical correlation. Foot Ankle 1991;11:289.

5. Brooks SC, Potter BT, Rainey JB. Treatment for partial tears of the lateral ligament of the ankle: a prospective trial. Br Med J 1981;282:606.

6. McCulloch PG, Holden P, Robson DJ, et al. The value of mobilization and nonsteroidal antiinflammatory analgesia in the management of inversion injuries of the ankle. Br J Clin Pract 1985;2:69.

7. Ruth C. The surgical treatment of injuries of the fibular collateral ligaments of the ankle. J Bone Joint Surg 1961;43A:229.

8. Jackson DW, Ashley RD, Powell JW. Ankle sprains in young athletes: relation of severity and disability. Clin Orthop 1974;101:201.

9. Smith RW, Reischl SF. Treatment of ankle sprains in young athletes. Am J Sports Med 1986;14:465.

10. Anderson ME. Reconstruction of the lateral ligaments of the ankle using the plantaris tendon. J Bone Joint Surg 1985;67A:930.

11. Freeman MAR. Instability of the foot after injuries to the lateral ligament of the ankle. J Bone Joint Surg 1965;47B:669.

12. Wolin I, Glassman F, Sideman S. Internal derangement of the talofibular component of the ankle. Surg Gynecol Obstet 1950;91:193.

13. Ferkel RD, Karzel RP, Del Pizzo W, et al. Arthroscopic treatment of anterolateral impingement of the ankle. Am J Sports Med 1991;19:440.

14. Liu SH, Raskin BS, Osti L, et al. Arthroscopic treatment of anterolateral ankle impingement. Arthroscopy 1994;10:215.

15. Martin DF, Baker CL, Curl WW, et al. Operative ankle arthroscopy: long-term follow-up. Am J Sports Med 1989;17:16.

16. Meislin RJ, Rose DJ, Parisien S, Springer S. Arthroscopic treatment of synovial impingement of the ankle. Am J Sports Med 1993;21:186.

17. Kapandji IA. The physiology of the joints. Edinburgh: Churchill Livingstone, 1987:164.

18. Hopkinson WJ, St. Pierre P, Ryan JB, Wheeler JH. Syndesmosis sprains of the ankle. Foot Ankle 1990;10:325.

19. Boytim MJ, Fischer DA, Neumann L. Syndesmotic ankle sprains. Am J Sports Med 1991;19:294.

20. Bassett FH, Gates HS, Billys JB, et al. Talar impingement by the anteroinferior tibiofibular ligament. A cause of chronic pain in the ankle after inversion sprain. J Bone Joint Surg 1990;72A:55.

21. Hamilton WG. Foot and ankle injuries in dancers. Clin Sports Med 1988;7:160.

22. Goldie I. A synopsis of surgery for rheumatoid arthritis (excluding the hand). Clin Orthop 1984;191:185.

23. Schoenholz GJ. Arthroscopic surgery of the shoulder, elbow and ankle. Springfield, IL: Charles C Thomas, 1987:59.

24. Aschan W, Moberg E. A long-term study of the effect of early synovectomy in rheumatoid arthritis. Bull Hosp Jt Dis Orthop Inst 1984;44:106.

25. Goldie IF. Synovectomy in rheumatoid arthritis: theoretical aspects and a 14-year follow-up in the knee joint. Reconstr Surg Traumatol 1981;18:2.

26. McEwen C. Multicenter evaluation of synovectomy in the treatment of rheumatoid arthritis: report of results at the end of 5 years. J Rheumatol 1988;15:765.

27. Granowitz SP, D'Antonia J, Mankin HJ. The pathogenesis and long-term end results of pigmented villonodular synovitis. Clin Orthop 1976;114:335.

28. Beltran J, Noto AM, Mosure JC, et al. Ankle surface coil MR imaging at 1.5 tl. Radiology 1986;161:203.

29. Schumacher HR, Lotke P, Athreya B, et al. Pigmented villonodular synovitis: light and electron microscopic studies. Semin Arthritis Rheum 1982;12:32.

30. Holm CL. Primary synovial chondromatosis of the ankle. J Bone Joint Surg 1976;58A:878.

31. Jeffreys TE. Synovial chondromatosis. J Bone Joint Surg 1967;49B:530.

32. Milgram JW. Synovial osteochondromatosis. J Bone Joint Surg 1977;59A:792.

33. Murphy FP, Dahlin DC, Sullivan CR. Articular synovial chondromatosis. J Bone Joint Surg 1962; 44A:77.

34. Goldman RL, Lichtenstein L. Synovial chondrosarcoma. Cancer 1964;17:1233.

35. Chen Y. Arthroscopy of the ankle joint. In Watanabe M, ed. Arthroscopy of small joints. New York: Igaku-Shoin, 1985.

36. Faller J, Thompson F, Hamilton W. Foot and ankle disorders resulting from Lyme disease. Foot Ankle 1991;11:236.

BIBLIOGRAPHY

Cetti R. Conservative treatment of injury to the fibular ligaments of the ankle. Br J Sports Med 1982;16:47.

Cox JS. Surgical and nonsurgical treatment of acute ankle sprains. Clin Orthop 1985;198:118.

Ferkel RD. Differential diagnosis of chronic ankle sprain pain in the athlete. Sports Med Arthroscopy Rev 1994;2:274.

Kleiger B. Anterior tibiotalar impingement syndromes in dancers. Foot Ankle 1982;3:69.

McMurray TP. Footballer's ankle. J Bone Joint Surg 1950;32B:68.

Rasmussen O, Tovburg-Jensen I, Boe S. Distal tibiofibular ligaments—analysis of function. Acta Orthop Scand 1982;53:681.

Arthroscopic Surgery: The Foot and Ankle,
by Richard D. Ferkel.
Lippincott-Raven Publishers, Philadelphia © 1996.

8

Articular Surface Defects, Loose Bodies, and Osteophytes

Osteochondral lesions of the ankle joint include many pathologic entities, including osteochondritis dissecans, chondral and osteochondral loose bodies, osteophytes, chondral and osteochondral fractures of the tibia and talus, cystic lesions of the talus, fracture defects, and arthritis. Many controversies and misconceptions persist regarding the etiology, treatment, and prognosis of osteochondral and chondral lesions of the ankle. In Section A of this chapter, the etiology, mechanism of injury, diagnosis, and treatment of osteochondral lesions of the talus will be discussed. In Section B, the arthroscopic treatment of osteophytes, loose bodies, and chondral lesions will be described.

A. *Osteochondral Lesions of the Talus*
Richard D. Ferkel

TERMINOLOGY

Multiple terms have been used to describe these lesions, including transchondral fractures, osteochondral fractures, osteochondritis dissecans, talar dome fractures, and flake fractures, but the best term to describe this problem is *osteochondral lesion of the talus* (OLT).

The controversy in terminology has resulted in part from a lack of a clearly defined and universally accepted etiology. The most common designation, osteochondritis dissecans, literally translated implies separation or an inflammatory lesion of cartilage and bone; this has very little relevance to the actual pathophysiology of this condition.

HISTORY

In 1856, Alexander Monro was the first to describe osteochondral loose bodies in the ankle joint and implicated trauma as the cause.[1] Konig coined the term *osteochondritis dissecans* when he noted loose bodies in other joints such as the knee, which he thought were due to spontaneous osteonecrosis.[2] He reasoned that these loose bodies were due to vascular occlusion. In 1898 Barth described the same lesion.[3] He thought it was due to an intraarticular fracture but was not sure whether trauma was the etiology. In 1922 Kappis first applied the term *osteochondritis dissecans* to the ankle joint.[4] This term was accepted and remained in use until Berndt and Harty's classic 1959 treatise, in which they postulated that the lesion had a traumatic etiology and coined the term *transchondral fracture of the talus* to describe the lesion.[5]

Later, O'Donoghue stated that these lesions were intraarticular fractures.[6] Davidson and associates agreed.[7] Campbell and Ranawat in 1966 concluded that OLTs were a disease process resulting in pathologic fractures through necrotic bone secondary to ischemia.[8] Since then, more papers have appeared that support the trauma etiology, including those of Alexander and Lichtman[9] and Canale and Belding.[10]

ETIOLOGY

The exact etiology of OLT has never been conclusively proved and remains controversial. The implication that idiopathic osteonecrosis may be the underlying pathologic process is supported by the fact that lower extremity trauma is not documented in all cases. Furthermore, some argue that history of an ankle injury may not be a statistically significant etiologic factor, because eliciting such a history is not uncommon. In addition, this lesion has been associated in the literature with alcohol abuse, use of steroids, emboli, and endocrine and some hereditary situations.

The trauma theory, however, remains the most popular as the etiology for OLT as it appears more feasible. This theory suggests that the lesion represents the chronic phase of a compressed or avulsed talar dome fracture. A distinct episode of macrotrauma or overuse constituting repetitive microtrauma may contribute to initiation of the lesion in a person with a predisposition to talar dome ischemia. An osteonecrotic process will result in subchondral fracture, and collapse may exist. Progression and symptomatology may result in alteration of joint biomechanics, with increased joint pressures resulting in the forcing of synovial fluid into the fracture site, preventing healing. (This subchondral fracture, having no soft-tissue attachments and no blood or nerve supply, is highly susceptible to subsequent avascular necrosis.)

INCIDENCE

OLTs are relatively uncommon. However, their exact incidence is probably underestimated because they may occur more commonly than clinically seen. X-ray identification may be subtle; in many instances, x-rays are not even taken because the trauma may seem insignificant. More than 700 cases have been reported in the world literature at present. The incidence of OLT has been reported as ranging from

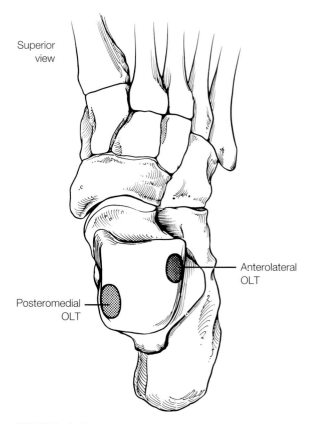

Superior view

Anterolateral OLT

Posteromedial OLT

FIGURE 8-1.
Location of osteochondral lesions of the talus. Most lesions are posteromedial or anterolateral, as seen on the axial view of the talus.

0.09% of all talar fractures compiled from a series reported during World War II to 6.5% of 133 sprains studied by Bosien and associates.[11] OLT reportedly represents 4% of all cases of osteochondritis dissecans.[12] Several series indicate that the incidence of bilateral lesions averages 10%. Most series report the average age between 20 and 30, with males slightly more predominant.

LOCATION

Osteochondral lesions on the medial aspect of the dome of the talus occur in the middle or posterior third; lateral lesions occur primarily in the middle or anterior portion (Fig. 8-1). There are exceptions: lesions in the anteromedial corner and posterolateral corner and central lesions also occur. On a few occasions, these lesions may occur in multiple sites. Medial OLT lesions are more common than lateral ones in most series; however, lateral lesions are ascribed to trauma in about 90% to 98% of cases, and medial lesions are ascribed to trauma in about 70%. Lateral lesions are usually shell- and wafer-shaped and are often displaced and elevated by the levering effect of the distal tibia (Fig. 8-2). Medial lesions are deeper

and cup-shaped and are usually not displaced (see Fig. 8-2).

MECHANISM OF INJURY

The mechanism of injury for OLTs appears to differ for medial, lateral, and central lesions. In addition, more than one mechanism is probably associated with similar-appearing lesions. Berndt and Harty used cadavers to try to reproduce the mechanisms of these lesions.[5] Lateral talar dome lesions were reproduced by a strong inversion force to a dorsiflexed foot with the tibia internally rotated. Medial dome lesions were reproduced by a strong inversion force to a plantarflexed foot with lateral rotation of the tibia on the talus (external rotation). They thought that the principal force causing medial and lateral talar dome lesions was torsional impaction. With the lateral lesions, as the foot is dorsiflexed and strongly inverted, the lateral talar margin is impacted and compressed against the medial articular surface of the fibula, causing a shearing and compressing component that could potentially displace the osteochondral fragment. Conversely, in medial talar dome lesions, when the foot was inverted and plantarflexed

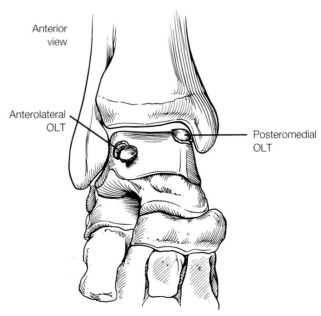

FIGURE 8-2.
The size of the osteochondral lesion varies by location. Lateral lesions tend to be shallower and wafer-shaped, medial lesions deeper and cup-shaped.

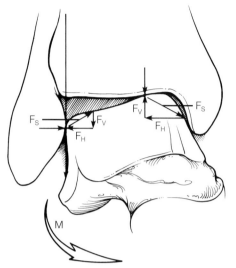

FIGURE 8-3.

Inversion stress on the ankle joint creates a moment of force (M) that can be resolved along coordinate axes as a vertical (F_v) and a horizontal (F_H) force. The result of these two forces is a shear force (F_S) along which the osteochondral lesion occurs. (Modified from Stauffer RN. Intraarticular ankle problems. In Evarts C. Surgery of the musculoskeletal system, vol. 3. New York: Churchill Livingstone, 1983. By permission of Mayo Foundation.)

resolved along coordinate axes (Fig. 8-3). A fracture may occur along the line of the shear force component (F_S). Whether the medial or lateral aspect of the dome is involved may depend on whether the ankle is in a dorsiflexed or plantarflexed position. The amount of displacement of the fragment that may occur depends on whether the shear stress is greater than the ultimate strength of the bone or cartilage. If the ultimate shear stress is greater than bone, articular cartilage may momentarily deform but will remain intact while the underlying bone fractures (Fig. 8-4A). However, if the magnitude of the resultant shear stress is greater than the ultimate strength of both articular cartilage and bone, a complete lesion is produced and displacement of the fragment from its bed may occur (see Fig. 8-4B).[13]

Yao and Weis reasoned that lateral lesions were caused by eversion of the foot with the ankle dorsiflexed and the tibia internally rotated on the talus.[14] In addition, they thought medial lesions were produced by inversion of the foot with the ankle plantarflexed. Clearly, no single mechanism can explain each case because many lesions, particularly on the medial side, occur without preceding known trauma.

Patients may develop this injury from a fall from a height or associated fractures or crushing-type trauma. In some patients, no specific mechanism of injury or associated etiologic factor can be documented. In this group, idiopathic osteonecrotic

with the tibia in external rotation, the posteromedial edge of the talar dome impacted against the posteromedial tip of the tibia, causing increased shear stress.

The shear stress that is the inversion stress on the ankle joint creates a moment of force that can be

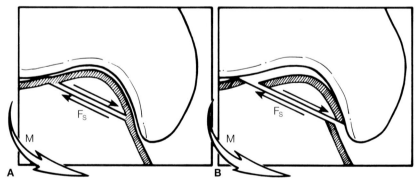

FIGURE 8-4.

Development of the osteochondral lesion. The articular cartilage may remain intact or may be injured along with the subchondral bone, depending on whether (**A**) the shear stress is greater than the ultimate strength of the bone, but less than that of the cartilage; or (**B**) the shear stress is greater than the ultimate strength of both cartilage and bone. (Modified from Stauffer RN. Intraarticular ankle problems. In Evarts C. Surgery of the musculoskeletal system, vol. 3. New York: Churchill Livingstone, 1983. By permission of Mayo Foundation.)

process versus repetitive microtrauma may be postulated.

CLINICAL PRESENTATION

The presentation of OLT can be acute after an injury, but more often it is associated with persistent ankle pain, particularly after a trauma such as inversion injury of the lateral ligamentous complex. A history of chronic lateral ankle pain or chronic ankle sprain pain is commonly noted. In addition, a history of associated injuries such as ankle or lower extremity fractures or falls from a height may be elicited. Usually symptoms are intermittent and can include stiffness, pain of a deep aching nature aggravated by weight bearing, swelling, catching, clicking, locking, and less commonly giving way.

The differential diagnosis of a patient with intermittent symptoms after an ankle sprain includes calcific ossicles beneath the medial or lateral malleolus, peroneal subluxation or tears, tarsal coalition, subtalar joint dysfunction, degenerative joint disease, soft-tissue impingement, infection, reflex sympathetic dystrophy, and OLT (see Chap. 7).

On physical examination, patients may have evidence of tenderness, either medially or laterally, pain with range of motion, limited range of motion, edema, weakness, or evidence of instability.

Different studies suggest that the average duration of symptoms before a definitive diagnosis is made ranges from 4 months to 2 years. Because of the nature of the problem, it is uncommon to diagnose this lesion acutely.

DIAGNOSIS

The diagnosis of OLT requires a high index of suspicion because in many cases the clinical symptoms and findings are so mild that routine radiographs are

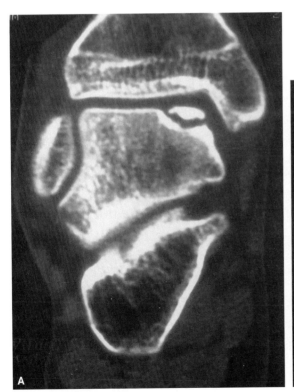
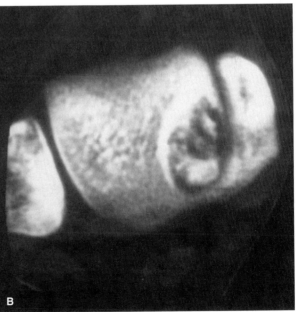

FIGURE 8–5.
Hindfoot CT scan in two planes. (**A**) Coronal plane demonstrates stage III lesion with lucency under the fragment. (**B**) Axial view shows that the lesion extends from the central to the posterior aspect of the medial talus.

not done. In addition, x-rays not infrequently do not reveal the osteochondral lesion.

After careful clinical examination, three views of the ankle should be done (AP, mortise, and lateral). Berndt and Harty in 1959 described a staging system, based on plain x-rays, for classifying these lesions; this is discussed further in the next section.[5] Other radiologic modalities include tomography and bone scan. Bone scans are a useful, inexpensive way to screen for OLT. Tomography has been replaced by more sophisticated modalities, such as CT and MRI scanning. CT scanning can be done with or without contrast and should always be done in two planes, both the axial (transverse) and coronal. I prefer to do bilateral hindfoot CT scans to assess both hindfeet at the same time, and also to determine if bilateral lesions are present. Contrast may assist in evaluating the articular surface, either pre- or postoperatively, and in determining healing. A CT scan also best localizes the lesion in three dimensions so the surgeon knows the exact extent of the lesion and where resection or surgical treatment should be done (Fig.

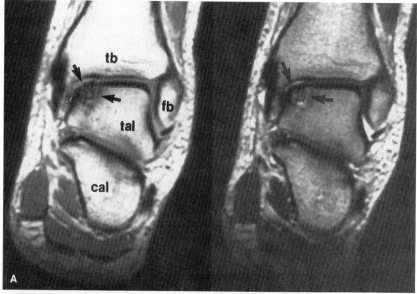

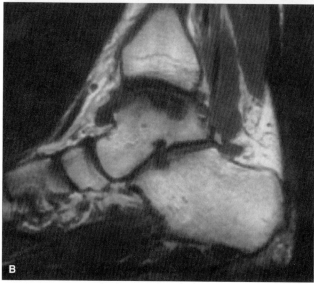

FIGURE 8-6.
MRI of osteochondral lesion of the talus. (**A**) Coronal T1- and T2-weighted images with the lesion well demonstrated. (**B**) Sagittal image demonstrating the large extent of the lesion in the anterior/posterior direction. tb, tibia; tal, talus; cal, calcaneus; fb, fibula.

8-5). More recently, MRI has been advocated as having diagnostic capabilities equal to those of CT scanning (Fig. 8-6).

CLASSIFICATION AND STAGING

Berndt and Harty's 1959 radiologic classification was based on plain x-rays of the ankle. More recently, Ferkel and Sgaglione have developed a CT classification considered to be more accurate and to correlate better with the arthroscopic picture and with subsequent results.[15] In this four-stage classification, CT scans are evaluated in two planes (Fig. 8-7; Table

8-1). Zinman and associates in 1988 reported on 32 patients with osteochondritis dissecans of the dome of the talus.[16,17] They found CT scans to be superior to x-rays for both diagnosis and follow-up.

MRI has also been advocated as a way to stage OLT.[18,19] Although MRI allows multiplanar imaging without the use of radiation, it is not as useful in showing cortical outlines; therefore, it sometimes gives a confusing picture as to the full extent of the lesion and whether it is loose. Anderson and colleagues compared CT with MRI results in 24 patients and developed an MRI classification system[20] (Table 8-2). In most cases, CT was comparable

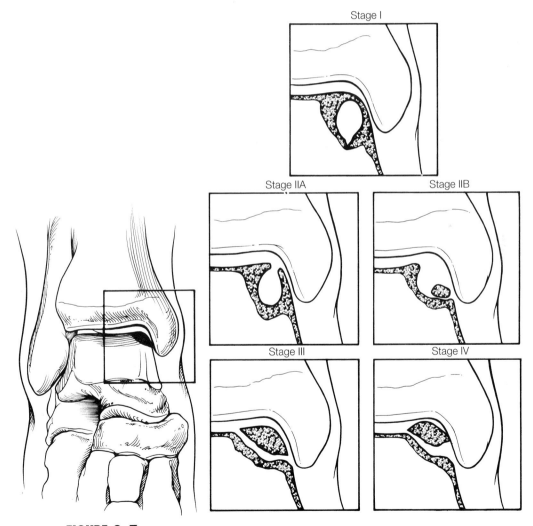

FIGURE 8-7.
CT scan classification. See also Table 8-1. (Modified after J. Daugherty and Richard Ferkel.)

TABLE 8-1.
CT CLASSIFICATION

Stage I	Cystic lesion within dome of talus, intact roof on all views
Stage IIA	Cystic lesion with communication to talar dome surface
Stage IIB	Open articular surface lesion with overlying nondisplaced fragment
Stage III	Undisplaced lesion with lucency
Stage IV	Displaced fragment

(From Ferkel RD, Sgaglione NA. Arthroscopic treatment of osteochondral lesions of the talus: long term results. Orthop Trans 1993–1994;17:1011.)

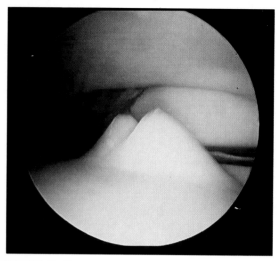

FIGURE 8-8.
Arthroscopic grade 3 lesion according to the Pritsch classification.

to MRI, but CT did not make the diagnosis in 4 patients with stage 1 lesions.

Pritsch and associates classified OLT lesions by the arthroscopic appearance of overlying cartilage into three grades: intact, firm, shiny articular cartilage; intact but soft cartilage; and frayed cartilage[21] (Fig. 8-8). They found some lesions that progressed from grade 1 to grade 3 during the course of treatment. They also noted a poor correlation between the x-ray appearance and arthroscopic findings, and considered the arthroscopic appearance to be the most important determinant for treatment.

Cheng, Ferkel, and Applegate studied 80 patients treated at the Southern California Orthopedic Institute between 1985 and 1994.[22] Their preoperative x-rays, CT or MRI, and intraoperative videotapes were reviewed and correlated, and the previously mentioned CT and MRI staging systems were corre-

lated with a new arthroscopic staging system (Table 8-3). The results indicated that CT is the scan of choice if there is a known diagnosis of OLT; however, if the x-ray and clinical findings are nondiagnostic, then an MRI may be more valuable because of its ability to image both soft tissue and bone.

TREATMENT INDICATIONS

The appropriate treatment for OLT is controversial. Some of the confusion is probably due to the uncertainty about the etiology and nature of this lesion. In addition, there is no long-term study of the natural

TABLE 8-2.
MRI CLASSIFICATION

Stage I	Subchondral trabecular compression
	Plain radiograph normal, positive bone scan
	Marrow edema on MRI
Stage IIA	Formation of subchondral cyst
Stage II	Incomplete separation of fragment
Stage III	Unattached, undisplaced fragment with presence of synovial fluid around fragment
Stage IV	Displaced fragment

(From Anderson IF, Crichton KJ, Grattan–Smith T, et al. Osteochondral fractures of the dome of the talus. J Bone Joint Surg 1989;71A:1143.)

TABLE 8-3.
Surgical Grade Based on Articular Cartilage

Grade A	Smooth, intact but soft or ballottable
Grade B	Rough surface
Grade C	Fibrillations/fissures
Grade D	Flap present or bone exposed
Grade E	Loose, undisplaced fragment
Grade F	Displaced fragment

(From Cheng MS, Ferkel RD, Applegate GR. Osteochondral lesions of the talus: a radiologic and surgical comparison. Presented at the Annual Meeting of the Academy of Orthopaedic Surgeons, New Orleans, February 1995.)

history of untreated OLT because patients rarely are seen for this problem unless they are symptomatic. With an average follow-up of 7 years, 7 of 11 patients in the series of Lindholm and associates were asymptomatic when treated conservatively.[23] Other studies have suggested that the lesion may show radiographic failure to heal over a long period of follow-up, but this is not incompatible with a successful outcome (asymptomatic ankle). However, because arthroscopy is not done on patients treated conservatively, one does not have a true assessment of the amount of articular damage that exists, nor can a determination be made as to whether a conservative treatment course in an ankle with a loose lesion may lead to accelerated degenerative changes in the future.

Berndt and Harty[5] and subsequently Canale and Belding[10] concurred that stage 1 and 2 lesions, whether medial or lateral, should be treated nonoperatively. They also advocated nonoperative treatment initially for stage 3 medial lesions and surgical treatment only if symptoms persisted. Surgical treatment is recommended in stage 3 lateral lesions and all stage 4 lesions, based on the Berndt and Harty classification.

Other authors have argued that surgical treatment is superior to conservative care. Blom and Strijk[24] stated that it was sometimes difficult to distinguish stage 2 from stage 3 Berndt and Harty lesions and advocated surgical treatment, as did Yvars,[25] Alexander and Lichtman,[9] O'Farrell and Costello,[26] and Flick and Gould.[27] The latter authors, in their review of the literature and of 22 patients with 2-year follow-up, argued that surgical treatment yielded superior results to conservative therapy, even with a number of stage 2 lesions.

Author's Indications

In CT scan stage 1 and 2 lesions, conservative treatment is initially advocated in both the acute and chronic situations. This should include 6 to 12 weeks of casting, with the length determined by the size of the lesion. At present there is no good evidence that non-weight bearing in a cast is any better than weight bearing, so it is not advocated. If the patient remains symptomatic after the proposed conservative program, then arthroscopic evaluation and treatment

are suggested. Arthroscopy is advocated for all symptomatic CT scan stage 3 and 4 lesions. The only exception is in children whose growth plates have not closed at the distal tibial and fibular epiphyses; for these patients, initial conservative treatment with casting before surgical intervention is recommended.

SURGICAL TREATMENT

Surgical treatment of OLT has traditionally been through extensive ankle arthrotomy with excision of loose bodies, joint debridement, and in certain cases drilling or abrasion at the site of the lesion. Loomer and associates found that 42% of patients had excellent and 32% had good results.[28] Initially, surgery was done by arthrotomy, but now most cases are performed arthroscopically. Methods for open treatment include grooving the anteromedial distal tibia, large soft-tissue arthrotomy, medial or lateral malleolar osteotomies, and percutaneous fluoroscopic drilling. These surgical approaches can all be associated with problems such as nonunion or malunion of the malleoli, postoperative joint stiffness and pain, prolonged rehabilitation time, scuffing of articular cartilage, neurovascular injury, degenerative joint disease, and inadequate posterior visualization.

Because of the problems associated with an open approach, more recently arthroscopy has been used to treat OLT. With the advent of new and improved arthroscopic techniques and equipment, more thorough arthroscopic visualization of the talar dome can be made and advanced treatment modalities used.

As detailed in Chapter 6, various arthroscopic approaches are available to treat these lesions. These include the supine position with an ankle and thigh holder, the supine position with a thigh holder and the table bent to allow the knee flexed to 90°, and the lateral decubitus position. Regardless of the method used, the therapeutic alternatives are the same. These include drilling the base of the lesion, excising the lesion with drilling, internally fixating a loose lesion, or bone graft with or without internal fixation.

Anterolateral lesions can usually be approached with the arthroscope in the anteromedial portal and surgical instrumentation through the anterolateral portal(s). Most medial lesions, however, are more difficult to approach because they are often in the middle or posterior region of the talar dome. Various distraction methods have been devised that permit easier access to these lesions (see Chap. 5).

PREFERRED APPROACH

Technique

The technique used to approach OLTs is the same as that described in Chapter 6. Small 2.7-mm 30° and 70° arthroscopes and small-joint instrumentation are particularly useful in treating these lesions because they enable the arthroscopist to see a wide angle of vision with minimal distraction and to work in small spaces.

Arthroscopic evaluation of osteochondral lesions starts with a complete 21-point examination, as discussed in Chapter 7. Care is taken to examine not only the talus but also the tibial articular surfaces, because some patients with OLT also have associated lesions on the tibia that are symptomatic and require treatment. The arthroscope must be placed in all three portals so that no area is left unvisualized.

Principles

The principles of treating acute osteochondral lesions are different than those for chronic lesions.

With acute OLT, the first priority is to identify

TABLE 8-4.
TREATMENT OF ACUTE OLT

1. Palpate the lesion with a small-joint probe.
2. Excise chondral fragment(s) with little or no bone and drill the base.
3. Reattach loose osteochondral fragments with absorbable pins, K-wire, or screws.
4. If lesion is displaced, reduce with probe or grasper gently and temporarily fixate with K-wire, then firmly fixate with absorbable pins, screws, or K-wire.

TABLE 8-5.
TREATMENT OF CHRONIC OLT

1. Probe with small-joint probe.
2. Evaluate with palpation whether lesion is loose; if there is any question, use dilute methylene blue to detect staining around the lesion that would suggest whether it is loose or not.
3. Drill the lesion if it is not loose.
4. Fixate the lesion if loose and if articular cartilage and underlying bone are healthy with absorbable pins, K-wires, or screws.
5. Excise the lesion if loose or displaced, then drill the base.
6. Bone-graft large cystic areas if cartilage is intact; otherwise, curette the cyst out and drill or abrade the base. (Bone-grafting of open defects can be considered.)

the lesion. CT or MRI may be used if needed to further visualize and distinguish the exact appearance and radiologic stage. If the acute lesion is displaced, arthroscopy should be done immediately, and the consent should read "arthroscopy with possible open pinning or removal of osteochondral lesion of the talus."

In the acute situation, the lesion should be palpated with a small-joint probe. Subsequent assess-

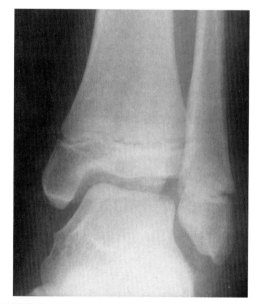

FIGURE 8-9.
Mortise x-ray demonstrating displaced osteochondral lesion from the anterolateral talar bed in an 11-year-old girl.

ment should be made as to whether the chondral fragment has enough bone to allow healing if it is reattached. If the lesion is primarily chondral in nature, excision is recommended, with subsequent debridement and drilling of the base to stimulate new vascularity and the formation of fibrocartilage. If the chondral fragment has enough underlying bone, the piece should be reattached with absorbable pins, K-wires, or screws. If the lesion is severely displaced, reduction with a probe or grasper is done gently

to reduce the fragment anatomically so it can be temporarily fixated with a K-wire. Then firm fixation can be accomplished with further K-wires, absorbable pins, or screws (Table 8-4).

With chronic OLT, it is again critical to identify the lesion correctly. CT or MRI should be done when indicated, as described previously. Generally, arthroscopy is performed on all stage 3 and 4 lesions, and stage 1 and 2 lesions that fail conservative treatment.

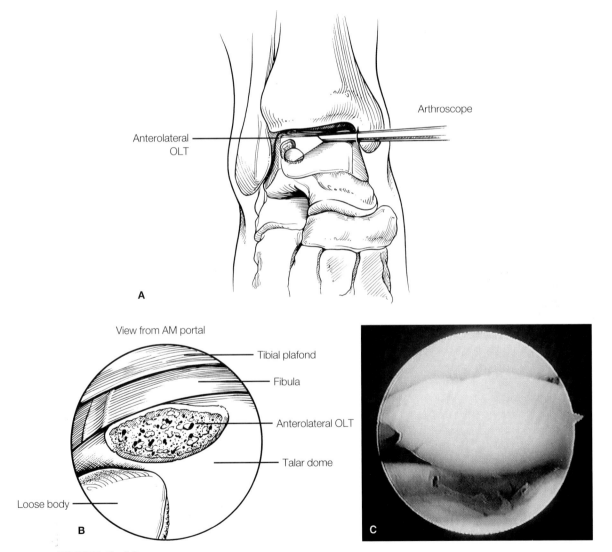

FIGURE 8–10.
Acute osteochondral lesion of the talus. (**A**) Displaced lateral talar dome lesion. (**B**) Bleeding osteochondral lesion bed along the anterolateral aspect of the talus, when viewed from the anteromedial portal. (**C**) Arthroscopic view of same patient. The osteochondral lesion is not only displaced but also upside-down in the joint.

There is controversy as to the best way to treat full-thickness loss of articular cartilage such as in OLT. Penetration of the subchondral bone disrupts subchondral blood vessels.[29–31] This leads to the formation of a fibrin clot, and a fibrocartilaginous repair tissue often forms over the surface if it is protected from excessive loading.[32,33] It has been shown experimentally that the cells responsible for the new fibrocartilaginous articular surface enter the fibrin clot from the marrow.[31,34] These cells start as undifferentiated mesenchymal cells and then differentiate into chondroblasts and chondrocytes.

Different methods have been developed for penetrating subchondral bone to perform cartilage repair, including resecting sclerotic subchondral bone, drilling through the subchondral bone, abrading the articular surface, and creating small-diameter defects with a sharp instrument. Although it is unclear which of these methods produces the best new articular surface, I prefer drilling through the subchondral plate. A recent comparison of abrasion with drilling for treatment of experimental chondral defects in rabbits demonstrated that the long-term results of drilling appear to be better than those of abrasion.[35] These findings support other works that have shown that cartilage surface can be repaired by tissue that grows up through the drill holes, then spreads to cover the exposed subchondral bone between the holes.[36]

In the chronic setting, the lesion should be carefully probed. If the lesion is posterior, visualization should be done through the posterolateral portal to facilitate complete assessment of the size, location, and looseness of the lesion. On occasion, a question still arises as to how loose the fragment is and its potential for healing. In this instance, a dilute methylene blue solution can be injected to detect staining around the lesion, which may suggest whether it is loose. If the lesion is not loose, transmalleolar or transtalar drilling can be done. If the lesion is loose, fixation can be accomplished with absorbable pins, K-wires, or screws if the articular cartilage is healthy. Usually, chronic lesions must be excised, as they are found to be loose and occasionally displaced. After excision, curettage and transmalleolar or transtalar drilling is done.

Rarely, a large cystic area is identified with an intact cartilage surface. If the cyst is symptomatic, it should be curetted out arthroscopically and a bone graft inserted. However, if the large cystic area does not have an intact cartilage, the entire cystic region, including the deformed loose cartilage, should be

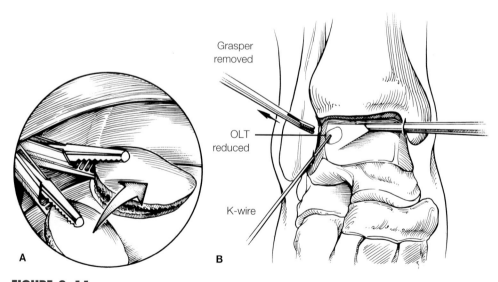

FIGURE 8–11.
Acute osteochondral lesion of the talus. (**A**) Loose body is located centrally in the joint and reduced back into the bleeding talar bed. (**B**) Once the loose lesion is reduced, it is held in place with a probe and can be temporarily fixated with a K-wire.

curetted out and the area debrided and drilled (Table 8-5). Some asymptomatic cystic lesions can be followed for years without adverse results.

SPECIFIC LESIONS

Anterolateral Lesions

Anterolateral lesions are usually displaced and may be upside-down in the joint (Fig. 8-9). Anterolateral lesions are best approached with the arthroscope in the anteromedial portal, inflow posterolaterally, and instrumentation anterolaterally (Fig. 8-10). Loose lesions can be reduced and fixated, or excised through the anterolateral portal (Fig. 8-11). A small-joint cannula can then be used to stabilize the K-wire while drilling into the base of the lesion to assist in fixation of the fragment. Fixation can be maintained with K-wires, screws, or absorbable pins. The Orthosorb pin, an absorbable pin, is made of polyglycolic acid and takes 6 months to absorb. Usually two or three pins are necessary for stable fixation (Fig. 8-12). If drilling is difficult from the anterolateral

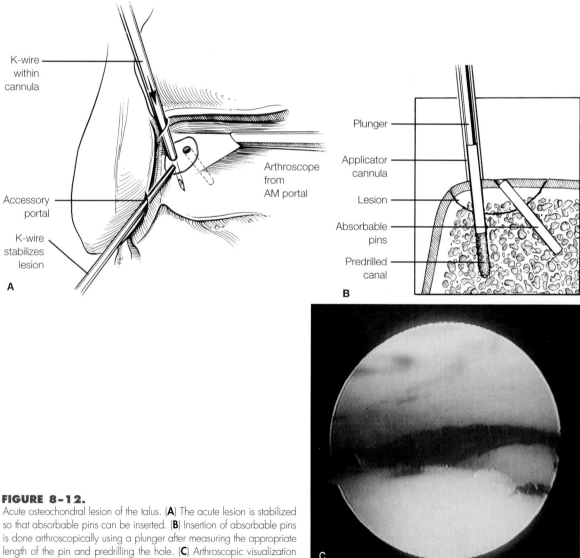

FIGURE 8-12.
Acute osteochondral lesion of the talus. (**A**) The acute lesion is stabilized so that absorbable pins can be inserted. (**B**) Insertion of absorbable pins is done arthroscopically using a plunger after measuring the appropriate length of the pin and predrilling the hole. (**C**) Arthroscopic visualization of the fragment after reduction and fixation with absorbable pins.

portal, the Micro Vector drill guide can be inserted through the anterolateral portal and drilling can be done from the medial portion of the talus across into the lateral talar dome lesion. Alternatively, the arthroscope can be inserted anterolaterally and the Micro Vector can be inserted anteromedially to drill into the anterolateral lesion. Postoperative x-rays at 4 months demonstrate excellent healing (Fig. 8-13).

Posterolateral Lesions

Posterolateral lesions are less common and more difficult to diagnose and treat. After accurate localization on CT scan, surgical planning can begin (Fig. 8-14). These lesions are best visualized through the posterolateral portal while a probe is inserted through the anterolateral portal. The anteromedial portal may be used for inflow. If the lesion is more in the middle to the posterolateral talus, visualization may be accomplished from the anterolateral portal with the probe inserted posterolaterally. Occasionally, the lesion is so posterior that the arthroscope is inserted through an accessory posterolateral portal and the primary posterolateral portal is used for in-

strumentation. The rest of the treatment principles are the same as previously discussed. Posterolateral lesions are best drilled by inserting a cannula onto the lesion through the posterolateral portal and then placing the K-wire through this portal (Fig. 8-15). Sometimes it is necessary to insert a Micro Vector drill guide through the posterolateral portal and perform transmalleolar drilling through the medial malleolus.

Anteromedial Lesions

These lesions, also less common than posteromedial lesions, can usually be approached alternating between the anteromedial and anterolateral portals, using the posterolateral portal for inflow. Most anteromedial lesions can be drilled through the anteromedial portal, but occasionally transmalleolar drilling is indicated through the medial malleolus using the Micro Vector drill guide.

Posteromedial Lesions

These are the most common lesions seen chronically and usually involve the middle or posteromedial dome of the talus. A preoperative CT scan in the coronal and transverse planes is particularly helpful to localize the lesion in an anterior-posterior direction and to plan the surgical approach (see Figs. 2-30, 8-5). In this lesion, the anteromedial portal must be placed in a more central location than usual to avoid abutment of the arthroscope and instruments against the medial malleolus. The groove of Harty permits the arthroscope to visualize most lesions in the midportion of the talus from the anteromedial portal; however, when the lesion is more posterior, the posterolateral portal provides better visualization. In the latter case, instrumentation is then brought through the anteromedial portal, with inflow through the anterolateral portal.

Posteromedial lesions should be palpated through the anteromedial portal; if stable, transmalleolar drilling is done (see below). If the lesion is loose, in most cases excision is necessary using small ring curettes, banana knives, motorized instrumentation, and small graspers (Fig. 8-16). Ring curettes may be used to debride and smooth the base (Fig.

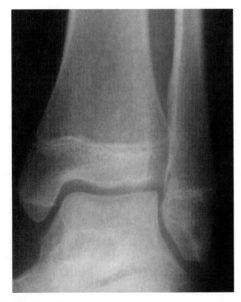

FIGURE 8-13.
Postoperative x-ray of the patient in Figure 8-9 4 months after surgery. The lesion is well incorporated into the anterolateral talar dome and appears healed.

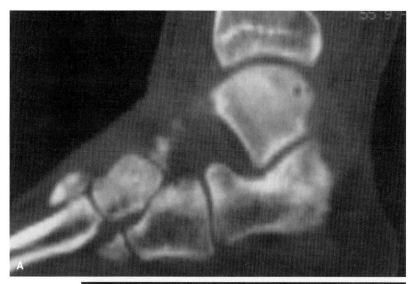

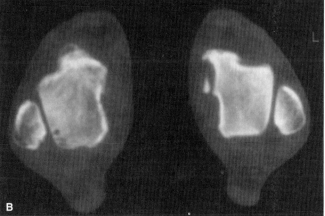

FIGURE 8-14.

CT scan of a posterolateral osteochondral lesion of the talus. (**A**) Sagittal CT scan shows multiple cystic lesions in the extreme posterior aspect of the talus. (**B**) Bilateral axial CT scan shows the lesions to be on the most posterolateral corner of the talus in the right ankle; the left ankle is normal.

8-17). Cartilage margins should be excised at 90° to the articular surface so as not to undermine or bevel these margins. This "quarry effect" may assist with better clot retention in the defect and subsequent metaplasia to fibrocartilage with the potential for reconstitution of the articular surface.[13]

Drilling of the medial talus can be done in four ways. First, a Micro Vector guide can be used to perform transmalleolar drilling. A small incision is made over the medial malleolus and the drill guide is inserted; 0.062 K-wires are used (Fig. 8-18). The drill holes are made in the medial malleolus in the area that provides the best direct angle into the lesion. Depending on the location of the lesion and the ease of distraction, visualization can be done through the anterolateral portal (Fig. 8-19) or the posterolateral portal (Fig. 8-20). Usually instrumentation is inserted through the anteromedial portal. A second method is to use an offset guide to place multiple holes; alternatively, the drill guide can be reinserted in a different position (Fig. 8-21). Drilling should be performed at 3- to 5-mm intervals to a depth of 10 mm to potentiate vascular access in the healing of new fibrocartilage. A third method is to flex and extend the ankle with the pin tip barely exposed from the distal tibia. If the pin is too prominent, scuffing will occur with flexion and extension. Once the pin is drilled into the talus, the ankle should never be moved until the pin is distracted (Fig. 8-22). Fluoroscopy is not routinely used because the lesion can be directly visualized as it is drilled. The 70° arthroscope may assist in visualizing

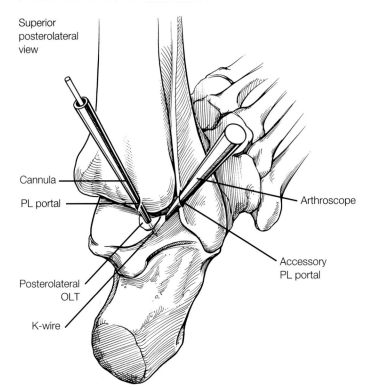

Superior
posterolateral
view

Cannula

PL portal

Arthroscope

Accessory
PL portal

Posterolateral
OLT

K-wire

FIGURE 8-15.
Posterolateral osteochondral lesions of the talus can be approached through two posterior portals. While visualizing from the accessory posterolateral portal, the usual posterolateral portal is used to drill the lesion through an arthroscopic cannula.

the most posterior lesions. A fourth method is to drill the osteochondral lesion from below, coming in through the anterolateral talus (see below).

In chronic OLT, the fragment rarely requires internal fixation. However, if this is required, it is best performed by making a small medial arthrotomy, unless the lesion is accessible through the anteromedial portal. In the unusual occasion when a large cyst is present with the overlying cartilage intact, a bone graft should be performed. One method advocated in the past was to ream a large enough hole through a transmalleolar approach to create a small window on the medial dome of the talus. The bone graft from the distal tibia can then be inserted and impacted through the transmalleolar approach. This is not recommended because of the morbidity associated with the large hole and the possible development of arthritic change. A preferred method is to insert a K-wire percutaneously near the sinus tarsi at the junction of the talar neck and body. Once the K-wire is verified to be in the posteromedial osteochondral defect, the hole is cored out and the bone

graft is inserted from the distal tibia and impacted with a plunger (Fig. 8-23).

Another alternative for bone grafting these lesions is to make a small window in the medial wall of the talus below the medial malleolus and to remove the cystic lesion using curved curettes. The bone graft can then be obtained from the distal tibia and inserted up into the cystic defect of the talus. This can usually be done only when the lesions are quite large and extend below the tip of the medial malleolus. Sometimes an arthroscopic approach to bone grafting is not feasible and an open approach should be used with bone grafting using tibial or iliac crest bone.

DISTRACTION DEVICES

The treatment of posterior osteochondral lesions almost always requires a distraction device, whether invasive or noninvasive. More anterior lesions may be approached successfully without distraction, de-

(*text continues on page 167*)

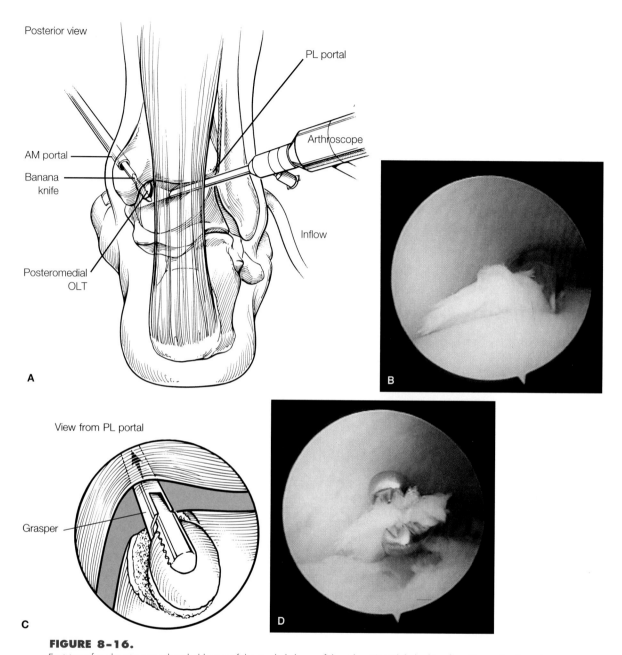

FIGURE 8-16.

Excision of a chronic osteochondral lesion of the medial dome of the talus. (**A**) While looking from the posterolateral portal, a banana knife is inserted through the anteromedial portal to excise the lesion. (**B**) While visualizing arthroscopically from the posterolateral portal, the banana knife is carefully brought into the joint and the blade is used to outline the extent of the lesion. (**C**) Once the lesion is loosened, it can be removed with a small-joint grasper. (**D**) A 2.7-mm grasper is very useful to remove the loose osteochondral lesion while visualizing arthroscopically from the posterolateral portal.

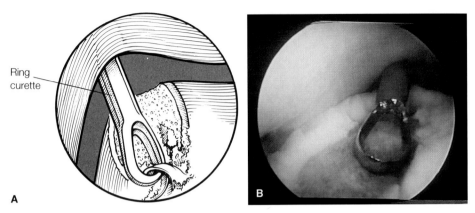

FIGURE 8-17.
Curettage of the osteochondral lesion base. (**A**) Use of a ring curette to remove any fibrous tissue from the underlying bony bed. (**B**) Arthroscopic view showing use of the curette intraarticularly.

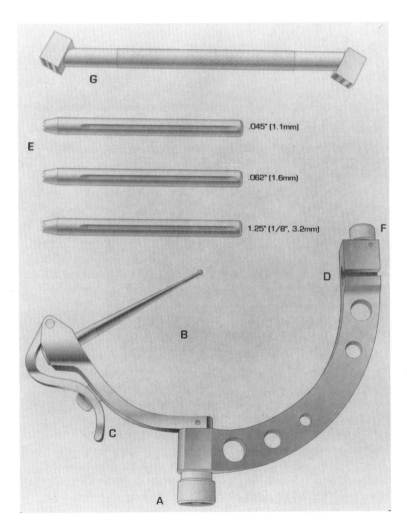

FIGURE 8-18.
The Micro Vector Drill Guide System has two articulating arms, ensuring that as the arm position changes, alignment between the distal ends remains constant. Different aspects of the drill guide are noted in letters A through G. The K-wire guides allow the use of different-sized K-wires. When multiple K-wire placement is indicated, the offset drill guide (G) allows a precisely patterned series of drill holes to be made.

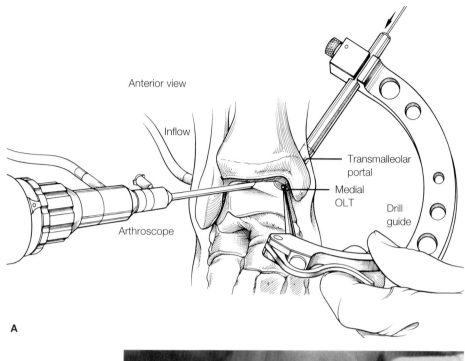

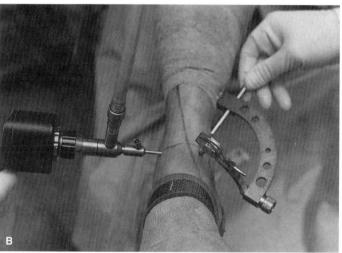

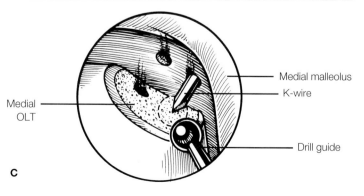

FIGURE 8-19.

Transmalleolar drilling with the arthroscope in the anterolateral portal. (**A**) If the lesion is anterior enough, it can be visualized through the anterolateral portal and the drilling commenced through the anteromedial portal. (**B**) Soft-tissue distraction device in place with the typical setup using small-joint instrumentation. (**C**) Once the K-wire is advanced through the distal tibia, the probe is retracted to allow the K-wire to pass into the talus.

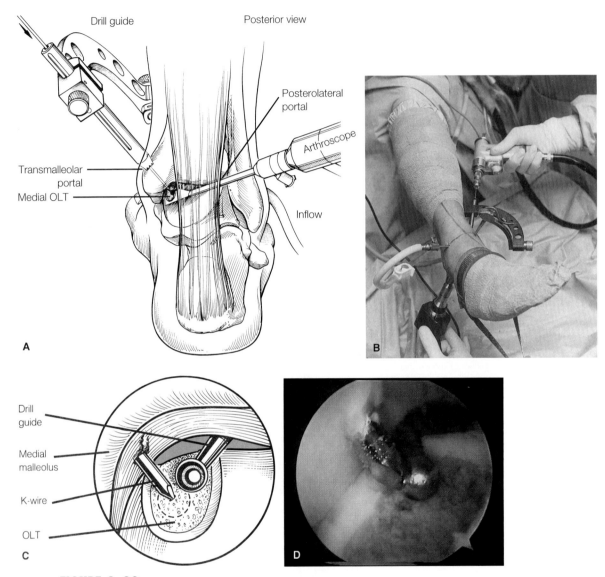

FIGURE 8-20.
Transmalleolar drilling with the arthroscope posterolaterally. (**A**) The arthroscope is positioned through the posterolateral portal and looks directly on the posteromedial osteochondral lesion. The drill probe is brought through the anteromedial portal. (**B**) Typical setup in the operating room with inflow through the anterolateral portal. (**C**) The probe is retracted as the K-wire enters the distal tibia before going into the talus. (**D**) The Micro Vector probe is retracted as the K-wire goes across the joint.

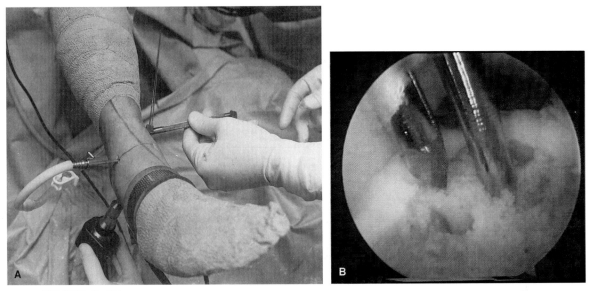

FIGURE 8-21.

Use of the offset drill guide. (**A**) The offset drill guide allows a parallel pin to be inserted next to a preexisting pin without reinserting the Micro Vector guide. (**B**) Note the position of the two pins using the offset guide and visualizing from the posterolateral portal.

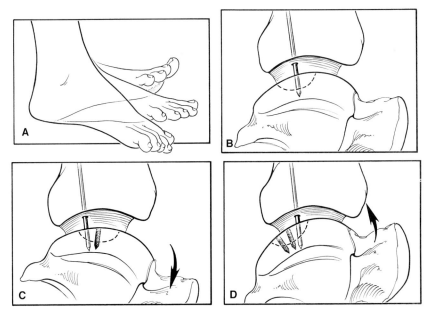

FIGURE 8-22.

(**A**) Flexion/extension of the ankle allows multiple drill holes to be made in the talus with limited holes through the tibia. (**B**) Initial drill hole made in talus. (**C**) Plantarflexion allows the same pin to drill a hole more posterolaterally in the talus. (**D**) Extreme dorsiflexion allows the same pin to drill a hole more anterolaterally into the talus.

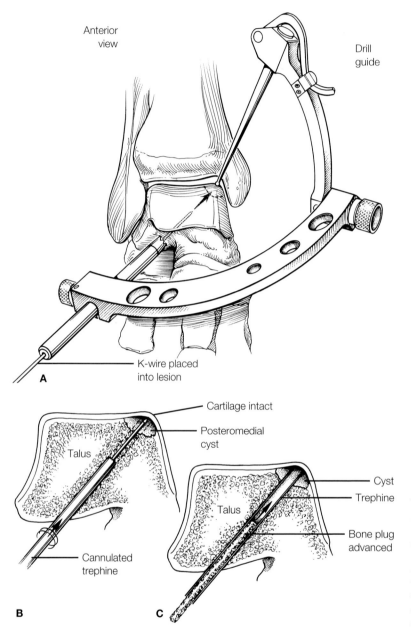

Anterior view

Drill guide

K-wire placed into lesion

A

Cartilage intact

Posteromedial cyst

Talus

Cannulated trephine

B

Cyst

Trephine

Talus

Bone plug advanced

C

FIGURE 8-23.

Transtalar drilling of an osteochondral lesion of the medial dome of the talus. (**A**) A K-wire is inserted using a drill guide by drilling from the sinus tarsi posteromedially. (**B**) A cannulated trephine is used to core out the bone from the lateral aspect of the talus into the area of the osteochondral defect. (**C**) Using a plunger, the bone plug is advanced into the area of the osteochondral lesion.

pending on the size and extent of the lesions. As previously mentioned, in children with open growth plates, distraction should be of a noninvasive nature; access usually is quite good because of ligamentous laxity. In adults, noninvasive distraction can be attempted, but if visualization is inadequate, invasive distraction should be done with a pin in the tibia and calcaneus as previously described.

POSTOPERATIVE CARE

If arthroscopic drilling has been performed, the tourniquet may be deflated (if used) and joint fluid flow turned off to allow visualization of the drilling sites and potential bleeding surfaces. Whether drilling or abrading using a burr, the subchondral surface of the lesion should demonstrate bleeding before wound closure (Fig. 8-24). The joint is then irrigated clear, the wounds are closed with 4-0 nylon suture, and a compression dressing is applied, as well as a posterior splint with the ankle at 90° to the tibia. The patient can usually be discharged home or is occasionally admitted to the hospital overnight, as needed. Postoperatively, the leg is elevated on a "leg elevator" and toe range of motion is encouraged immediately.

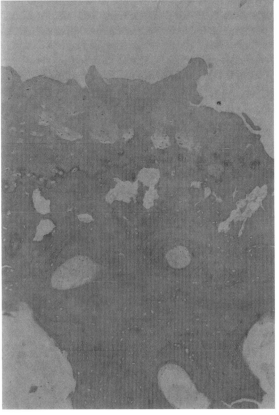

FIGURE 8-25.
Osteochondral fragment showing devitalized bone covered by degenerated articular cartilage. (Hematoxylin and eosin × 50.)

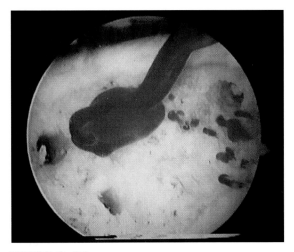

FIGURE 8-24.
After transmalleolar drilling of an osteochondral lesion of the posteromedial dome of the talus, a good bleeding bed is seen.

At 1 week, the stitches are removed and a removable posterior splint is made so the patient can initiate range of motion exercises at least three or four times a day while continuing non-weight bearing. Formal physiotherapy is usually started after the wounds are healed, with pool therapy and subsequent gentle range of motion exercises and dorsi- and plantarflexion. Inversion and eversion are restricted for about 6 weeks.

Debate exists as to the appropriate amount of time the patient should be non-weight-bearing. Some authors advocate weight bearing as early as 2 weeks; others wait 8 to 12 weeks. My patients are kept on non-weight-bearing status for 4 weeks if the lesion is less than 1.5 cm in diameter. If the lesion is more than 1.5 cm in diameter, non-weight bearing is prolonged for 8 weeks.

Rehabilitation is discussed in Chapter 14. Run-

TABLE 8-6.
Comparison of Arthrotomy Treatment Results

STUDY	CASES	F/U (MO)	AVERAGE AGE (YR)	TRAUMA (%)	GOOD RESULTS (%)
Berndt[5] (1959)	56	—	35	90	79
Muktherjee[37] (1973)	10	17	28	100	90
Alexander[9] (1980)	25	65	22	92	88
Naumetz[38] (1980)	31	—	24	84	63
Canale[10] (1980)	15	134	23	83	73
O'Farrell[26] (1982)	24	47	24	92	63
Flick & Gould[27] (1985)	19	24	28	91	79
Pettine[39] (1987)	30	90	12–66	85	33
Zinman[16] (1988)	28	62	14–60	21	82

ning activities are avoided for at least 3 months. Cutting and jumping-type sports are not permitted for about 4 to 6 months.

PATHOLOGIC APPEARANCE

When the histologic specimens are examined, they display segments of articular cartilage with fibrillation and cracks (degenerative change) as well as some new cartilage proliferation. Essentially, there is dead bone, and the overall appearance of the fragment is consistent with osteochondritis dissecans. The synovium often shows marked hypervas-

cularity in a superficial position, which is consistent with irritation from the injury (Fig. 8-25).

RESULTS

Open versus arthroscopic results are summarized in Tables 8-6 and 8-7. The arthroscopic results appear to be as good as or better than the open results reported.

Author's Results

To date, more than 100 patients have been treated arthroscopically for OLT.[15] This series is larger than any we have found reported. Sixty-six percent in-

TABLE 8-7.
COMPARISON OF ARTHROSCOPIC TREATMENT RESULTS

STUDY	CASES	F/U (MO)	AVERAGE AGE (YR)	TRAUMA (%)	GOOD RESULTS (%)
Baker[40] (1986)	10	12.5	29	100	90
Pritsch[21] (1986)	24	30	28	75	75
Parisien[41] (1986)	10	24	14–40	89	88
	8	6.5			
Van Buecken[42] (1989)	15	26	23	93	87
Frank[43] (1989)	9	10–24	24	66	89
Loomer[44]*	19	19	31	—	74
Ferkel & Sgaglione[15]† (1992)	59	40	30	83	83

* In this group, 51 patients were treated surgically, with 32 via arthrotomy and 19 arthroscopically.
† Currently, 104 patients have been treated arthroscopically for OLT, with 86 patients having greater than 2 years of follow-up. In this group, the results are similar to the previous group of 59 patients.

volved the medial dome, 27% involved the lateral dome of the talus, and 7% were central lesions. Overall results were 83% good to excellent, graded by three different methods. The two poor patients had CT scan stage 3 lesions that were drilled but not excised; subsequently, one of the patients had excision and further drilling with resolution of his symptoms. The lateral lesions that were acute were either excised and drilled or internally fixated. The medial lesions were either drilled or excision and drilling was performed. The average follow-up was 50 months. Outcome was not significantly affected by a delay in diagnosis.

CONCLUSION

Successful treatment of OLT requires a high index of suspicion for patients who have both acute and chronic sprain pain. These lesions can be missed in many patients with no history of trauma if they are not suspected. Newer techniques have evolved for OLT treatment, using ankle arthroscopy and a comprehensive approach to diagnosis, staging, debridement, and drilling of specific lesions of the talar dome. Such an approach can provide good to excellent results in many patients with either acute or chronic ankle pain secondary to these lesions. Imaging techniques such as CT and MRI are particularly helpful in the diagnosis and treatment of these lesions, although arthroscopic staging probably is the best way to determine treatment. When arthroscopic intervention is indicated, newer techniques provide results that are equal to or better than management by arthrotomy. The advantages of arthroscopy include minimal morbidity, shortened hospitalization, earlier range of motion and strengthening, and quicker overall rehabilitation time.

REFERENCES

1. Monro A. Microgeologie. Berlin: Th. Billroth, 1856:236.
2. Konnig F. Veber freie Korper in den Gelenken. Dtsch Z Chir 1888;27:90.
3. Barth A. Die Enstehung und das Wachsthum der Frein Gelenkkor per. Arch Klin Chir 1898;56:507.
4. Kappis M. Weitere Beitrage zu traumatisch—mechanischen Enstehung der "spontanen" Knorpelablosungen sogen. (Osteochondritis dissecans). Dtsch Z Chir 1922;171:13.
5. Berndt AL, Harty M. Transchondral fractures (osteochondritis dissecans) of the talus. J Bone Joint Surg 1959;41A:988.
6. O'Donoghue DH. Chondral and osteochondral fractures. J Trauma 1966;6:469.
7. Davidson AM, Steele HD, MacKenzie DA. A review of 21 cases of transchondral fracture of the talus. J Trauma 1967;7:378.
8. Campbell CJ, Ranawat CS. Osteochondritis dissecans: the question of etiology. J Trauma 1966;6:201.
9. Alexander AH, Lichtman OM. Surgical treatment of transchondral talar dome fractures (osteochondritis dissecans). J Bone Joint Surg 1980;62A:646.
10. Canale ST, Belding RH. Osteochondral lesions of the talus. J Bone Joint Surg 1980;62A:97.
11. Bosien WR, Staples OS, Russell SW. Residual disability following acute ankle sprains. J Bone Joint Surg 1955;36A:1237.
12. Thompson JP, Loomer RL. Osteochondral lesions of the talus in a sports medicine clinic. Am J Sports Med 1984;12:460.
13. Stauffer RN. Intraarticular ankle problems. In Evarts CM. Surgery of the musculoskeletal system, vol 3. New York: Churchill Livingstone, 1983.
14. Yao I, Weis E. Osteochondritis dissecans. Orth Rev 1985;14:190.
15. Ferkel RD, Sgaglione NA. Arthroscopic treatment of osteochondral lesions of the talus: long-term results. Orth Trans 1993–1994;17:1011.
16. Zinman C, Wolfson N, Reis ND. Osteochondritis dissecans of the dome of the talus. J Bone Joint Surg 1988;70A:1017.
17. Zinman C, Reis ND. Osteochondritis dissecans of the talus: use of the high-resolution computed tomography scanner. Acta Orthop Scand 1982;53:697.
18. Dipaola JD, Nelson DW, Colville MR. Characterizing osteochondral lesions by magnetic resonance imaging. Arthroscopy 1991;7:101.
19. Nelson DW, Dipaola J, Colville M, Schmidgall J. Osteochondritis dissecans of the talus and knee: prospective comparison of MR and arthroscopic classifications. J Comp Assist Tomography 1990;14:804.
20. Anderson IF, Crichton KJ, Grattan-Smith T, et al. Osteochondral fractures of the dome of the talus. J Bone Joint Surg 1989;71A:1143.
21. Pritsch M, Horoshouski H, Farine I. Arthroscopic treatment of osteochondral lesions of the talus. J Bone Joint Surg 1986;68A:862.
22. Cheng MS, Ferkel RD, Applegate GR. Osteochon-

dral lesions of the talus: a radiologic and surgical comparison. Presented at the Annual Meeting of the Academy of Orthopaedic Surgeons, New Orleans, February 1995.

23. Lindholm TS, Osterman K, Vankka E. Osteochondritis dissecans of the elbow, ankle, and hip. Clin Orthop 1980;148:245.

24. Blom JMH, Strijk SP. Lesions of the trochlea tali. Radiol Clin 1975;44:387.

25. Yvars MF. Osteochondral fractures of the dome of talus. Clin Orthop 1976;114:185.

26. O'Farrell TA, Costello BG. Osteochondritis dissecans of the talus—the latest results of surgical treatment. J Bone Joint Surg 1982;64B:494.

27. Flick AB, Gould N. Osteochondritis dissecans of the talus (transchondral fractures of the talus): review of the literature and new surgical approach for medial dome lesions. Foot Ankle 1985;5:165.

28. Loomer R, Fisher C, Lloyd-Smith R, et al. Osteochondral lesions of the talus. Am J Sports Med 1993;21:13.

29. Buckwalter JA, Cruess RL. Healing of the musculoskeletal tissues. In Rockwood CA Jr, Green DP, Bucholz RW, eds. Fractures in adults. Philadelphia: JB Lippincott, 1991:181.

30. Buckwalter JA, Mow VC. Cartilage repair in osteoarthritis. In Moskowitz RW, Howell DS, Goldberg VM, Mankin HJ, eds. Osteoarthritis: diagnosis and medical/surgical management. Philadelphia: WB Saunders, 1992:71.

31. Buckwalter JA, Rosenberg LC, Hunziker EB. Articular cartilage: composition, structure, response to injury, and methods of facilitating repair. In Ewing JW, ed. Articular cartilage and knee joint function: basic science and arthroscopy. New York: Raven Press, 1990:19.

32. Johnson LL. Arthroscopic abrasion arthroplasty, historical and pathologic perspective: present status. Arthroscopy 1986;2:54.

33. Johnson LL. The sclerotic lesion: pathology and the clinical response to arthroscopic abrasion arthroplasty. In Ewing JW, ed. Articular cartilage and knee joint function, basic science and arthroscopy. New York: Raven Press, 1990:319.

34. Shapiro E, Koide S, Glimcher MJ. Cell origin and differentiation in the repair of full-thickness defects of articular cartilage. J Bone Joint Surg 1993;75A:532.

35. Frenkel SR, Menche DS, Blair B, Watnik NF, Toolan BC, Pitman ML. A comparison of abrasion burr arthroplasty and subchondral drilling in the treatment of full-thickness cartilage lesions in the rabbit. Trans Orthop Res Soc 1994;19:483.

36. Mitchell N, Shepard N. The resurfacing of adult rabbit articular cartilage by multiple perforations through the subchondral bone. J Bone Joint Surg 1976;58A:230.

37. Muktherjee SK, Young AB. Dome fractures of the talus—a report of ten cases. J Bone Joint Surg 1973;55B:319.

38. Naumetz VA, Schweigel JF. Osteocartilaginous lesions of the talar dome. J Trauma 1980;20:924.

39. Pettine KA, Morrey BF. Osteochondral fractures of the talus, a long-term follow-up. J Bone Joint Surg 1987;69B:89.

40. Baker CL, Andrews JF, Ryan JB. Arthroscopic treatment of transchondral talar dome fractures. Arthroscopy 1986;2:82.

41. Parisien JS. Arthroscopic treatment of osteochondral lesions of the talus. Am J Sports Med 1986;14:211.

42. Van Buecken KP, Barrack MD, Alexander AH, Ertl J. Arthroscopic treatment of transchondral talar dome fractures. Am J Sports Med 1989;17:350.

43. Frank A, Cohen P, Beaufils P, Lamare J. Arthroscopic treatment of osteochondral lesions of the talar dome. Arthroscopy 1989;5:57.

44. Loomer RL. Personal communication, January 1995.

BIBLIOGRAPHY

Bruns J, Rosenbach B. Osteochondrosis dissecans of the talus: comparison of results of surgical treatment in adolescents and adults. Arch Orthop Trauma Surg 1992;112:23.

Dickson KF, Sartoris DJ. Injuries to the talus—neck fractures and osteochondral lesions. J Foot Surg 1991;30:310.

Shea MP, Manoli A. Osteochondral lesions of the talar dome. Foot Ankle 1993;14:48.

B. *Osteophytes, Loose Bodies, and Chondral Lesions of the Ankle*

James W. Stone
James F. Guhl
Richard D. Ferkel

This section will discuss the arthroscopic evaluation and treatment of other chondral and osteochondral lesions of the ankle.

Common indications for ankle arthroscopy have included osteochondral fragments or loose bodies, posttraumatic or degenerative arthritis, and persistent ankle pain or limitation of motion after trauma.[1-3] Several long-term follow-up studies are now available and help to place the role of arthroscopic treatment into perspective. Martin and associates found good or excellent results in 71% of ankles treated arthroscopically for transchondral defects of the talar dome, but only 12% good or excellent results in patients with degenerative joint disease.[4] In seven ankles with osteophytes or loose bodies, only 57% good or excellent results were obtained. The authors suggested that such ankles may have a greater degree of degenerative joint disease than anticipated preoperatively. In two papers, Ferkel and associates have suggested that arthroscopy is useful in treating osteophytes or early degenerative joint disease, in removal of loose bodies, and in debridement of osteochondral fragments.[5,6]

LOOSE BODIES

Etiology

Loose bodies may be either chondral or osteochondral and may arise from defects in the talus or tibia, osteophytes, or degenerative joint disease.[7] They may result from major trauma to the ankle joint, or from a relatively innocuous injury such as a lateral ligament sprain. In either case, an unsuspected chondral or osteochondral lesion may occur and result in a loose body floating within the joint (Figs. 8-26, 8-27).

Multiple loose cartilaginous or osteocartilaginous bodies may also form in synovial chondromatosis. This disorder is more common in the larger joints, but it can occur in the ankle. In this disorder, metaplastic mesenchymal cells in the joint capsule develop into chondroblasts, which produce small clusters of cartilage. These nodules of cartilage can protrude into the joint and break off to form small loose bodies. As the cartilage mass grows, the central portion may become necrotic and calcify. The loose bodies then become visible on routine radiographs (see Chap. 7).

Symptoms and Signs

A small loose body may cause catching symptoms with joint motion along with pain, swelling, and limitation of motion. Symptoms of internal derangement may resolve if a small loose body becomes fixed to the synovial lining, ceasing to cause joint irritation. A loose body may grow by proliferation of chondroblasts/osteoblasts, or may shrink due to the action of chondroclasts/osteoclasts.

The physical examination may not be very revealing, with vague areas of tenderness, possible limitation of motion, and catching. Rarely is a loose body palpable. As with all ankle problems, a careful physical examination must rule out extraarticular entities that can cause symptoms similar to intraarticular lesions. Peroneal tendon subluxation, posterior tibial tendon attrition or rupture, tarsal tunnel syndrome, sinus tarsi syndrome, stress fracture, and tendinitis must be carefully excluded by both physical examination and ancillary studies.

Diagnostic Evaluation

Plain radiographs usually reveal an osseous loose body, but chondral loose bodies are not visible on routine studies. The arthrogram, especially when combined with CT, usually reveals the loose bodies. Bone scans are rarely informative, although MRI holds promise for showing chondral lesions not seen on other types of studies. The plain radiographs, arthrogram, CT scan, or MRI scan should be scrutinized to discover the origin of the loose body, such as a defect of the talar dome, tibial plafond, or osteophyte.

Lesions that appear on routine radiographs to be loose bodies may actually be intraarticular, intracapsular, or extraarticular in location, particularly in the posterior ankle joint compartment. The location of the lesions should be determined preoperatively to avoid the embarrassment of performing an arthroscopic examination for loose body removal, only to find the joint free of any abnormality. An arthrogram, an arthrogram/CT scan, or an MRI study is best suited to make the distinction between an intraarticular versus an extraarticular or intracapsular abnormality.

Treatment

The arthroscopic approach to loose bodies is straightforward, but the procedure can be complicated by difficulties in the triangulation techniques

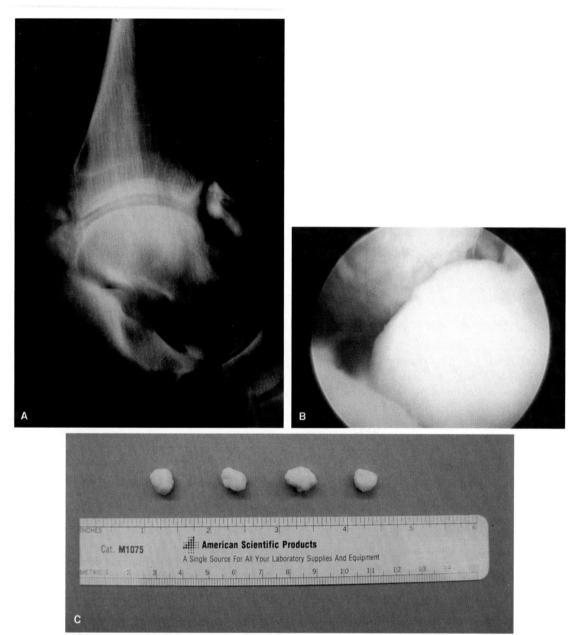

FIGURE 8–26.

(**A**) Lateral arthrotomogram shows loose bodies in the anterior and posterior recesses of the ankle joint. (**B**) Arthroscopic view of loose body in anterior ankle joint. Medial malleolus above, talus below. (**C**) Specimen: four large osteochondral loose bodies.

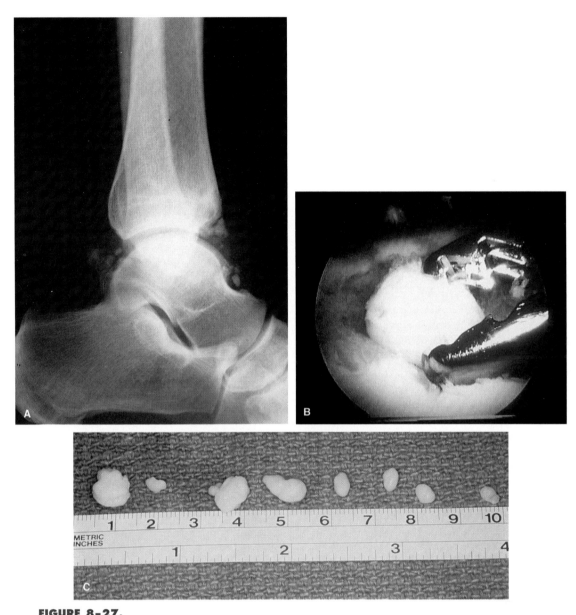

FIGURE 8-27.
(**A**) Lateral radiograph shows numerous loose bodies in the anterior and posterior recesses of the ankle joint. (**B**) Arthroscopic view shows removal of loose body with a grasper. (**C**) Specimen: eight osteochondral loose bodies removed from the ankle joint arthroscopically.

required to retrieve them. Loose bodies localized to the anterior compartment, particularly in patients with ligamentous laxity, can be approached with a routine setup using anteromedial and anterolateral portals. However, the posterior joint should also be examined for the presence of loose bodies, which

can hide in the posterior recess of the joint. Joint distraction is helpful to visualize this area. In the case of an ankle with tight ligamentous support, joint distraction may be mandatory[8] (see Chap. 5).

Loose bodies in the anterior joint can generally be retrieved from anterior portals. However, if there is instrument crowding, then the arthroscope can be placed in the posterolateral portal and the loose bodies removed using the anteromedial or anterolateral portal. Retrieval of loose bodies in the posterior aspect of the joint can be more problematic. Rarely, a carefully placed anterocentral portal may be used to triangulate into the posterior joint. This portal should be placed directly through the common toe extensor tendons. With the arthroscope placed in either of the anterior portals, removal may be best accomplished with the loose body forceps placed in the posterolateral portal.

After the loose bodies are retrieved, a careful evaluation of the joint surfaces should be performed to find their source. If a chondral or osteochondral defect is found, it should be debrided as described below. If an osteophyte is responsible for the loose body, it should be debrided with an arthroscopic burr, an osteotome, or a pituitary rongeur.

Postoperatively, a bulky compressive dressing with a posterior splint is applied. We use a cold-therapy cooling pad under the splint to minimize postoperative swelling and pain. The splint is removed 5 to 7 days postoperatively and exercises to regain range of motion are begun. The exercise regimen then advances to include strengthening and proprioceptive training.

The clinical results after loose body removal are quite good in patients who do not have associated abnormalities. When degenerative or posttraumatic arthritic changes or significant chondral defects are present, the results are less predictable.

OSTEOPHYTES

Etiology

Osteophytes may form as a consequence of degenerative joint disease of the ankle, or they may be associated with posttraumatic conditions. They are most commonly seen with a beak-like prominence of bone at the anterior lip of the tibia, usually associated with a corresponding area over the anterior neck of the talus. The talar abnormality may be a defect or an opposing osteophyte ("kissing lesion"). The lesions may form as a result of direct trauma following forced dorsiflexion injuries of the ankle, or they may form after forced plantarflexion trauma that causes capsular avulsion injury. Osteophytes causing anterior impingement are probably common after athletic trauma. O'Donoghue[9] reported a 45% incidence of osteophytes in football players, and Stoller[10] reported a 59.3% incidence in dancers. These osteophytes can impinge on each other, especially with ankle dorsiflexion, and may actually limit motion. The patient may complain of pain, catching, limitation of motion, and joint swelling.[11] Rarely, anterolateral exostoses between the talus and the lateral malleolus can occur and cause disability in the athlete.[12] Alternatively, osteophytes have been noted on the anterior aspect of the medial malleolus and may cause pain when they abut the talus. Posterior ankle joint osteophytes may also form and cause greatest symptoms with plantarflexion.

As with loose bodies, osteophytes may be intraarticular, intracapsular, or extraarticular in location. The preoperative workup should attempt to distinguish among these possibilities to guide the surgical procedure. In addition, the osteophytes should be carefully evaluated to determine their relative medial or lateral extent. Doing so preoperatively will avoid confusion at the time of surgery, when their exact location and extent may be difficult to determine.

Symptoms and Diagnostic Evaluation

Clinically, the patient may complain of anterior joint pain made worse with walking up stairs or hills, squatting, or running. Tenderness is localized over the bony prominence of the anterior ankle joint, and it may be made worse by passive ankle dorsiflexion. Ankle motion, particularly dorsiflexion, may be limited. Plain radiographs most often demonstrate anterior osteophytes, and a lateral stress radiograph taken in maximum dorsiflexion may demonstrate physical impingement of the two osteophytes. A bone scan shows significant increased radiotracer uptake in the area of the osteophytes in symptomatic lesions. The arthrogram, MRI, and bone scan are helpful mainly in ruling out other pathologic entities.

Surgery

Surgical resection of ankle osteophytes is reasonable in patients with pain well localized to a palpable bony prominence, limited range of motion docu-

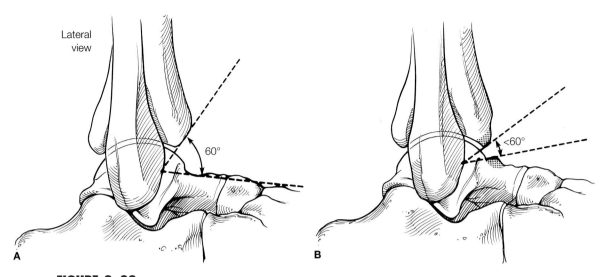

FIGURE 8-28.
(**A**) The normal angle between the distal tibia and the talar neck should be 60° or greater. (**B**) The presence of osteophytes on the distal tibia or talus can narrow the angle to less than 60°.

mented on radiographs, and mild coexisting degenerative changes in the rest of the joint. Preoperatively, the amount of bone resected can be judged by remembering that the normal angle formed by lines tangent to the talar neck and the anterior tibia should be about 60° or greater. Osteophytes in either location decrease this angle to less than 60°, and their removal should restore this angle (Fig. 8-28). Alternatively, a lateral x-ray of the normal, opposite ankle can be used to assist in determining the amount of bone to be resected. Visualization of the anterior ankle joint and particularly the inferior and superior confines of the osteophyte can be improved with mechanical distraction. However, sometimes distraction makes the anterior capsule more tense over the osteophyte. When this problem occurs, distraction should be decreased to allow the anterior capsule to relax and provide more working room anteriorly. It is critical to identify the anterior and superior borders of the osteophyte, and this often requires careful elevation or peeling off of the soft tissues from the confines of the osteophyte. The neurovascular structures *must not* be injured during this process (Fig. 8-29). Once the osteophyte's borders have been defined, it can be removed with a small burr, pituitary rongeur, or osteotome. The surgical instruments should be alternated between both the anteromedial and anterolateral portals to obtain a complete resection. Attention should then be directed to the anterior talar neck to ensure it is smooth. An intraoperative lateral x-ray is recommended before completion of the procedure to confirm that the osteophyte resection is complete and the normal angle between the talar neck and the anterior tibia has been reestablished (Fig. 8-30). Occasionally, visualization through the posterolateral portal is necessary to verify complete anterior osteophyte removal. The osteophytes are then resected with a motorized burr, osteotome, or rongeur placed in either the anterolateral or anteromedial portal (Fig. 8-31*A,B*). It may be helpful during the procedure to switch the arthroscope to the anterior portals to determine the extent of the osteophyte excision and to avoid removing excessive bone (see Fig. 8-31*C*). To use this posterior approach, mechanical distraction of the joint is necessary. In addition, damage to the articular surfaces due to arthroscopic instruments is minimized with the joint distracted mechanically. During the procedure, the joint must be fully explored to rule out coexisting intraarticular pathology, such as the presence of loose bodies or chondral injury. As the presence of osteophytes may induce a significant inflammatory synovial reaction, a partial synovectomy may be required in the initial phase of the arthroscopic procedure to gain visualization of the lesion. Rarely, an osteophyte may have to be resected by an open surgical procedure.

Postoperatively, patients are managed similar to those who have had loose bodies removed (see above). A splint to eliminate ankle motion reduces postoperative pain, allows healing of the arthroscopic portals, and discourages the formation of a synovial sinus. After 5 to 7 days of immobilization, the patient is encouraged to rehabilitate the ankle with active range of motion exercises. In general, patients whose symptoms are due to impinging osteophytes have significant pain relief after arthroscopic resection and often have increased ankle motion in dorsiflexion. The actual result in a given patient depends on the other ankle pathology coexisting with the osteophytes.

Martin and colleagues suggested that patients with isolated osteophytes were more amenable to arthroscopic debridement than were patients with generalized degenerative joint disease.[4] The former condition may represent a less severe or less advanced stage of the degenerative process. Hawkins reported on three athletes with anterior ankle osteophytes.[11] After arthroscopic osteophyte excision, each had symptomatic relief and could return to sports. One might hypothesize that these relatively young patients had osteophytes related primarily to athletic-induced trauma rather than a generalized degenerative process and, therefore, had a better prognosis for good results after simple excision of the osteophytes. Ogilvie-Harris and associates reported on 17 patients after arthroscopic resection for anterior bony impingement of the ankle.[13] At 39 months, significant improvements were seen in levels of pain, swelling, stiffness, limping, and activity, as well as improvement in dorsiflexion. Scranton and McDermott

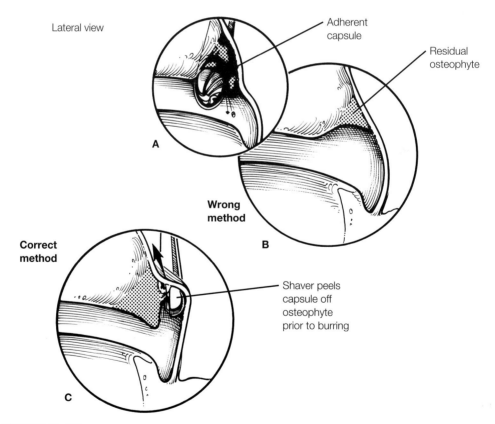

FIGURE 8-29.
Removal of osteophyte with burr. (**A**) Incorrect removal of osteophyte secondary to the adherent capsule to the distal tibia. (**B**) Residual anterior distal tibial osteophyte is present after burring because the anterior aspect of the spur is not visualized. (**C**) Correct method of removing an osteophyte using a shaver to peel the anterior capsule off the anterior border of the osteophyte.

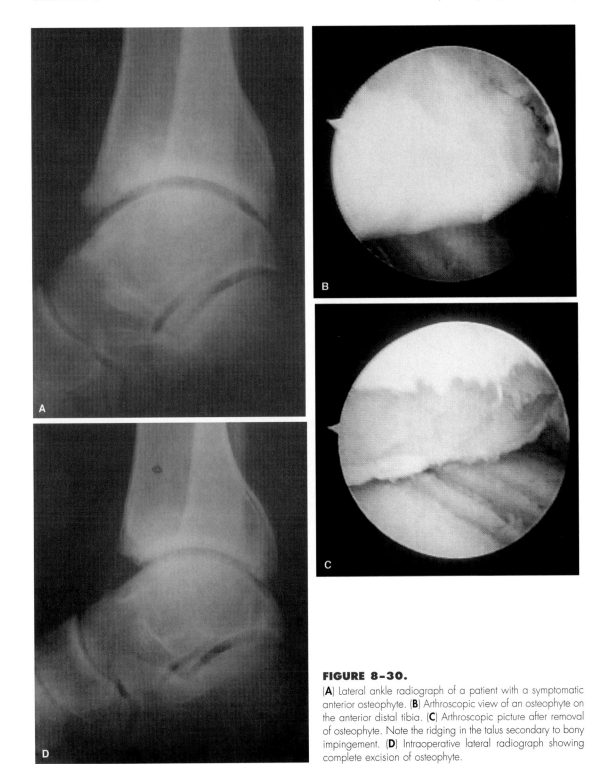

FIGURE 8-30.

(**A**) Lateral ankle radiograph of a patient with a symptomatic anterior osteophyte. (**B**) Arthroscopic view of an osteophyte on the anterior distal tibia. (**C**) Arthroscopic picture after removal of osteophyte. Note the ridging in the talus secondary to bony impingement. (**D**) Intraoperative lateral radiograph showing complete excision of osteophyte.

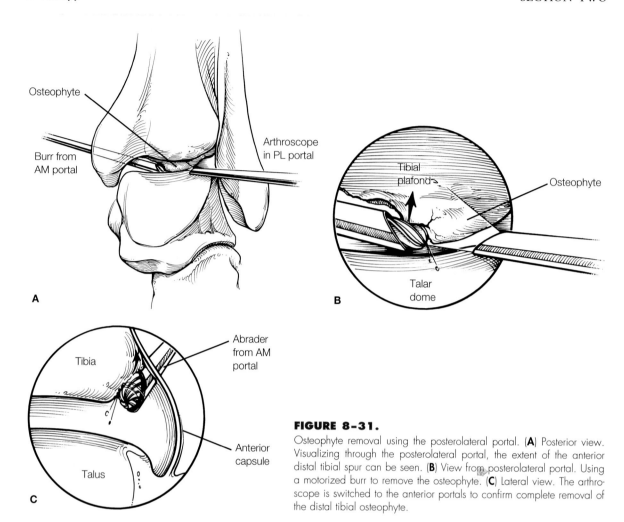

FIGURE 8-31.
Osteophyte removal using the posterolateral portal. (**A**) Posterior view. Visualizing through the posterolateral portal, the extent of the anterior distal tibial spur can be seen. (**B**) View from posterolateral portal. Using a motorized burr to remove the osteophyte. (**C**) Lateral view. The arthroscope is switched to the anterior portals to confirm complete removal of the distal tibial osteophyte.

compared open resection with arthroscopic resection of painful anterior impingement spurs.[14] They categorized ankle spurs from grades 1 through 4, according to the size of spurs and degree of involvement of the ankle, and showed that the treatment and recovery correlated with the grade (Fig. 8-32). Grades 1, 2, and 3 spurs could be resected arthroscopically or by arthrotomy. However, the patients who had arthroscopic resection recovered in about half the time of those managed with arthrotomy. Grade 4 spurs initially were not thought to be appropriate for arthroscopic resection. However, as experience has increased, grade 4 spurs can also be resected using great care and patience not to injure the surrounding neurovascular structures. St. Pierre

and associates reported on less common impingement exostoses of the talus and fibula, which were removed by an open technique.[12] These same lesions can also be approached arthroscopically with similarly good results expected.

CHONDRAL LESIONS

Etiology

Chondral injury to the articular surface of the talus or the tibia may occur after acute trauma, or with repetitive overuse injury to the joint (Fig. 8-33). The injury to the joint surface can range from softening of

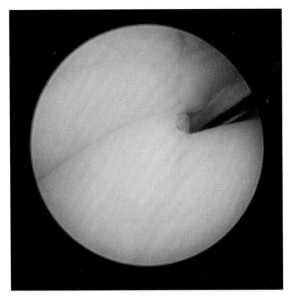

FIGURE 8-34.
Arthroscopic view of separated chondral fragment from talar dome.

to encourage vascular invasion and the formation of a fibrocartilage surface (Fig. 8-35).[15]

In the case of a posteromedial lesion, drilling may be performed using a transmalleolar approach, as previously described. An alternative approach that is rarely used is to insert a guide pin across the medial malleolus into the lesion. The accuracy of the guide pin's position is confirmed with anteroposterior and lateral fluoroscopic views. The placement of the guide pin can be facilitated with an arthroscopic anterior cruciate ligament reconstruction guide or a specially designed ankle guide, as described earlier. The guide pin is then overdrilled with a 4- or 5-mm cannulated drill, and multiple drill holes are placed into the lesion through this hole with a 0.062 Kirschner wire. Postoperatively, the ankle is immobilized for 5 to 7 days in a posterior splint. Active motion is then begun, but weight bearing is delayed for 6 weeks to optimize conditions for fibrocartilaginous overgrowth of the lesion. Ankle joint rehabilitation, as noted in previous sections, is then pursued.

CYSTS OF THE TALUS

Talar dome cysts are rare but can be found as isolated entities or in association with degenerative changes in the ankle joint. They are also seen in posttraumatic

conditions such as ankle sprains or fractures (Fig. 8-36). As isolated entities, they may be similar to intraarticular ganglion cysts. A patient who presents with ankle pain may be noted to have a talar cyst on radiographs, and have no other explanation for the ankle discomfort. Tomography, CT, MRI, or bone scanning may be useful to delineate the presence and extent of the lesion.

The cyst should be approached arthroscopically, and the position accuracy confirmed using intraoperative radiographs or an image intensifier. The cyst is debrided using a curette or abrader and then drilled. Small cysts may simply be drilled to encourage healing. In contrast, some large lesions may require an arthrotomy for adequate debridement, and possibly bone grafting. If a transmalleolar approach is used, the channel should be placed low on the malleolus so as to approach it from the side rather than from the weight-bearing surface.

TRAUMATIC AND DEGENERATIVE ARTHRITIS

The experience with arthroscopy in treating degenerative joint disease of the ankle has paralleled that of other joints. Initial hopes for long-lasting pain

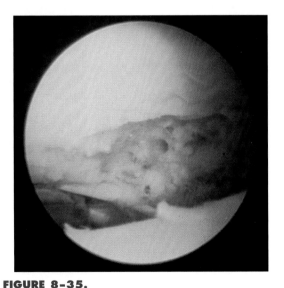

FIGURE 8-35.
Arthroscopic view after debridement and drilling of a chondral defect of the plafond. The patient had significant postoperative pain relief.

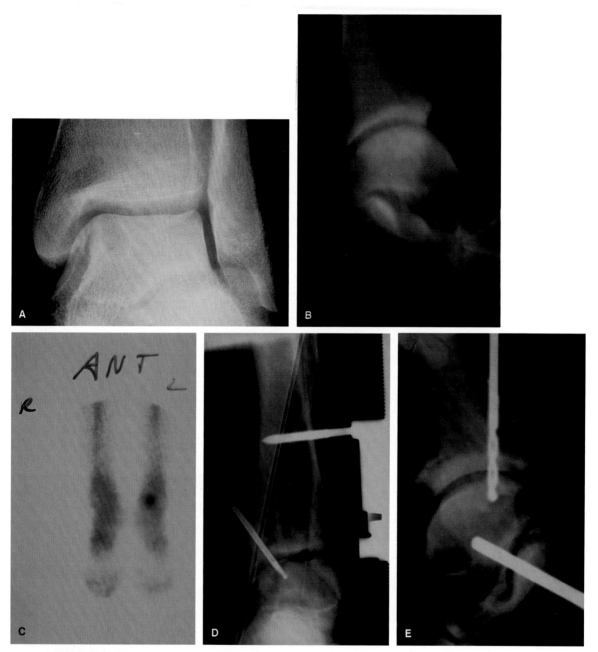

FIGURE 8-36.

Treatment of posttraumatic talar cyst. (**A**) Anteroposterior radiograph shows symptomatic posttraumatic cyst of talus. (**B**) Lateral tomogram of talar dome cyst. (**C**) Bone scan shows increased radiotracer uptake at the site of the cyst. (**D**) Intraoperative anteroposterior view shows small reamer entering the cyst through the transmalleolar approach. (**E**) A lateral view shows the transmalleolar drill within the cyst. It was further debrided with a burr and then drilled with fine wires. Complete clinical and radiographic healing occurred. The patient has remained asymptomatic for the past 3 years with recent follow-up.

relief have been tempered by the results of long-term studies that suggest little benefit in cases of generalized joint degeneration. Some pathologic entities associated with degenerative joint disease, however, may be treated arthroscopically.

In eight ankles treated by arthroscopic debridement, only one had a good or excellent result in a study by Martin and colleagues.[4] However, arthroscopy may still be indicated to evaluate the relative degree of degenerative changes suggested on radiographic studies.

Arthroscopic treatment of the arthritic ankle was initially considered effective. Experience with arthritic knees generated much initial enthusiasm and later disappointment. It became evident that with proper selection, some indications could be developed. Cases of arthritis of the ankle that should be excluded from arthroscopic intervention are those with advanced destruction, marked joint-line narrowing, extensive fibrosis, and significant instability or deformity. Patients presenting with ankles having some limited motion due to capsulitis; a minimal to moderate degree of fibroarthrosis, osteophytes, chondral defects, or loose bodies; or only minimal instability can be candidates for arthroscopic surgery. Also to be considered when contemplating arthroscopic treatment of degenerative arthritis of the ankle are the degree of disability, alternative forms of treatment, results of previous treatment, type of job demand, and expected result. Finally, a cooperative patient with a positive attitude and reasonable expectations should be considered a candidate for this type of surgery.

Some results may be very favorable, but in other patients improvement may be limited. Partial recovery may be much appreciated and may allow continued function and employment. The result may be further enhanced with the aid of anti-inflammatory medications, or other means to keep these patients comfortable. Overtreatment should be carefully avoided.

The radiographic picture of degenerative arthritis of the ankle does not always correlate with the symptoms. Some patients with advanced radiographic findings and longstanding involvement may be relatively asymptomatic.

The pathologic components of the arthritic ankle, as viewed from the arthroscopic standpoint, should be considered separately for treatment and the total picture assessed. Defects of the surface include chondromalacia, osteophytes, loose bodies, and chondral and osteochondral defects. Of additional consideration is extensive chronic synovitis, synovial impingement lesions (local or general), adhesions, fibroarthrosis, and in some cases capsulitis. Initial debridement with motorized equipment and lavage is required. The mechanical distraction method has further contributed to the treatment of capsulitis with limited motion; this is done along with manipulation and excision of osteophytes. In advanced cases, double-heavy skeletal distraction may be required. We have had two such patients, who did moderately well.

Finally, careful remodeling of the articular cartilage with small-joint instruments (rasps, burrs, arthroscopic osteotomes, baskets, and knives) is important. Areas of degenerative cartilage require more extensive debridement, abrasion, and drilling in some cases. The immediate postoperative use of ice packs and early motion, plus heat modalities later for rehabilitation, are suggested. Range of motion, strengthening, and stretching exercises in a progressive manner should be performed daily. Continuous passive motion for the ankle may be advisable for selected cases. Patients should be well selected and properly informed to achieve reasonable results. Limited arthroscopic abrasion arthroplasty may be efficacious in some patients; extensive abrasions are not recommended. With severe degenerative changes, joint arthrodesis should be performed either arthroscopically or by an open procedure, if necessary.

REFERENCES

1. Drez DJ. Symposium: arthroscopy of joints other than the knee. Contemp Orthop 1984;9:4.
2. Drez D Jr, Guhl JF, Gollenhon DL. Ankle arthroscopy: technique and indications. Clin Sports Med 1982;1:35.
3. Parisien JS, Shereff MJ. The role of arthroscopy in the diagnosis and treatment of disorders of the ankle. Foot Ankle 1981;2:3.
4. Martin DF, Baker CL, Curl WW, et al. Operative ankle arthroscopy, long-term follow-up. Am J Sports Med 1989;17:16.
5. Ferkel RD, Fischer SP. Progress in ankle arthroscopy. Clin Orthop 1989;240:210.
6. Strafford BS, Ferkel RD. Arthroscopic approach to the degenerative ankle (in press).

7. Milgram JW. The classification of loose bodies in human joints. Clin Orthop 1977;124:282.

8. Yates CK, Grana WA. A simple distraction technique for ankle arthroscopy. Arthroscopy 1988;4:103.

9. O'Donoghue DH. Chondral and osteochondral fractures. J Trauma 1966;6:469.

10. Stoller SM. A comparative study of the frequency of anterior impingement exostosis of the ankle in dancer and nondancer. Foot Ankle 1984;4:201.

11. Hawkins RB. Arthroscopic treatment of sports-related anterior osteophytes in the ankle. Foot Ankle 1988;9:87.

12. St. Pierre RK, Velazco A, Fleming LL. Impingement exostoses of the talus and fibula secondary to an inversion sprain—a case report. Foot Ankle 1983; 3:282.

13. Ogilvie-Harris DJ, Mahomed N, Demaziere A. Anterior impingement of the ankle treated by arthroscopic removal of bony spurs. J Bone Joint Surg 1993;75B:437.

14. Scranton PE, McDermott JE. Anterior tibiotalar spurs: a comparison of open versus arthroscopic debridement. Foot Ankle 1992;13:125.

15. Cheung HS, Cottrell WH, Stephenson K, Nimni ME. In vitro collagen biosynthesis in healing and normal rabbit articular cartilage. J Bone Joint Surg 1978;60A:1076.

Arthroscopic Surgery: The Foot and Ankle,
by Richard D. Ferkel.
Lippincott-Raven Publishers, Philadelphia © 1996.

9

Arthroscopic Treatment of Acute Ankle Fractures and Postfracture Defects

Richard D. Ferkel and John F. Orwin

Fractures of the ankle are relatively common and occur in all age groups. Evidence of healed ankle fractures has been found in the remains of ancient Egyptian mummies.[1] Hippocrates suggested that closed fractures be reduced by traction of the foot, but that open fractures should not be reduced or the patient would die from "inflammation and gangrene" within several days.[2,3] Unfortunately, until the mid–18th century there were few advances in the understanding and treatment of ankle injuries. Closed treatment of ankle fractures was recommended in the 18th and 19th centuries.[4–6] Subsequently, interest in operative treatment of ankle injuries arose, due to the unsatisfactory results of closed treatment of some fractures, as well as the evolution of x-rays, anesthesia, and surgical asepsis.[7] In 1894, Lane was the first to recommend surgical treatment to anatomically reduce fractures of the ankle.[8,9] In a series of articles in the 1950s, Lauge-Hansen developed a classification system based on clinical, radiographic, and experimental observations.[10–14] More recently, Weber developed a different classification system modified from Danis, which was based on the level of the fibular fracture.[15–18]

Although the long-term results of ankle fractures treated in either closed or open fashion have significantly improved over the last 50 years, problems still exist with postfracture stiffness, pain, swelling, and discomfort. In the past, the extent of the intraarticular injury had not been comprehensively studied because there was no method to look at the entire ankle joint. Even with extensive open reduction and internal fixation, not all areas of the intraarticular surface of the ankle are well seen. Recent excellent results with arthroscopic reduction and stabilization of tibial plateau fractures has stimulated the development of similar techniques in the ankle.

ACUTE ANKLE FRACTURES

Advantages of Arthroscopy

The advantages of arthroscopic evaluation and treatment of ankle fractures include minimal surgical trauma (compared with open techniques) and excellent visualization of the joint surfaces for assessment of intraarticular damage. Arthroscopy also permits evaluation of injured ligaments and removal of loose debris that may cause eventual articular damage. It is also helpful in facilitating open reduction and internal fixation in certain types of ankle fractures, and allows the surgeon to understand and correct the full extent of the damage that has occurred after such a significant injury.

Indications

Indications for arthroscopy of the ankle in the acute setting include all intra- and extraarticular ankle fractures where there is any likelihood of articular damage. In addition, arthroscopically assisted reduction and internal fixation can be accomplished in certain fractures with minimal to mild displacement, easily reducible by manipulation, where minimal to mild

ankle swelling has occurred and there is no neurovascular injury. Arthroscopy can also be used to treat syndesmosis disruptions, to evaluate posterior malleolar fixation of the tibial plafond, and to assist in the removal of debris and reduction of talus fractures.[19–21]

Contraindications

Ankle arthroscopy is contraindicated in an open fracture, with preexisting neurovascular injury, and with moderate to severe ankle swelling. However, fracture-dislocation is considered a relative contraindication, and ankle arthroscopy can be used for reduction in this situation in selected cases.

Arthroscopic Appearance

Arthroscopic evaluation and reduction of acute ankle fractures is best done immediately when feasible. After the ankle becomes more swollen, conservative treatment for any ankle fracture usually involves a bulky dressing and posterior splint with strict elevation before initiating surgery. This period of conservative care can last 7 to 14 days. Many different

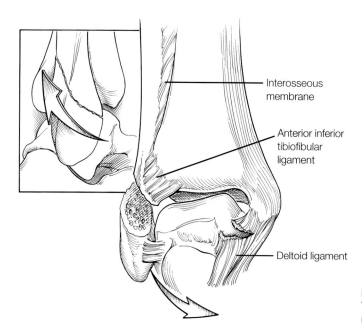

Interosseous membrane

Anterior inferior tibiofibular ligament

Deltoid ligament

FIGURE 9-1.
Weber type B fracture/subluxation of the right ankle (see Fig. 9-9).

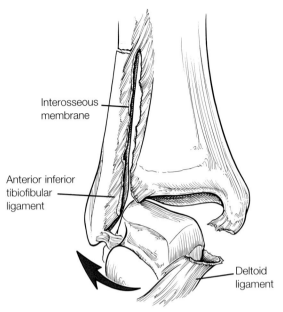

FIGURE 9-2.
Weber type C fracture/subluxation. Note the tear of the anterior inferior tibiofibular ligament, interosseous membrane, and deltoid ligament.

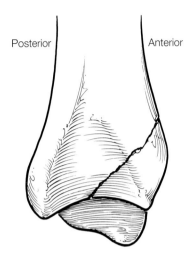

FIGURE 9-4.
Anterior tubercle fracture of the tibia.

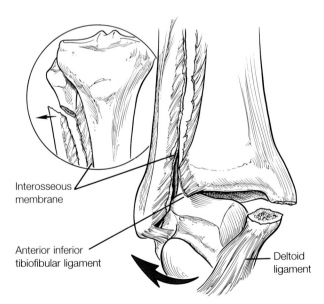

FIGURE 9-3.
Maisonneuve fracture with an associated medial malleolar fracture.

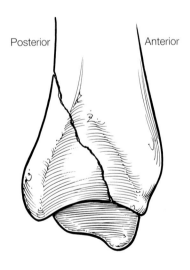

FIGURE 9-5.
Posterior tubercle fracture of the tibia.

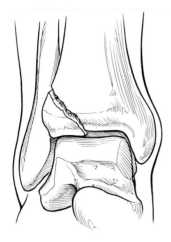

FIGURE 9-6.
Tillaux fracture of the anterolateral corner of the tibia.

fracture patterns are encountered; some of the more common patterns treated arthroscopically are illustrated in Figures 9-1 through 9-8.[22]

Treatment

After satisfactory anesthesia, the fracture can be assessed using a fluoroscope. This allows the surgeon to gain insight into how difficult the reduction will be once surgery is performed, and whether arthroscopically assisted reduction and internal fixation is feasible. Arthroscopy should be performed with caution in an acutely fractured ankle, and care must be taken to avoid excessive fluid extravasation, swelling, and potential compartment problems. In our experience, fluid extravasation has not caused a problem as long as good inflow and outflow are maintained.

In the acute fracture setting, an invasive distractor is not indicated; manual distraction or non-invasive devices can be used to permit adequate visualization and reduction. A small-joint probe should be inserted and the fracture lines identified and studied. The intraarticular shaver is inserted to remove hematoma, debris, and frayed cartilage and bone. Graspers are used as needed to remove loose fragments.

When the arthroscope is initially inserted, visualization is difficult because of the amount of frac-

ture debris, hematoma, and cartilage and bony fragments that exist. Once the joint is completely clean and all damage has been assessed, including capsular and ligamentous injury, a plan can be developed as to the best way to accomplish reduction and internal fixation. If a loose fragment is identified, it should be pinned back in place if a large enough piece of bone remains with the chondral fragment. This can usually be accomplished with absorbable pins, K-wires, or screws (see Chap. 8). If the osteochondral fragment is devoid of significant bone and has primarily cartilage, it should be removed and the bed from which it came should be curetted, debrided, and possibly drilled (Fig. 9-9).

If arthroscopic reduction and internal fixation can be done, K-wires are usually inserted. The fracture fragments are reduced either manually or with reduction forceps. Another method to obtain and maintain reduction is to skewer the fracture fragment with one or two K-wires and then to use these K-wires under arthroscopic visualization to reduce the fracture fragment. Once the fracture fragment is reduced, the K-wires can be advanced across the fracture site. Cannulated screws can then be inserted after checking for adequate reduction by arthroscopic and fluoroscopic means.

In some instances, both arthroscopic reduction and open reduction may be used on different portions of the ankle. It is important not to prolong the arthroscopic procedure so as to prevent excessive fluid extravasation and tourniquet time. A video re-

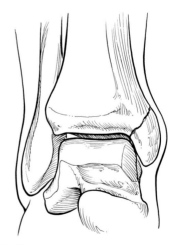

FIGURE 9-7.
Medial malleolar fracture.

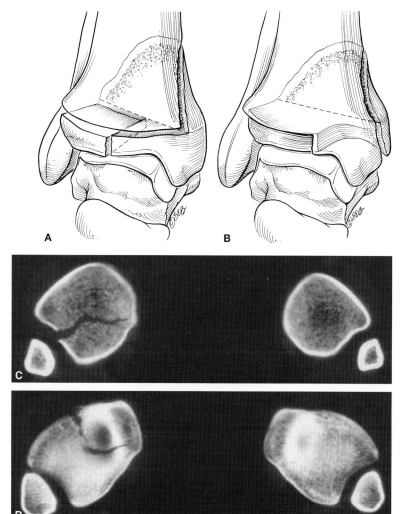

FIGURE 9-8.

Triplane fractures of the ankle. (**A**) Three-part triplane fracture. (**B**) Two-part triplane fracture. (**C**) Axial CT scan of a triplane fracture showing the fracture of the posterior distal tibia. (**D**) Axial CT scan of the same patient done more distally, showing the fracture through the anteromedial distal tibia. (**A** and **B** from Whipple TL, Martin DR, MacIntyre LF, Meyers JF. Arthroscopic treatment of triplane fractures of the ankle. Arthroscopy 1993;9:456.)

cord is always taken during the procedure to document the extent of the damage for the patient to review at the first postoperative visit and to facilitate analysis if the patient develops subsequent problems. Sometimes K-wire insertion can be performed more accurately with the use of a Micro Vector drill guide (Fig. 9-10).

If the fracture fragments cannot be reduced, then a standard open reduction and internal fixation of the fracture is undertaken. However, the arthroscope can still be used to confirm the anatomic reduction of the fracture fragments on the fibular, posterior malleolar and medial malleolar articular surfaces.

Stable internal fixation is always desirable to allow early postoperative mobilization. Postopera-

tively, most patients are immobilized in a bulky dressing and posterior splint, and gentle range of motion and strengthening exercises are started at 4 to 7 days postoperatively, depending on the stability of the fracture and the amount of soft-tissue damage.

Preferred Method

All intra- and extraarticular fractures should undergo arthroscopy, even if open reduction and internal fixation is planned, to look for loose bodies, osteochondral lesions, ligament damage, and other unsuspected injuries. The patient is brought to the operating room and placed on the operating table

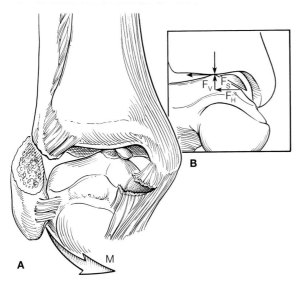

FIGURE 9-9.
Weber type B fracture/subluxation of the right ankle. (**A**) As the fracture occurs in the distal fibula, the talus tilts, tearing the deltoid ligament and producing an osteochondral lesion of the medial talar dome. (**B**) Inversion stress on the ankle joint creates a moment of force (M) that can be resolved along coordinate axes as a vertical (F_V) and a horizontal (F_H) force. The resultant of these two forces is a shear force (F_S), along which the osteochondral lesion occurs (see Fig. 8-3). (Stauffer RN. Intraarticular ankle problems. In Evarts C. Surgery of the Musculoskeletal System, vol. 3. New York: Churchill Livingstone, 1983.)

after the fluoroscopic attachment has been applied. Satisfactory general, epidural, or spinal anesthesia is then administered, and the foot is prepared and draped in the usual manner. All external landmarks are carefully palpated and marked, as well as the neurovascular structures. Generally, the tourniquet is not used unless excessive bleeding prohibits adequate visualization.

The anteromedial portal is established first. The anterolateral portal is then made, with care taken not to injure the superficial peroneal nerve. With inflow through the anterolateral portal, the posterolateral portal is then established using an 18-gauge spinal needle. The inflow is transferred to the posterolateral portal and the joint is lavaged thoroughly to remove all clots, fibrin, cartilage debris, and bone crumbs.

After adequate visualization is attained, a probe is inserted through the anterolateral portal while visualizing anteromedially, and the fracture fragments are palpated. If necessary, fragments can be

disimpacted with a Freer dissector by gently placing the edge of the Freer between the fracture lines. The arthroscope is transferred into the anterolateral portal to permit a different perspective of the fracture alignment. Visualization should also be done from the posterolateral portal.

Treatment of Specific Fractures

Fracture patterns vary greatly depending on the nature of the injury. Arthroscopic treatment of some of the more common fracture patterns is described below.

Medial Malleolar Fracture

Medial malleolar fractures can be evaluated arthroscopically to help assess the amount of intraarticular damage and to assist in fracture reduction (Fig. 9-11*A,B*). The fracture site can be debrided and curetted clear of hematoma arthroscopically and two K-wires inserted from the cannulated screw set percutaneously into the tip of the medial malleolus. These K-wires are then used to manipulate the fracture fragment into place while visualization is done arthroscopically to verify reduction (see Fig. 9-11*C,D*). Once adequate reduction has been verified arthroscopically, the pins are drilled across the fracture site. After fluoroscopy is used to confirm the appropriate position and reduction, two cannulated 4.0-mm cancellous screws are inserted (see Fig. 9-11*E*). If the reduction is stable and the patient is reliable, guided range of motion can be started with the use of a removable splint after the soft tissues have healed and the swelling has resolved. In Figure 9-11*F*, follow-up x-rays at 9 months postoperatively show excellent healing with anatomic reduction.

Fibular Fracture with Osteochondral Lesion of the Talus

Osteochondral lesions of the medial dome of the talus can occur in conjunction with fibular fractures, particularly with supination/external rotation injuries (see Figs. 9-9, 9-12*A*). After the patient is taken to the operating room, arthroscopy is initially performed before open reduction and internal fix-

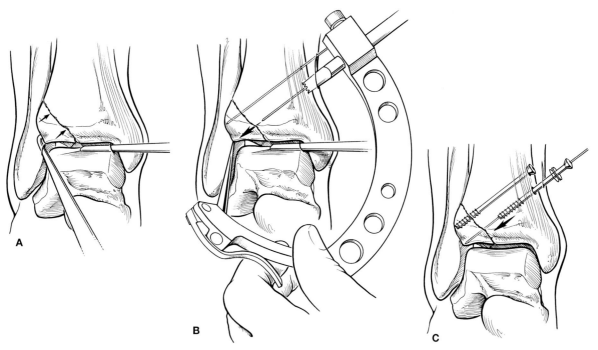

FIGURE 9–10.
Arthroscopic reduction and internal fixation of an anterolateral fracture of the tibia. (**A**) Reduction of fracture with probe or Freer with arthroscope inserted anteromedially. (**B**) Insertion of drill guide and passage of two K-wires to secure fixation of the fracture. (**C**) Insertion of two cannulated screws. Care must be taken not to violate the articular surface when screws are inserted from this direction.

ation. After removal of the fracture debris and hematoma, arthroscopic visualization can demonstrate an acute osteochondral or chondral fracture of the medial dome of the talus (see Fig. 9-12*B*). If the fragment is devoid of bone, it is removed and a gentle abrasion arthroplasty performed. Otherwise, an attempt can be made at internally fixating the fragment as previously described. Subsequently, an open reduction and internal fixation is performed after additional Betadine prepping and changing of gloves and instrumentation. In Figure 9-12*C*, at 11 months follow-up, the fracture is completely healed and the alignment is satisfactory.

Tillaux Fracture

This injury is a Salter-Harris type 3 fracture in which the lateral portion of the distal tibial physis is injured. The distal tibial physis initially closes in the middle and medial regions and subsequently in the lateral region, a factor predisposing to this type

of injury. It usually occurs in patients ages 12 to 14. The mechanism of injury is forced external rotation of the foot with the lateral physeal fragment pulled by the anterior tibiofibular ligament. Closed reduction is usually successful, but when more than 2 mm of displacement is present, surgical reduction is necessary (Fig. 9-13*A,B*). If the fracture is treated immediately, arthroscopic fixation is often possible. After removing the fracture debris arthroscopically, a Freer is used to reduce the fracture under direct vision (see Fig. 9-13*C*). Because the distal tibial epiphyseal plate is still open, a Micro Vector can be inserted through the posterolateral portal along the posteromedial corner of the tibia. A K-wire can then be drilled through the anterolateral portal into the fracture site while it is held reduced (see Fig. 9-13*D*). The drill guide is then removed and fluoroscopic reduction verifies appropriate position below the epiphyseal plate. A cannulated screw is then inserted while visualizing from the anteromedial portal with inflow from the postero-

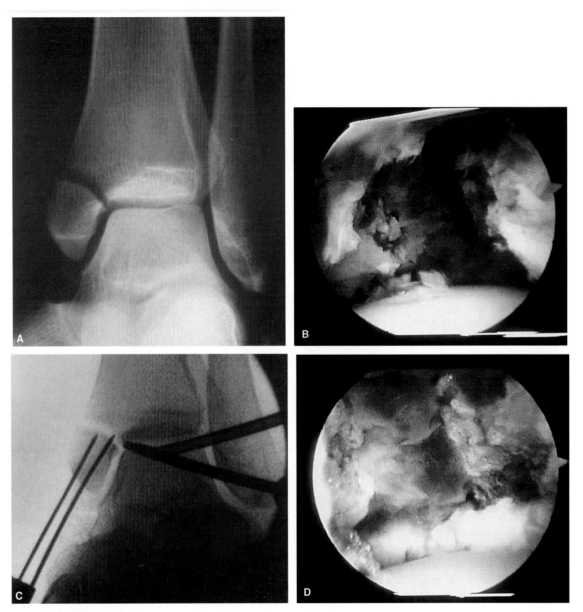

FIGURE 9-11.
Medial malleolar fracture. (**A**) Preoperative x-ray shows displaced medial malleolar fracture with malrotation. (**B**) Arthroscopic view of left medial malleolar fracture. There is a fragment missing from the anterior portion of the fracture that had to be removed. (**C**) Intraoperative fluoroscopic view of K-wire insertion used to reduce the fracture. (**D**) After the fracture is reduced, the K-wires are advanced proximally and the fracture reduction is assessed arthroscopically. (**E**) Fracture reduction verified with fluoroscopy. (**F**) Postoperative x-ray at 9 months showing healed medial malleolar fracture.

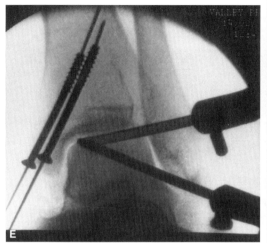 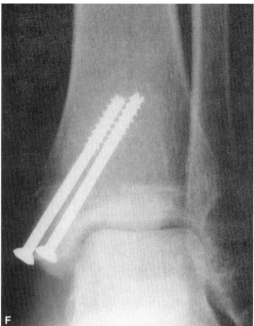

FIGURE 9–11. (Continued)

lateral portal. As the screw is tightened, the fracture will compress and anatomic alignment can be obtained (see Fig. 9-13E). In Fig. 9-13F, subsequent follow-up at 4 months postoperatively demonstrates anatomic healing.

Clinical Results

Our initial report consisted of 16 patients who underwent ankle arthroscopy and operative fixation in conjunction with an acute ankle fracture.[23] Our current study includes 33 patients (21 males, 12 females). The average age at the time of injury was 36 years (range 12 to 77 years). The mechanism of injury was a fall in 19 patients, sporting activity in 11 patients, and a motor-vehicle accident in 3 patients. The average time from injury to surgery was 6 days (range 2 to 17 days). A tourniquet was used in 30 of the 33 patients, with an average tourniquet time of 81 minutes. In the first 25 patients, distraction was performed manually as needed; on the last 8 patients distraction was done using a noninvasive strap when neces-

sary. The average follow-up was 38 months (range 24 to 100 months).

The operative lesions identified in this group were chondromalacia of the tibia and talus, osteochondral lesions of the tibia and talus, and loose bodies within the ankle joint. Chondromalacia was identified in seven ankles at surgery (21%). Three ankles had a lesion only on the tibia, while three had lesions only on the talus. One ankle had lesions on both articular surfaces. Osteochondral lesions were identified in 26 of 33 ankles (79%), with nine lesions found on the tibia, 16 on the talus, and one on the fibula. The osteochondral lesions of the talus included 13 medial and three lateral. Loose bodies were identified in 18 of 33 ankles (55%).

CHRONIC ANKLE FRACTURES

Numerous problems have been documented in patients with previous ankle fractures. These postfracture problems include chronic pain, swelling, catching, and stiffness. Conservative treatment is initially

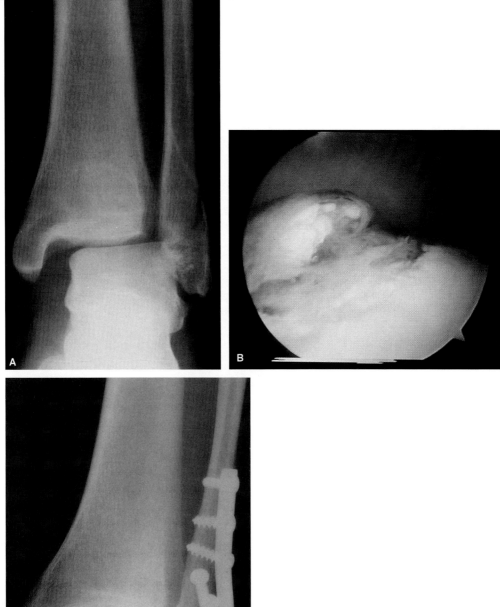

FIGURE 9-12.

Weber type B fracture/subluxation of the ankle. (**A**) Pre-operative x-ray of fracture with lateral talar shift. (**B**) Arthroscopic view demonstrating acute osteochondral fracture of the medial dome of the talus. (**C**) Postoperative x-ray at 11 months.

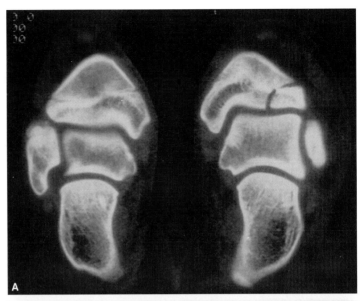

FIGURE 9-13.

Tillaux fracture. (**A**) Preoperative coronal CT scan showing fracture of the anterolateral corner of the distal tibia. (**B**) Axial CT scan demonstrating fracture with mild external rotation. (**C**) Arthroscopic view of Tillaux fracture. (**D**) Under direct vision, the fracture is reduced and stabilized with a K-wire. The guide pin is then inserted in the appropriate position next to the K-wire. (**E**) Arthroscopic insertion of a cannulated screw across the fracture site. (**F**) Postoperative x-ray at 9 months showing the fracture completely healed.

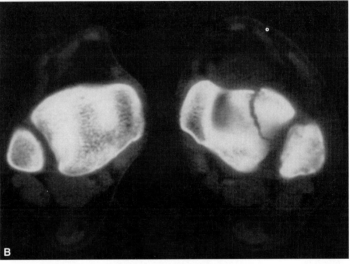

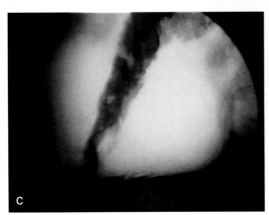

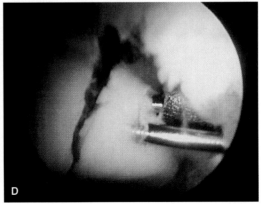

(*continues*)

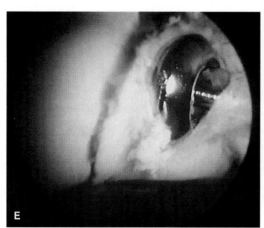

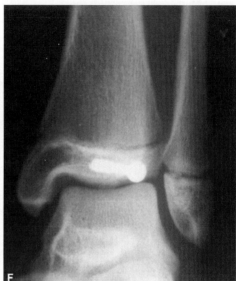

FIGURE 9-13. (Continued)

indicated for swelling reduction, range of motion and strengthening exercises, proprioceptive training, and occasionally orthotic management. However, for patients who fail conservative treatment, arthroscopic surgery is indicated. At surgery, debridement of chondromalacia, removal of osteophytes, excision of scar and synovitis, and removal of loose bodies can be done. If the articular cartilage is severely damaged, then arthrodesis may be considered.

Arthroscopic Treatment

The most difficult aspect of arthroscopic surgery in chronic ankle fracture patients is visualization. Often the ankle has abundant scar tissue and fibrosis and joint contracture, thereby restricting visualization and limiting range of motion and distraction. Sometimes the surgeon cannot be sure whether he or she is in the joint, and the only way to verify this is to place cannulae through the anteromedial and anterolateral portals and triangulate the tips posteriorly to ensure the cannulae are intraarticular. It is critical to verify that the arthroscopic instruments are intraarticular to prevent shaving the soft-tissue structures, including the neurovascular bundle. Once the joint space is well visualized, the appropriate arthroscopic

techniques can be used to further debride the joint, remove adhesions, excise fibrosis and osteophytes, and remove loose bodies.

The patient is taken to the operating room and an examination under anesthesia is done before initiating surgery to determine the amount of stiffness in the joint and the amount of contracture, if any, in the surrounding soft tissues. Anteromedial and anterolateral portals are then established. Care must be taken when entering the joint and triangulation techniques are used to confirm placement of the cannulae safely within the joint and not in the subcutaneous tissue. Adequate flow is always a problem with chronic ankle fractures because the ankle joint is small and contracted and numerous scar bands may inhibit the flow. A noninvasive distractor is applied; if adequate separation and visualization cannot be obtained, an invasive distraction device is then used. The posterolateral portal is established using a spinal needle and verified by inflowing from the anterolateral portal and seeing outflow through the needle.

Once adequate irrigation has been established, arthroscopic evaluation is performed anteriorly and posteriorly. Arthroscopic shavers, scissors, and baskets are used to debride the scar and to enlarge the visualization area until the entire joint is free of scar, fibrotic material, and synovitis. Care is taken to remove any loose bodies and to address any cartilaginous or osteochondral lesions identified (Fig. 9-14). Caution must be used at all times to avoid injury to the dorsal neurovascular structures.

Once the procedure is complete, the joint is irrigated clear and the arthroscopic portals are closed with one 4-0 nylon suture. A soft compression dressing with a plaster splint is applied. When possible, early range of motion is started 1 week postoperatively, with weight bearing as tolerated. Physiotherapy is initiated as soon as swelling and discomfort are diminished, starting with pool therapy and progressing to land therapy.

Preferred Method

The patient is taken to the operating room and placed in the supine position, and satisfactory general or regional anesthesia is administered. The thigh is secured on the thigh holder and the ankle is prepared and draped in the usual manner. All areas are carefully marked with a marking pen, including neurovascular structures and bony landmarks. The standard anteromedial, anterolateral, and posterolateral portals are established in the usual manner. As stated above, sometimes additional patience is necessary to

establish all the portals. Visualization is usually started through the anteromedial portal and the shaver is inserted anterolaterally. Because visualization is initially difficult, the shaver should be kept in one quadrant of the ankle, cutting a hole in the scar until the anatomy is completely visualized—this is usually on the anterolateral corner of the ankle and the lateral gutter. After adequate visualization is obtained in this area, the middle quadrant and then the anteromedial quadrant of the ankle are debrided of all scar tissue, adhesions, and fibrous material.

Arthrofibrosis

Patients with arthrofibrosis after traumatic injuries pose a difficult problem arthroscopically (Fig. 9-15*A*). At arthroscopy, significant scarring and fibrosis are seen and initial visualization is very difficult (see Fig. 9-15*B*). Large and smaller shavers, suction baskets, and burrs are used to perform extensive debridement and removal of associated osteophytes, fibrosis, and synovitis (see Fig. 9-15*C*). Postoperatively, the patient is immobilized in a posterior splint for a minimal period to allow the soft tissues to heal; then

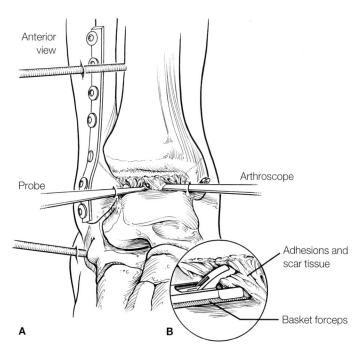

FIGURE 9-14.
Arthrofibrosis of the ankle. (**A**) Debridement of scar tissue, chondromalacia, and loose bodies in an ankle with a healed fibular fracture. The arthroscope is anteromedial and the instruments are anterolateral with invasive distraction in place. (**B**) Excision of thick bands with basket forceps.

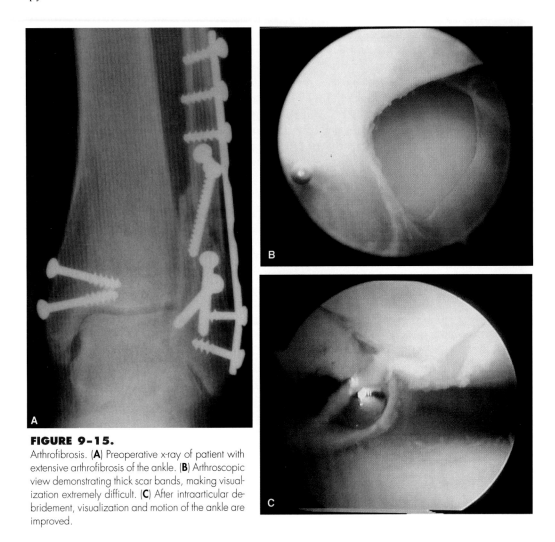

FIGURE 9–15.
Arthrofibrosis. (**A**) Preoperative x-ray of patient with extensive arthrofibrosis of the ankle. (**B**) Arthroscopic view demonstrating thick scar bands, making visualization extremely difficult. (**C**) After intraarticular debridement, visualization and motion of the ankle are improved.

range of motion and strengthening exercises are started.

Results

Initially, 12 patients who presented with postfracture problems subsequently underwent arthroscopic evaluation of the ankle.[23] The present study includes 25 patients (14 males, 11 females). The mechanism of injury was a fall in 13 patients, a motor-vehicle accident in 6, and a sporting accident in 6. There were 23 closed fractures and two open fractures. Eighty-four percent of the patients had open reduction and internal fixation of their fractures; the other 16%

were treated with casting. The time from the initial injury until subsequent arthroscopic debridement averaged 35 months (range 3 to 240 months). A tourniquet was used in all but 2 patients, with an average tourniquet time of 68 minutes. The invasive ankle distractor was used in 8 of the 25 patients, noninvasive distraction in the rest. The indication for surgery in all patients was chronic ankle pain, with 8 of the 25 patients also complaining of loss of motion in the affected ankle. Follow-up averaged 36 months (range 24 to 100 months).

All 25 ankles were found to have significant scar-like adhesions, which were debrided at surgery. Chondromalacia of the tibia or talus was identified in 20 of the 25 ankles. Three ankles had large osteochondral lesions of the talus, and three ankles had a loose body.

The average arc of tibial-talar motion was 35° preoperatively, with an average dorsiflexion of 8° and an average plantarflexion of 27°. At follow-up, the tibial-talar arc of motion was increased by an average of 15° to 50°. There was an average increase in dorsiflexion of 4° and an average increase in plantarflexion of 11°. Five patients regained ankle motion equivalent to that of the nonoperative side.

Only 1 patient developed loss of motion in follow-up. This patient had sustained a bimalleolar fracture initially treated with open reduction and internal fixation. At arthroscopy, this patient was found to have a large osteochondral lesion of the talus as well as advanced fibrous scar within the ankle joint. This patient underwent scar debridement and abrasion of the articular lesion but continued to have pain and limited motion. At 8 months follow-up, the patient subsequently underwent tibial-talar arthrodesis, which successfully relieved the pain.

Of the 2 patients who initially sustained open fractures, one patient had improved motion at follow-up, and her procedure was considered to be successful because she also obtained significant pain relief. The other patient thought that his surgery was successful because he obtained adequate pain relief from the surgery. This patient's postoperative motion was not well documented.

Overall, 19 of 25 patients were considered to have excellent or good results, with a decrease in ankle pain and an increase in activity. Two patients had only fair results, and 4 had poor results.[24] Of these 4, 1 used an AFO-type brace, 1 patient had a subsequent tibial-talar fusion for pain relief, and 2 had no pain relief and redeveloped arthrofibrosis of the ankle joint, necessitating a second debridement arthroscopically.

There were no infections or neurovascular injuries in this series. No patient developed reflex sympathetic dystrophy. There were no refractures, and only 1 patient developed persistent swelling postoperatively.

SUMMARY AND CONCLUSIONS

Ankle arthroscopy has become a valuable procedure in the diagnosis and treatment of various disorders of the ankle. Until recently, its use in acute ankle fractures or chronic ankle fractures with postfracture defects has been uncommon. In the acutely fractured ankle, arthroscopy enables the surgeon to examine the articular surface of the tibia and talus carefully, and aids in the reduction and internal fixation of the fracture fragments. Arthroscopy also helps identify different types of pathology within the ankle, such as cartilaginous lesions, osteochondral defects, and loose bodies. It is unclear whether addressing these issues in this setting will affect the outcome or treatment of these fractures. It is quite possible, however, that these lesions do contribute to the overall morbidity associated with the treatment of ankle fractures. Although not proved, we suspect that after lavage and debridement of an acute ankle fracture, the postoperative range of motion improves more quickly.

In the chronic fracture with postfracture defects, arthroscopy is helpful to remove scar and adhesions, to debride chondromalacia and osteochondral lesions, and to remove loose bodies. However, numerous factors affect the results of arthroscopic surgery in this group, including the age of the injury, the amount of articular cartilage damage and arthritic changes, and the degree of arthrofibrosis and joint contracture. The primary indication for surgery in the chronic fracture patient is pain and loss of motion. Loss of motion is usually more of a problem in dorsiflexion than in plantarflexion. Motion can be improved by debridement, as documented by our studies. Dorsiflexion is improved about 4°, plantarflexion about 13°. From following these patients over a long period, it is apparent that an improvement of only a few degrees from their preoperative setting is necessary to allow them to walk and perform activities more comfortably. Overall, patient satisfaction is high, with minimal risk and good pain relief.

In the future, as more acute fractures are arthroscopically evaluated, perhaps fewer chronic postfracture problems will develop in the ankle.

REFERENCES

1. Elliot S, Wood J. The archaeological survey of the Nubia report, 1907–1908, vol 2. Cairo, 1910.
2. Hippocrates; Adams F (trans). The genuine works of Hippocrates. London: C and J Adlard, 1849.

3. VanderGriend RA, Savoie FH, Hughes JL. Fractures of the ankle. In Rockwood CA Jr., Green DP, Bucholz RW, eds. Fractures in adults, 3rd ed. Philadelphia: JB Lippincott, 1991.

4. Cooper AP. On dislocation of the ankle joints. In A treatise on dislocations and on fractures of the joints. London: E Cox and Son, 1822.

5. Maisonneuve JG. Recherches sur la fracture du perone. Archives of General Medicine 1840;165:433.

6. von Volkman R. Beitrage zur Chirurgie. Leipzig: Breitkopf and Hartel, 1875.

7. Hughes SPF. A historical review of fractures involving the ankle joint. Mayo Clin Proc 1975;50:611.

8. Lane WA. The operative treatment of fractures. London: Medical Publishing Co, 1910.

9. Lane WA. The operative treatment of simple fractures. London: Medical Publishing Co, 1914.

10. Lauge-Hansen N. "Ligamentous" ankle fractures: diagnosis and treatment. Acta Chir Scand 1949;97:544.

11. Lauge-Hansen N. Fractures of the ankle. II. Combined experimental-surgical and experimentalroentgenologic investigations. Arch Surg 1950;60:957.

12. Lauge-Hansen N. Fractures of the ankle. IV. Clinical use of genetic roentgen diagnosis and genetic reduction. Arch Surg 1952;64:488.

13. Lauge-Hansen N. Fractures of the ankle. V. Pronation-dorsiflexion fracture. Arch Surg 1953;67:813.

14. Lauge-Hansen N. Fractures of the ankle. III. Genetic roentgenologic diagnosis of fractures of the ankle. AJR 1954;71:456.

15. Danis R. Theorie et pratique de l'osto-synthese. Paris: Masson & Cie, 1947.

16. Weber BG. Die Verletzungen des oberen Sprunggelenkes, Aktuelle Probleme in der Chirurgie, 1st ed. Bern: Verlag Hans Huber, 1966.

17. Weber BG. Die Verletzungen des oberen Sprunggelenkes, Aktuelle Probleme in der Chirurgie, 2d ed. Bern: Verlag Hans Huber, 1972.

18. Lindsjo U. Classification of ankle fractures: the Lauge-Hansen or AO system? Clin Orthop 1985;199:12.

19. Ogilvie-Harris DJ, Reed SC. Disruption of the ankle syndesmosis: diagnosis and treatment by arthroscopic surgery. Arthroscopy 1994;10:561.

20. Holt ES. Arthroscopic visualization of the tibial plafond during posterior malleolar fracture fixation. Foot Ankle 1994;15:206.

21. Saltzman CL, Marsh JL, Tearse DS. Treatment of displaced talus fractures: an arthroscopically assisted approach. Foot Ankle 1994;15:630.

22. Whipple TL, Martin DR, McIntyre LF, Meyers JF. Arthroscopic treatment of triplane fractures of the ankle. Arthroscopy 1993;9:456.

23. Ferkel RD, Orwin JF. Ankle arthroscopy: a new tool for treating acute and chronic ankle fractures. Arthroscopy 1993;9:352.

24. Phillips WA, Spiegel PG. Evaluation of ankle fractures: nonoperative vs. operative. Clin Orthop 1979;138:17.

BIBLIOGRAPHY

Guhl JF, Ferkel RD, Stone JW. Other osteochondral pathology—fractures and fracture defects. In Guhl JF, ed. Foot and ankle arthroscopy, 2d ed. Thorofare, NJ: Slack, 1993.

Ogilvie-Harris DJ, Reed SC. Disruption of the ankle syndesmosis: biomechanical study of the ligamentous restraints. Arthroscopy 1994;10:558.

Arthroscopic Surgery: The Foot and Ankle,
by Richard D. Ferkel.
Lippincott-Raven Publishers, Philadelphia © 1996.

10

Arthroscopic Approach to Lateral Ankle Instability

Richard B. Hawkins and Richard D. Ferkel

*L*ateral ankle sprains caused by forced inversion are the most common of all ankle injuries, and one of the injuries most frequently seen by orthopedists.[1] Usually these inversion injuries heal uneventfully with appropriate conservative treatment of rest, ice, anti-inflammatory medication, and physiotherapy. However, repeated ankle sprains may lead to chronic ankle instability that cannot be controlled by conservative methods. Once a person suffers repeated lateral sprains, the progression in severity may lead to increased laxity, pain, and swelling that eventually interferes with normal daily activities[1,2] (Fig. 10-1). With chronic instability, minor provocations can lead to a significant inversion injury and ultimately an unpredictable convalescence and chronic pain secondary to repeated chondral and osteochondral injuries.[1,3]

When conservative treatment of lateral ankle sprains fails and chronic recurrent instability persists, the method of treatment changes and surgical repair is necessary to stabilize the ankle. In recent years, as equipment has improved and experience has increased, indications for ankle arthroscopy have broadened.

HISTORY

One of the earliest reports on reconstruction of lateral ankle ligaments for chronic lateral instability was that of Nilsonne in 1949.[4] He described transposing the tendon of the peroneus brevis muscle into a subperiosteal groove behind the lateral malleolus. Peroneus brevis tendon transfers of various types were developed by Elmslie, Watson-Jones, and Evans; later, numerous modifications of these classic repair procedures were presented by other authors.

In contrast, Brostrom in 1966 studied a large group of patients with ankle ligament injuries and concluded that direct suture could be accomplished, even years after an initial injury.[5] If ligaments have been elongated or are difficult to distinguish from scar tissue, then imbrication could be

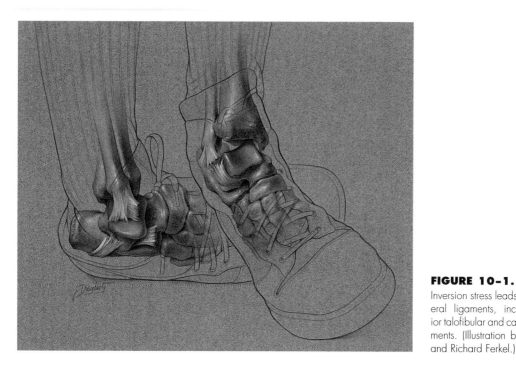

FIGURE 10-1.

Inversion stress leads to tears of the lateral ligaments, including the anterior talofibular and calcaneofibular ligaments. (Illustration by John Daugherty and Richard Ferkel.)

used to allow direct suture into bone. The direct repair concept has appealed to many surgeons in recent years as it avoids disturbing and rerouting healthy adjacent structures such as the peroneal tendons. In 1993 Hamilton and colleagues reported their results with the modified Brostrom procedure in 27 patients: overall, the results were 93% good or excellent.[6]

With the advent of arthroscopic techniques, such direct repair procedures with imbrication and tightening of lateral ligament structures are feasible.

BIOMECHANICS

Strain gauge analysis of normal ankle ligaments and biomechanical testing indicate that the anterior talofibular ligament is a primary restraint to anterior translocation, internal rotation, and inversion of the talus at all angles tested. Cadaver stress tests have shown that the anterior talofibular ligament always fails before the calcaneofibular ligament. Studies by Brostrom showed that rupture of the calcaneofibular ligament is rare in chronic lateral instability.[5]

The ideal ligament reconstruction would recreate the anterior talofibular ligament in an anatomic fashion without restricting subtalar motion.[7] Procedures that restrict subtalar motion are thought to be less desirable than those that correct the laxity of the anterior talofibular ligament per se.

ANATOMY

A detailed description of the ligaments of the ankle was presented in Chapter 5. The tibiofibular syndesmosis includes the anterior and posterior inferior tibiofibular ligaments, the transverse tibiofibular ligament, and the interosseous membrane. The anterior portion is injured after an inversion ankle sprain more often than is commonly appreciated, but instability at this syndesmosis is rare. Damage to the posterior syndesmotic ligament is less common after a soft-tissue injury (Figs. 10-2, 10-3).

The lateral ligaments of the ankle most commonly damaged after a soft-tissue injury to the ankle include the anterior talofibular, calcaneofibular, and posterior talofibular ligaments (see Figs. 10-2, 10-3). The anterior talofibular ligament arises from the anterior border of the lateral malleolus and passes

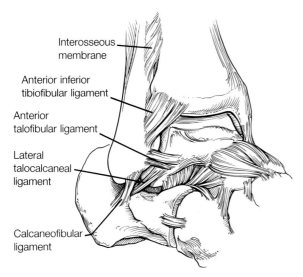

FIGURE 10-2.
Anterolateral view of the ligaments of the ankle.

arises from the posterior aspect of the lateral malleolus and runs almost horizontally to insert on the posterior talus. This ligament is the strongest and most deeply seated of the lateral ligaments, and the least commonly injured.

CLINICAL PRESENTATION

The major complaint of patients with chronic instability of the ankle is pain and swelling after each episode of injury. The second most frequent complaint is giving way or a sense of instability. The problem of not being able to predict when the ankle will "give out" adds a sense of insecurity and inability to rely on the ankle. Other complaints include weakness, stiffness, tenderness, a sense of looseness, sensitivity to damp or cold weather, and giving way unexpectedly.

Physical examination reveals a wide variety of signs with related symptoms. Most frequently, there is a positive anterior drawer test caused by rupture or laxity of the anterior talofibular ligament. By grasping the patient's heel, the examiner can slide the entire foot forward at the tibiotalar joint while using the opposite hand to anchor the leg (Fig. 10-4). The examiner may also elicit tenderness over

obliquely forward and somewhat medially to insert on the talus just anterior to the lateral articular facet. The calcaneofibular ligament is a strong, large ligament that originates from the lower segment of the anterior border of the lateral malleolus and courses inferiorly and slightly posterior to its insertion on the calcaneus. The posterior talofibular ligament

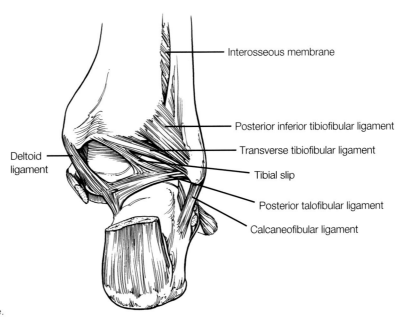

FIGURE 10-3.
Posterior view of the ligaments of the ankle.

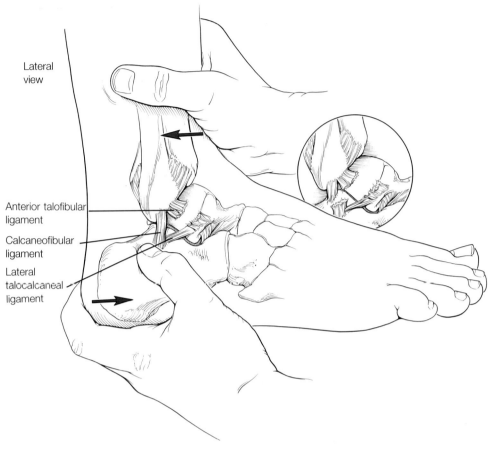

Lateral
view

Anterior talofibular
ligament

Calcaneofibular
ligament

Lateral
talocalcaneal
ligament

FIGURE 10-4.

Anterior drawer stress test. With a tear of the anterior talofibular ligament, the talus will slide anteriorly on the distal tibia, but with a tear of both the anterior talofibular and calcaneofibular ligaments, the anterior translation of the talus will be significantly increased (*inset*).

the anterior talofibular ligament and note related swelling and crepitus with motion. Another excellent test to determine lateral ankle instability is the inversion stress test. This test is done by stabilizing the distal tibia with one hand while plantarflexing and inverting the foot and ankle with the other. As the ankle tilts and subluxates anteriorly, pain is often elicited (Fig. 10-5). Most patients had a normal gait pattern, with only an occasional patient favoring the affected ankle while walking. Although one may expect to find a combination of these symptoms and signs, sometimes patients with chronic lateral laxity have only subtle signs of instability on examination.

The radiographic lateral stress view should be an essential part of the examination when evaluating ankle instability.[1,2] Many patients show an increased

"talar tilt" on stress inversion radiographs, ranging from 6° to 17°. It is important to compare the ankles simultaneously to determine whether the talar tilt is marked in relation to the unaffected side. Rarely, patients have questionably positive stress tests and still have chronic lateral instability; the actual result can be subtle unless the calcaneofibular ligament and the anterior talofibular ligament are both torn.[1,8,9] (For further details, see Chapter 2.)

ARTHROSCOPIC APPEARANCE

Patients with chronic lateral ankle instability demonstrate at arthroscopy an attenuated anterior talofibular ligament with scarring of the lateral gutter and

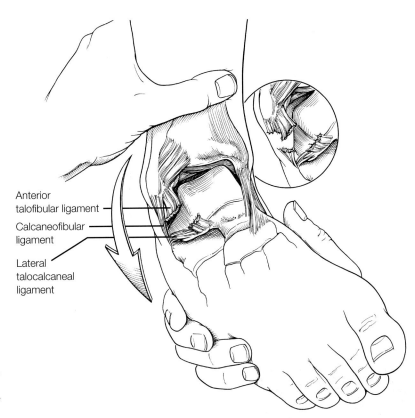

FIGURE 10–5.
Plantarflexion inversion stress test. With a tear of the anterior talofibular ligament, the talus will invert; if both ligaments are torn (*inset*), talar tilt will be increased.

Anterior talofibular ligament

Calcaneofibular ligament

Lateral talocalcaneal ligament

syndesmosis (Fig. 10-6). There may be associated loose bodies or ossicles. Occasionally, with recurrent instability, chondromalacia may be seen, both on the talus and the distal tibia. Although most of the pathology is in the anterolateral corner, additional abnormalities can be seen on the medial side as the talus tilts, abutting the medial dome against the surface of the tibia. Pathology and synovitis are sometimes seen in the posterior ankle as well.

TREATMENT

Arthroscopic lateral ankle stabilization is a technically difficult procedure that requires skill in arthroscopic surgery. Careful patient selection and preoperative assessment are of the greatest importance. Practicing on an ankle model with instruments and a video monitor and cadaver dissection can enhance the

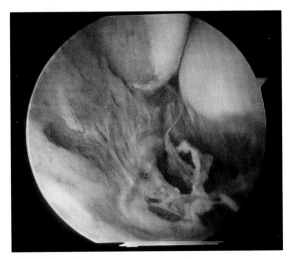

FIGURE 10-6.
Arthroscopic view of a right ankle demonstrating the lateral gutter. The fibula is to the left, the talus to the right. The anterior talofibular ligament is thinned with scarring at its attachment to the talus.

arthroscopist's skills and enable the procedure to be successfully performed at the time of surgery.

In 1983, an arthroscopic staple was first used to repair chronic laxity of the lateral ligamentous structures. Beginning in 1990, the Mitek suture anchor has been used as an improved method of fixation of sutures for tightening the lateral ankle structures.

Preferred Method
(Method of R. B. Hawkins)

The patient is placed in the supine position on the operating table under general or regional anesthesia. The leg is elevated by the circulating nurse while the surgeon applies the tourniquet to midthigh. The leg is exsanguinated from midthigh to toes with the tourniquet. The leg is held in position just distal to midcalf with a surgical assistive device. It is important to avoid undue pressure over the proximal calf near the fibular neck, as this could lead to peroneal palsy (Fig. 10-7).

Portal Placement

The patient is prepared and draped in the usual manner for routine ankle arthroscopy. Portal placement is exceedingly important for ankle ligament reconstruction. Four portals are established. The first, the anteromedial, is for water inflow. The anterolateral portal (2) is used for the arthroscope and camera. The lateral, posterior portal (3) is used for instrumentation, and the lateral, anterior portal (4) is used for insertion of the staple or suture anchor. It is extremely important to choose the most accurate position for this fourth portal because the reconstruction is performed through it[10] (Fig. 10-8).

Patients with true lateral instability of the ankle often show relative laxity or ballooning of the entire lateral capsule or anterior talofibular ligament. Hemorrhagic synovitis and loose bodies are common. Damage to the articular cartilage, if present, is generally found at the medial corner of the tibia. This results from frequent subluxation, during which the medial talus abuts the medial tibia.

Once the diagnostic part of the surgery is fin-ished, the procedure begins, but first a thorough debridement of the entire joint is necessary.

Ligamentous Reconstruction

A favorable environment is created for the insertion of the staple or Mitek anchor by inserting an abrader at a 45° angle to the area on the vertical surface of the talus. The abrader is advanced and used to denude the articular cartilage down to bleeding bone on the vertical surface of the talus about 1 cm anterior to the tip of the fibula. An area about 6 to 8 mm in diameter is created to accommodate the repair (Fig. 10-9). The synovial resector helps smooth the outer dimensions of the crater, making a gradual transition to healthy cartilage. Once the joint is adequately prepared for stapling or Mitek insertion, the fourth portal, also lateral, is made directly over the anterior talofibular ligament.

The knife blade creates an incision for the percutaneous insertion of the staple or the Mitek anchor. The arthroscopic staple is inserted so that it enters the talus at a right angle. While viewing arthroscopically, the small 5.5-mm staple is brought into the joint, gathering the talofibular ligament and contiguous capsule along the way (Figs. 10-10A,B). The ligamentous contents are then plicated into the abraded area on the talus. The foot is held in the neutral position to allow sufficient tightening of the lateral structures. The staple is inserted into the talus with a mallet until it is well seated (see Fig. 10-10C,D). The inserter device, used to advance the staple, is unscrewed and removed from the joint and the procedure is completed. Viewing into the fourth portal ensures proper advancement of the ligamentous tissue and secure fixation into the talar bed. A final probing of the staple head confirms secure fixation. Postoperative x-rays demonstrate the appropriate position of the staple in two planes (see Fig. 10-10E,F).

The Mitek suture anchor system is inserted using a similar technique. The four portals are created as in Figure 10-8. The lateral dome of the talus is identified, and a small 2.9-mm shaver is used to remove damaged tissue. An abrader is then advanced to denude the vertical surface of the talus 1 cm anterior to the tip of the fibula. An oval site about 4 mm × 6 mm is abraded down to bleeding bone for tissue reattachment (see Fig. 10-9).

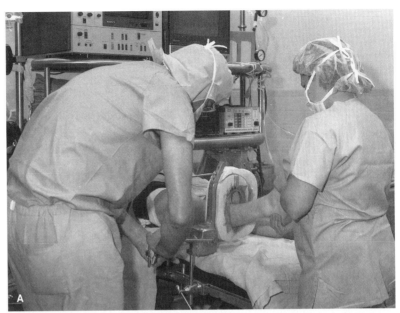

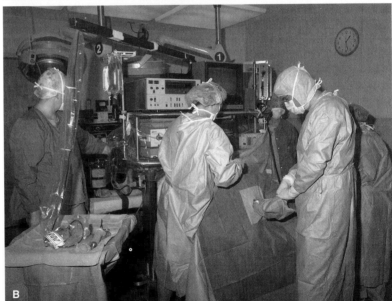

FIGURE 10-7.
Arthroscopic setup of Dr. Hawkins. (**A**) Patient is placed in the supine position. The arthroscopic support is well padded and placed below the knee. (**B**) The foot of the table is then released and the ankle is draped to allow free access to the anterior and posterior aspects of the joint.

Two or three Mitek G-2 anchors are prepared by attaching #2 nonabsorbable suture to the anchor. Under arthroscopic control, a $^5/_{32}$" × 9" (4 mm in diameter) Steinmann pin is used to pierce the capsuloligamentous complex over the reattachment site and to facilitate placement of the drill guide. The Mitek drill guide is then advanced over the pin to the insertion site for the first Mitek anchor, and the pin is removed. The teeth on the drill guide are then impacted at the reattachment site to stabilize the drill and to preserve access to the insertion hole. The drill is then placed through the drill guide and oriented toward the competent talar bone, and a hole is drilled up to the chamfer edge (Fig. 10-11*A*). The scribe line on the drill shank aligns with the drill guide once the correct depth is achieved. All this is done through the fourth portal.

With the drill guide held in a stable position, the

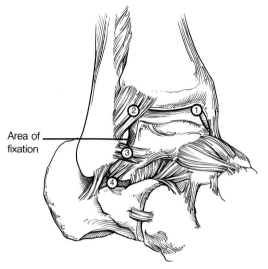

FIGURE 10-8.

Anterolateral view of the right ankle demonstrating proper portal placement. The anteromedial portal (*1*) is used for water inflow, the anterolateral portal (*2*) for viewing with the arthroscope and camera. The lateral posterior portal (*3*) is used for instrumentation; the lateral anterior portal (*4*) is used for insertion of the staple or Mitek anchor.

drill is carefully removed. The first Mitek G-2 anchor with attached nonabsorbable suture is advanced through the drill guide. The anchor is inserted fully within the drill hole and the inserter is withdrawn without twisting or sawing the anchor (see Fig. 10-11*B*). The superior sutures are labeled AA′ and exit through the lateral skin incision. The anchor is set by first applying gentle traction to the AA′ suture pair to pull the anchor 1 to 2 mm to a set position. A pause is made, and then further traction of about 6 to 8 pounds is used to verify stable position. If the anchor fails to engage and pulls out, the drill guide is reinserted and the hole redrilled.

To create the second parallel BB′ suture track, the Steinmann pin is inserted below the AA′ suture pair through the capsuloligamentous complex and a second hole is drilled. The Mitek G-2 anchor is then inserted with BB′ suture. The surgeon verifies the suture pairs are not tangled or twisted, and performs a final arthroscopic check in the joint. The water inflow is then shut off and the arthroscope and cannulae are removed.

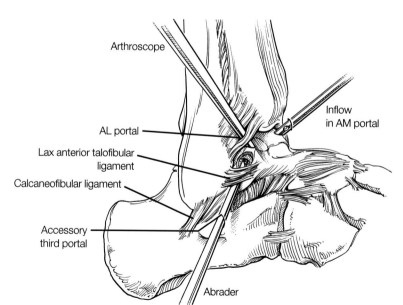

FIGURE 10-9.

An abrader is used to denude the articular cartilage on the vertical surface of the talus 1 cm anterior to the tip of the fibula.

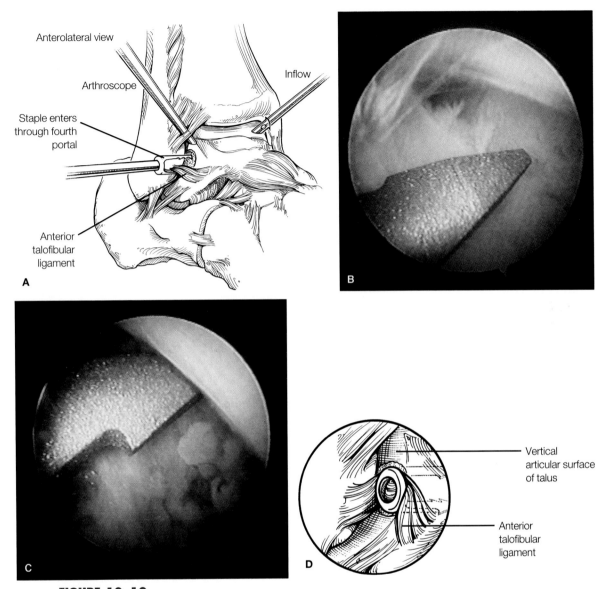

FIGURE 10-10.

Staple insertion. (**A**) While visualizing from the anterolateral portal, the staple is brought through portal 4 and gathers the anterior talofibular ligament and the contiguous capsule. (**B**) Arthroscopic view of a right ankle demonstrating the position of the staple before insertion into the talus. (**C**) As the staple is advanced in the talus, it should be carefully visualized to verify correct insertion. (**D**) The staple is advanced all the way down to plicate the ligamentous tissue onto the talus. (**E**) Postoperative AP x-ray demonstrating the position of the staple. (**F**) Postoperative lateral x-ray demonstrating the position of the staple.

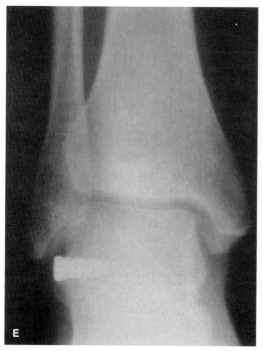

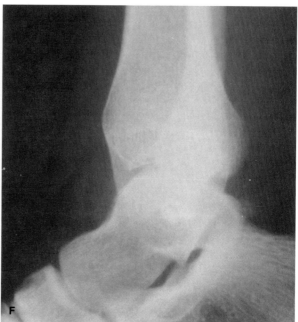

FIGURE 10-10. (Continued)

The ankle is then held in neutral dorsi- and plantarflexion and neutral inversion/eversion. One strand of A and B is selected from each suture pair, and a surgeon's knot is placed to press the capsuloligamentous tissue bridge against the reattachment site. Locking throws are placed to secure the first AB knot. The remaining A'B' sutures are tied and the excess length cut off (see Fig. 10-11C). The portals are injected with bupivacaine 0.25% with epinephrine. This decreases postoperative bleeding and increases comfort once the patient awakens from anesthesia. No sutures are used; instead, a bulky dressing is applied with an ankle orthosis with a fixed hinge in neutral position. A postoperative x-ray may be taken to confirm accurate staple or Mitek placement (see Fig. 10-11D,E). All procedures are done on an outpatient basis, and patients are sent home after being stabilized.

POSTOPERATIVE TREATMENT

Touch-down weight bearing is allowed immediately, with full weight bearing in about 1 week. The orthosis is used for 4 weeks to protect the repair. A graduated rehabilitation program is started, stressing cycling and swimming. A lightweight brace with medial and lateral supports is recommended for sports or physical activity after the ankle has been fully rehabilitated.

CLINICAL RESULTS

A group of 25 patients with ankle instability treated by arthroscopic stapling has been followed for an average of 6 years with generally satisfactory results. Two patients returned with a history of additional trauma, both playing softball. One responded to conservative treatment and did not wish to undergo additional surgery, although his ankle was mildly unstable to clinical testing. The other patient had a repeat arthroscopic stapling with alleviation of symptoms and returned to sports. The findings at the second-look arthroscopy indicated that the staple was secure in the talus, with soft-tissue avulsion from the staple.

Only a small group of patients has been followed since the Mitek anchor sutures have been available.

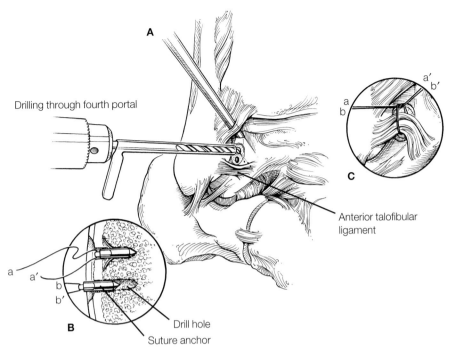

Drilling through fourth portal

Anterior talofibular ligament

Drill hole

Suture anchor

FIGURE 10–11.
Mitek anchor insertion. (**A**) After the talar bed is prepared, two drill holes are made using the appropriate instrumentation. (**B**) After the holes are drilled, a nonabsorbable suture is placed through the Mitek and the anchor is inserted all the way into the bone. The superior sutures are labeled AA', the inferior sutures BB'. (**C**) The sutures are tied with the ankle held in neutral position. Strand A is tied to strand B, strand A' to strand B'. (**D**) Postoperative AP x-ray demonstrating the position of the anchors. (**E**) Postoperative lateral x-ray demonstrating the position of the anchors.

All have maintained a stable ankle and are carrying on normal activities, including sports. Follow–ups are short, so long-term conclusions cannot yet be reached about the efficacy of suture anchor versus staple.

SECOND-LOOK ARTHROSCOPIES

A few patients early in the stapling series were brought back for elective staple removal and second-look arthroscopies. Entry into the anterolateral ankle joint was difficult because scar tissue obliterated the area of the previous staple insertion. Extraction of the staple was performed easily through a lateral cut-down incision.

COMPLICATIONS

No neurovascular complications were noted in either the staple series or the anchor suture series. No infections occurred. One staple was inserted too vigorously in the talus in a patient with relatively soft bone. It was immediately withdrawn and repositioned more proximally without difficulty. Several thin patients could palpate the staple head and wanted it removed electively several months after the initial surgery.

SUMMARY

Arthroscopic repair of chronic lateral ankle instability is a new and developing technique. Follow-ups are short and only a small number of patients

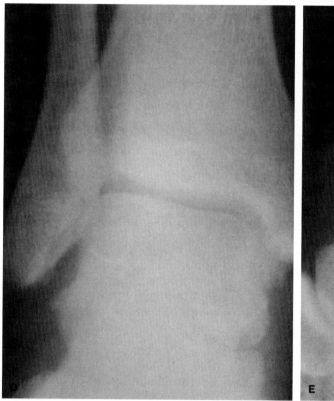
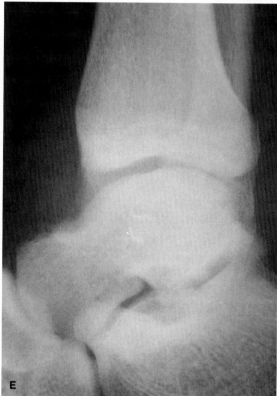

FIGURE 10-11. (Continued)

have undergone this type of surgery, so it will take some time to see where the procedure fits in the spectrum of ankle reconstructive procedures. The arthroscopic repair procedure has several advantages, including the fact that it is minimally invasive, with rapid healing and rehabilitation. Direct repair and tightening of anatomic structures to bone is possible, much like the Brostrom procedure that has become so popular among the open procedures.

REFERENCES

1. Glasgow M, Jackson A, Jamieson AM. Instability of the ankle after injury to the lateral ligament. J Bone Joint Surg 1980;62B:196.
2. Sefton GK, George J, Fitton JM, McMullen H. Reconstruction of the anterior talofibular ligament for the treatment of the unstable ankle. J Bone Joint Surg 1979;61B:352.
3. Hawkins RB. Arthroscopic repair for chronic lateral ankle instability. In Guhl JF, ed. Foot and ankle arthroscopy. Thorofare, NJ: Slack, 1993:155.
4. Nilsonne H. Making a new ligament in ankle sprain. J Bone Joint Surg 1949;31A:380.
5. Brostrom L. Sprained ankles: VI. Surgical treatment of "chronic" ligament ruptures. Acta Chir Scand 1966;132:551.
6. Hamilton WG, Thompson FM, Snow SW. The modified Brostrom procedure for lateral ankle instability. Foot Ankle 1993;14:1.
7. Colville MR, Marder RA, Zarins B. Reconstruction of the lateral ankle ligaments—a biomechanical analysis. Am J Sports Med 1992;20:594.
8. Johnson EE, Markolf KL. The contribution of the anterior talofibular ligament to ankle laxity. J Bone Joint Surg 1983;65A:81.
9. Ruth CJ. The surgical treatment of the fibular collat-

eral ligament of the ankle. J Bone Joint Surg 1961;43A:229.

10. Gollehon DL, Drez D. Ankle arthroscopy—approaches and technique. Orthopedics 1983;6:1150.

BIBLIOGRAPHY

Boruta PM, Bishop JO, Braly WG, et al. Acute lateral ankle ligament injuries: a literature review. Foot Ankle 1990;11:107.

Chen YC. Arthroscopy of the ankle joint. In Watanabe M, ed. Arthroscopy of small joints. Tokyo: Igaku-Shoin, 1985:104.

Gould N, Seligson D, Gassman J. Early and late repair of the lateral ligaments of the ankle. Foot Ankle 1980;1:84.

Johnson LL. Ankle joint. In Klein EA, Falk KH, O'Brien T, eds. Arthroscopic surgery: principles and practice, 3rd ed, vol 2. St. Louis: CV Mosby, 1986:1517.

Karlsson J, Bergsten T, Lansenger O, et al. Reconstruction of the lateral ligaments of the ankle for chronic instability. J Bone Joint Surg 1988;70A:581.

Sammarco GJ, DiRaimondo CV. Surgical treatment of lateral ankle instability syndrome. Am J Sports Med 1988;16:501.

Arthroscopic Surgery: The Foot and Ankle,
by Richard D. Ferkel.
Lippincott-Raven Publishers, Philadelphia © 1996.

11

Arthroscopic Ankle Arthrodesis

James M. Glick and Richard D. Ferkel

Arthrodesis is the procedure of choice for salvaging debilitating conditions of the ankle associated with pain and instability. With a successful fusion, the patient usually can return to work (including heavy labor) and some sports with close to a normal gait. Numerous open surgical procedures have been described for fusion of the tibiotalar joint. In reviewing the literature, postoperative discomfort is often prolonged and the complication rate may be as high as 60%, with an average rate of pseudarthrosis of about 20% and an infection rate of 5% to 25%.[1-6] In contrast, Morgan and colleagues in 1985 reported a 96% rate of successful fusion, with excellent or good functional clinical results in 90% of 101 fusions, followed for an average of 10 years.[7] The complication rate in this series was 6%, including pseudarthrosis. His fusion method differed from others in that it included a debridement that maintained the normal bony contour of the talar dome and tibial plafond instead of squaring it off. In addition, the ankle was placed in a neutral position and transmalleolar cross-screw internal fixation was used.

With the advent of improvements in arthroscopic technique and instrumentation of the ankle, it has become possible to apply open arthrodesis techniques using minimal incisions. The use of invasive or noninvasive distraction has permitted easier access to both the anterior and posterior aspects of the tibiotalar joint to facilitate the arthrodesis procedure. Schneider[8] was the first to describe an arthroscopic technique for ankle arthrodesis, and Morgan[9] published the first report on this method. Myerson described his experience with arthroscopic ankle fusion and compared it with open arthrodesis.[10,11] The mean time for arthrodesis in patients done arthroscopically was 8.7 weeks; with the open method it was 14.5 weeks. Ogilvie-Harris and colleagues reported 19 fusions done arthroscopically, with an 11% (2/19) nonunion rate and 88% (15/17) healed by the third postoperative month.[12] The results were excellent or good in 84% (16/19). Dent and associates described 8 patients treated by arthroscopic ankle arthrodesis.[13] Clinical ankylosis was achieved in all cases, but radiologic evidence of bone fusion was seen in only 4.

ADVANTAGES AND DISADVANTAGES

The advantages of arthroscopic ankle arthrodesis include reduced morbidity, reduced hospitalization, a rapid fusion rate, better cosmesis, decreased complications, and an optional tourniquet. Disadvantages include a difficult learning curve for the surgeon; the need for expensive arthroscopic equipment; and the inability to correct significant varus, valgus, or rotational problems.

INDICATIONS AND CONTRAINDICATIONS

Indications for arthroscopic ankle arthrodesis include significant, unrelenting pain at the tibiotalar joint that does not respond to conservative measures. Etiology of the pain can include traumatic arthritis, hemophilic arthropathy, congenital deformity, rheumatoid arthritis, old osteochondritis dissecans, and previous ankle infection now eradicated. Contraindications include varus or valgus malalignment greater than 15°, malrotation of the ankle, significant bone loss, active infection, previous failed fusion, reflex sympathetic dystrophy, a neuropathic destructive process in the tibiotalar joint, and anterior-posterior translation of the tibiotalar joint requiring correction to planar joint surfaces (Fig. 11-1).

FUSION POSITION

The optimal position for arthrodesis of the ankle is neutral for dorsiflexion and plantarflexion.[14] Equinus, especially more than 10°, should be avoided unless the patient has poliomyelitis, in which case 10° to 15° degrees of equinus helps stabilize the knee joint (Fig. 11-2). Normally, fusions done in more than 10° of equinus produce a significant loss of dorsiflexion that is compensated for by external rotation of the limb and a back-knee thrust into hyperextension that is uncomfortable for the patient.[14] The calcaneus should be in about 5° of valgus and the transverse plane rotation should be equivalent to that of the uninvolved side, usually 5° to 7° of external rotation.[14]

Case studies demonstrate that when the ankle is fused in neutral position, patients can walk with

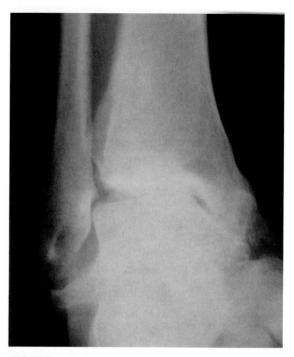

FIGURE 11–1.
Mortise x-ray of the right ankle demonstrating significant talar tilt and varus angulation. This ankle should not be fused arthroscopically.

good velocity and without unusual movements of the limbs or trunk.[15] However, after ankle fusion, most patients show some minor gait irregularities while walking, running, climbing stairs, and particularly walking on inclines.[16] Morgan and associates demonstrated through motion studies that there is an average 58°±7° of combined tibiotalar-tarsal motion in normal controls and 18°±3° in securely fused ankles, a loss of 70% of the total motion arc with a fused ankle.[7] In the same study, the authors demonstrated that compensatory tarsal hypermobility was increased 85%.

OPERATIVE TECHNIQUE

Arthroscopic ankle arthrodesis is performed using the same instrumentation and techniques as described in the first section of this book. Like the open method, the arthroscopic procedure includes three basic steps: (1) removal of all hyaline cartilage

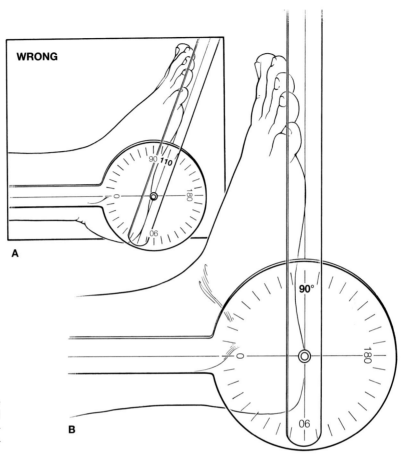

FIGURE 11-2.
Fusion position. (**A**) In most cases, more than 10° of equinus should be avoided with ankle arthrodesis. (**B**) The optimal position for ankle arthrodesis is neutral dorsi- and plantarflexion.

and avascular subchondral bone, (2) fusion reduction in the neutral position, and (3) internal fusion fixation in a neutral position with two (occasionally three) transmalleolar screws.

The equipment commonly used includes a 30° oblique 4-mm or 2.7-mm arthroscope with camera, monitor, and video equipment; high-speed motorized suction shaver and abrader; cup curettes; fluoroscope; invasive or noninvasive distraction systems; and cannulated compression screws. Optional equipment includes a 70° degree oblique 4-mm or 2.7-mm arthroscope, small-joint osteotomes, and a small-joint drill guide.

The patient is positioned supine on a standard operating table. The procedure can be done under general or regional anesthesia. There are two methods for patient positioning. In the first, the patient is placed in the supine position on a standard operating table with the knee bent well over a padded

support and the end of the table bent 90° (Fig. 11-3). In the second method, the patient is placed in the supine position with a fluoroscopic attachment to the foot of the table. Thigh and ankle supports are used (Fig. 11-4).

Distraction

Distraction can be applied by an invasive or noninvasive device. With the knee flexed over the end of the table, a distraction strap is placed around the foot and ankle and a hole is cut in the drape so that 20 to 25 pounds of weight can be applied to distract the tibiotalar surfaces (Fig. 11-5). If the patient is in the supine position, a similar strap is applied but is attached to a distraction device that generates a force by pulling against a loop in the strap (see Fig. 11-4).

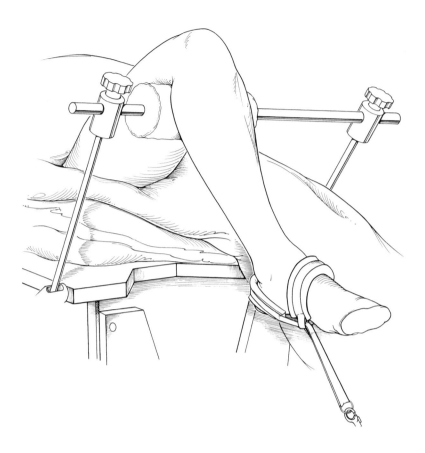

FIGURE 11-3.
With this technique, the patient is positioned supine with the knee bent over a padded support and the end of the table bent 90°.

If noninvasive distraction does not provide adequate separation of the joint surfaces, an invasive distractor can be applied (see Chap. 3). The invasive distractor can be placed either medially with 5-mm ($^{3}/_{16}''$) pins in the tibia and talus, as described by Morgan (Fig. 11-6), or laterally with 5-mm ($^{3}/_{16}''$) pins placed in the tibia and os calcis, as described by Guhl (Fig. 11-7).

The advantages of medially based distraction include easier dorsiflexion and plantarflexion of the ankle while maintaining parallel separation of the joint surfaces rather than lateral talar tilting, which occasionally occurs with laterally based distraction, and easier access to the posterolateral and anterolateral portals. The advantages of lateral pin distraction include avoidance of injury to the calcaneal branches of the posterior tibial nerve, easier access to the anteromedial portal of the ankle, and less difficulty inserting the guide pins for screw insertion.

Portals

Three arthroscopic portals are used: anterolateral, anteromedial, and posterolateral. Initially, a complete arthroscopic examination is done and the entire anterior portion of the ankle is visualized. With increased distraction, the arthroscope can be maneuvered through the medial notch of the tibia and the posterolateral portal established under direct vision. Fluid inflow can be delivered by gravity or a mechanical pump that functions through the sheath that houses the arthroscope or through a posterolateral cannula. If a pump is used, the amount of fluid extravasation must be monitored at all times to avoid complications. Alternatively, good inflow and outflow can usually be maintained by using a large-bore cannula for fluid inflow through the posterolateral portal.

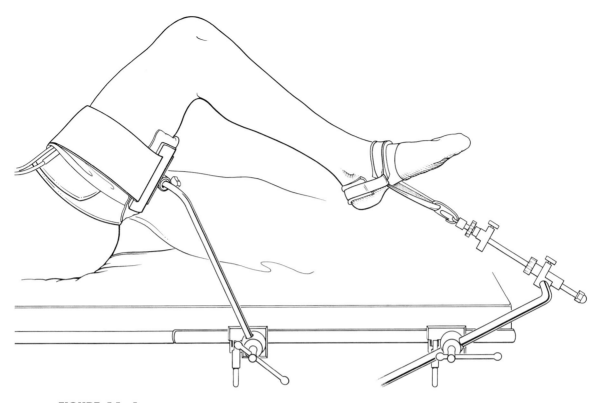

FIGURE 11-4.
Patient positioning can also be done using a thigh support with a noninvasive strap attached to a distraction device (see Chap. 3).

Procedure

The key factor in establishing a complete, rapid union is to remove as little subchondral bone as possible. Before beginning surgery, the preoperative x-ray should be studied to assist in surgical planning (Fig. 11-8*A,B*). Most cases demonstrate at least partial loss of the articular cartilage and some synovitis (see Fig. 11-8*C*). The shape of the talus and tibial surfaces should be maintained. Initially, the soft tissues obstructing visualization are removed with the intraarticular shaver. All remaining hyaline cartilage is removed systematically from the articular surfaces of the talus, tibial plafond, and medial and lateral gutters, thus exposing the subchondral plate in these areas. Hand-held ring and cup curettes are best for removing the hyaline cartilage (Fig. 11-9*A–C*). Periodically, the floating loose pieces of cartilage are removed using a grasper or shaver, or by suctioning through the arthroscopic cannula.

Next, the articular surfaces of the tibial plafond, talar dome, and medial and lateral transmalleolar spaces are abraded systematically, with the motorized abrader alternating between the anteromedial and anterolateral portals. The subchondral plate is denuded to a bleeding surface throughout the fusion area (see Fig. 11-9*D,E*). During debridement, care should be taken to maintain the normal bony contour of the talar dome and tibial plafond (ie, talar convexity and concavity). To prevent a varus/valgus deformity and delayed union, the surgeon must not remove too much bone or square off the tibiotalar surfaces (Fig. 11-10).

In most cases, the posterior compartment of the ankle can be abraded from the anterior portals. If the motorized abrader and curettes do not reach far enough back posteriorly, then these instruments can be used through the posterolateral portal. Using both the 30° and 70° arthroscopes, it becomes easier to visualize these areas, thus facilitating the complete

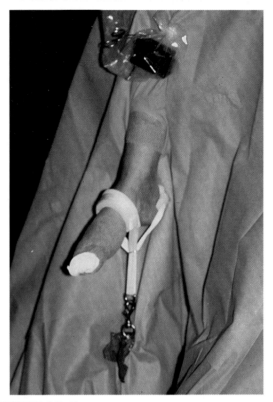

FIGURE 11-5.
When the patient is positioned as in Figure 11-3, a hole in the drape is made and nonsterile weights are applied to the end of the sterile distraction strap.

removal of hyaline cartilage. The medial half of the debridement process is usually performed with the arthroscope placed anterolaterally and the abrader placed anteromedially; conversely, the lateral half is easier to do with the arthroscope placed anteromedially and the abrader anterolaterally.

The final step in the debridement process involves removing the usually large anterior "lip osteophyte" so it will not block reduction of the talar dome convexity into the concavity of the tibial plafond. This is accomplished by abrading while viewing through the anterior portals (Fig. 11-11). The anterior capsule sometimes adheres to the osteophyte, and great caution must be exercised in peeling the capsule off the anterior distal tibia so as not to injure the neurovascular structures (see Chap. 8). In addition, visualizing through the posterolateral portal sometimes makes it possible to assess the required amount of bone to be removed. The osteophyte can

be removed with either a small-joint osteotome or abrader (Fig. 11-12).

Once viable bleeding cancellous bone is visualized throughout the fusion area, the fusion site can be internally fixated. Two guide pins from a cannulated 6.5-mm or 7.0-mm cancellous screw set are placed percutaneously, one from the metaphyseal area of the fibula and the other from the metaphyseal area of the tibia, into the body of the talus. One pin is drilled from the proximal portion of the medial malleolus just above the joint line and is angled 45° inferior and 45° anterior, which allows maximum purchase into the body of the talus. The positioning of this guide pin can be facilitated by the use of a small-joint drill guide (Fig. 11-13*A*). The tip of the guide is placed at the junction of the tibial plafond and the medial malleolus, sufficiently posterior so that good purchase is obtained into the talus. The drill sleeve is placed on the more posterior aspect of the medial tibia and the guide pin is inserted under direct arthroscopic visualization (see Fig. 11-13*B*). The lateral pin is inserted through the fibula so it enters the lateral dome of the talus at the intersection between the horizontal and vertical walls, and is also angled 45° inferior and 45° anterior. The small-joint drill guide can be used to place the pin in the appropriate position, and the pin should be started at the posterior aspect of the fibula (see Fig. 11-13*C*). The pin should be visualized arthroscopically and its position verified. Subsequently, both pins are backed out so the tips are level with the denuded surfaces of the tibial plafond.

The next step is to release the distraction and to remove the arthroscopic instruments. The fusion surfaces are then reduced under image intensification by manual posterior displacement of the hindfoot and dorsiflexion of the ankle and foot to a neutral position. While holding the foot in this position, the medial guide pin is placed into the talus and image intensification is used to ensure the pin does not enter the subtalar joint in both the anteroposterior and lateral planes. Next, the screw length is determined and the appropriate-length screw is inserted under fluoroscopic guidance. This step can be facilitated by using a self-tapping and self-cutting screw. Placing the medial screw in first, with the lateral pin out of the talus, allows for some medial translation and compression. The lateral pin is then advanced and the screw inserted (see Fig. 11-13*D*). The posi-

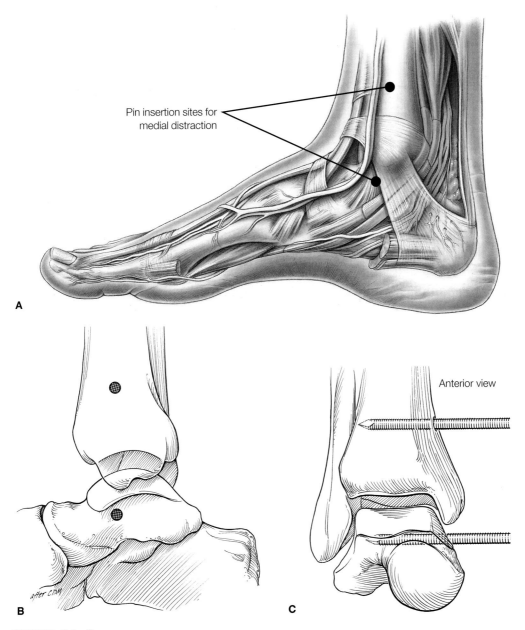

Pin insertion sites for
medial distraction

Anterior view

A

B

C

FIGURE 11-6.

Medial pin distraction. (**A**) When inserting the pins into the tibia and talus, care must be taken to avoid injury to the neurovascular structures and surrounding tendons. (**B**) Medial view of the pin insertion sites with bony anatomy demonstrated. (**C**) Both pins should be inserted unicortically to avoid potential stress risers.

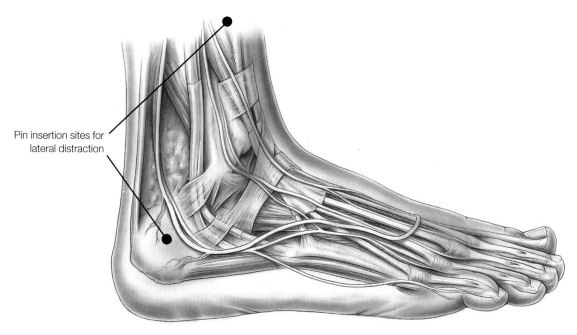

FIGURE 11-7.
Lateral pin distraction is done through the distal tibia and calcaneus. Extreme caution is needed to avoid injury to neurovascular structures.

Pin insertion sites for lateral distraction

tion of the fusion, reduction, and screw placement should be verified with image intensification; if there are any questions, permanent roentgenograms should be obtained in both the anteroposterior and lateral planes (see Fig. 11-13*E–G*). If the bone is soft and screw purchase is suboptimal, an additional screw can be inserted from the medial side and angled less anteriorly to provide more stable fixation.

Occasionally it may be difficult to achieve neutral position of the ankle after removal of the articular surfaces and debridement of the gutters. If a significant contracture of the Achilles tendon exists, either percutaneous or open Achilles lengthening can be performed to facilitate placing the ankle in neutral position.

POSTOPERATIVE CARE

The wounds are closed with nylon sutures, and a compression dressing and well-padded posterior splint is applied with the foot in the appropriate position. At 1 week, the posterior splint and the stitches are removed and the patient is placed in a short-leg, non-weight-bearing cast for 3 weeks. Four weeks after surgery, x-rays are taken out of plaster; if fusion appears to be progressing and position is satisfactory, a walking cast is applied for another 4 to 6 weeks (Fig. 11-14*A,B*). In compliant patients who will exert low stress across the fusion site, a removable cast boot can be used 2 weeks postoperatively if excellent fixation at the fusion site was obtained at surgery. Once a solid arthrodesis is achieved, the screws can be removed if they are causing pain (see Fig. 11-14*C,D*).

RESULTS

We have performed 34 arthroscopically assisted ankle fusions. One of us (JMG) first performed the procedure in February 1984. Crossed, threaded Steinmann pins were used for fixation. We tried alternate methods of debridement and fixation to develop a simple technique that produced a consistent fusion rate, and the best results were achieved with the technique described in this chapter.

Thirty-three patients were followed for 1 year

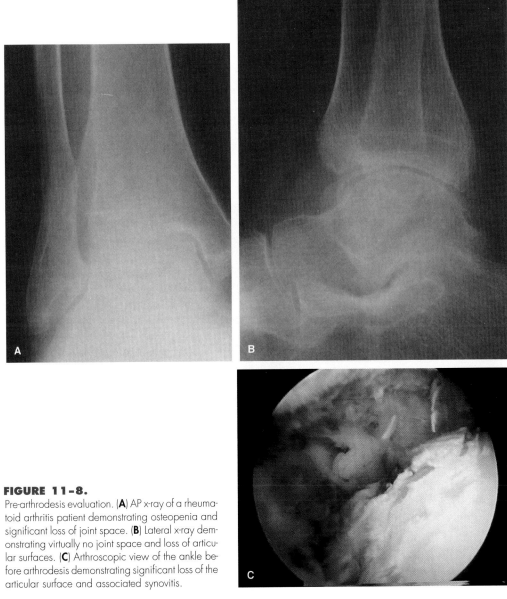

FIGURE 11-8.
Pre-arthrodesis evaluation. (**A**) AP x-ray of a rheumatoid arthritis patient demonstrating osteopenia and significant loss of joint space. (**B**) Lateral x-ray demonstrating virtually no joint space and loss of articular surfaces. (**C**) Arthroscopic view of the ankle before arthrodesis demonstrating significant loss of the articular surface and associated synovitis.

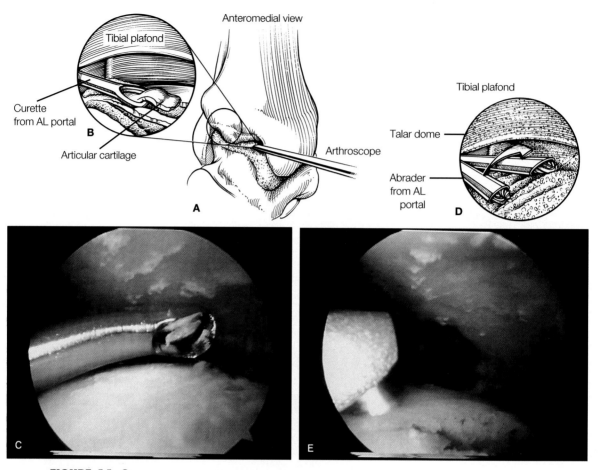

(see Chap. 15)

FIGURE 11-9.
Preparing the joint surfaces for fusion. (**A**) The arthroscope is inserted anteromedially and instruments are inserted anterolaterally. (**B**) Strong ring curettes are used to remove the remaining diseased articular cartilage. (**C**) Arthroscopic view demonstrating the use of a curved curette on the distal tibia. (**D**) The subchondral plate is denuded to a bleeding surface using a motorized burr. (**E**) Arthroscopic view using 5.5-mm burr.

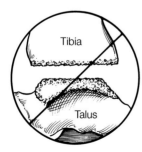

FIGURE 11-10.
With arthroscopic arthrodesis, it is critical not to "square off" the tibiotalar surfaces, but rather to maintain the normal contour of the distal tibia and talus.

or more. One died from an unrelated cause. The average age was 50 years, and males dominated. Most patients had traumatic arthritis. Several had rheumatoid arthritis, and one had an equinus deformity from residuals of polio. There were six nonunions; four of the six were the fault of the technique used at the time. The following is an explanation of each of these four.

There were two errors in the first case. A central portal was used to reach the joint, and smooth Steinmann pins were used for fixation. A pseudoaneurysm of the dorsalis pedis artery developed postoperatively because of its close proximity to the central portal (see Chap. 15). To repair the aneurysm,

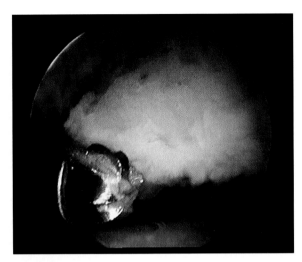

FIGURE 11-11.
Distal tibial spurs are removed using the motorized burr to permit dorsiflexion of the ankle to the neutral position.

a cast immobilizing the ankle was removed and the smooth pins fell out. All immobilization was lost. Eventually, a successful fusion was accomplished using an open conventional technique.

In the next case, a Charnley compression device was used for fixation. Solid fixation could not be accomplished because it is impossible to shape the joint surfaces properly for stability when viewing through the arthroscope. In the other two nonunions, a laser was used to debride the joint surfaces.

The laser worked efficiently, the blood supply appeared to be maintained, and the shapes of the tibia and talus were not altered, but nonunion occurred in both. Bone necrosis from the effects of the laser appeared to be the reason.

The four techniques that caused nonunions have not been considered in the overall results. We do not suggest the use of the central approach, Charnley fixation, or laser. With these techniques excluded, there were two nonunions in 29 patients for a 93% fusion rate. In one nonunion, the lateral and medial gutters were not debrided. In the other, the patient was obese, a heavy smoker, and uncooperative. He removed his cast shortly after it was applied and returned to work as a truck driver.

The average number of days until union occurred was 63 days or 9 weeks. In four cases, fusion was sufficient enough to discontinue immobilization in 6 weeks. The cause of prolonged union in three cases was, in one case, the removal of too much bone in an attempt to square off the surfaces and, in two cases, an apparent lack of stability following Achilles lengthening. Two screws were used for fixation after the Achilles lengthenings. We now think that a third screw is indicated if the patient's bone is soft and simultaneous Achilles lengthenings are performed.

The average time to union after traditional open ankle arthrodesis has been cited in the orthopedic

(*text continues on page 229*)

FIGURE 11-12.
Osteophyte excision while visualizing from the posterior portal. (**A**) Using the posterolateral portal, the distal tibial osteophyte is well visualized and removed with a burr or osteotome. (**B**) After removal of the osteophytes, the ankle moves without bony impingement.

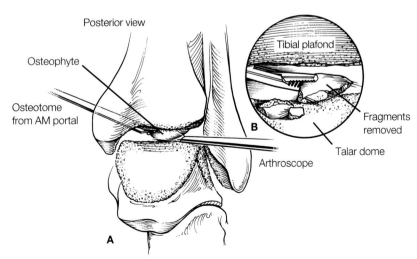

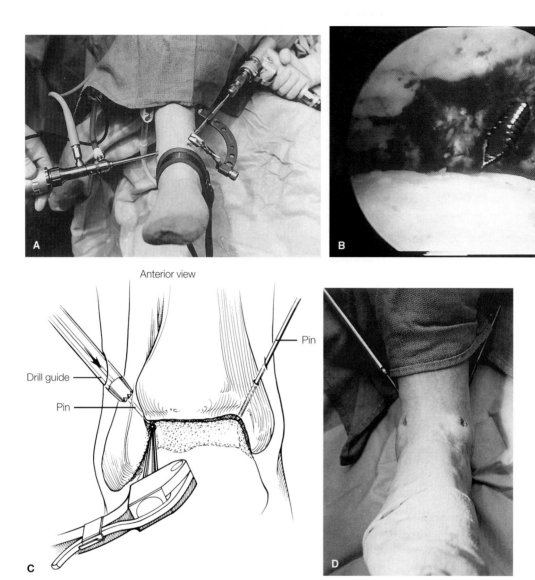

Anterior view

Pin

Drill guide

Pin

FIGURE 11-13.

Inserting the cannulated screws. (**A**) A small-joint drill guide can be used to assist in the accurate placement of the guide pin in the medial malleolus. (**B**) Visualizing from the anterolateral portal, the guide pin position can be assessed as it enters the medial ankle joint. (**C**) Both pins are inserted from the posterior aspect of the malleoli and angled 45° inferior and 45° anterior. (**D**) With the ankle stabilized in the neutral position, a 6.5-mm self-drilling, self-tapping screw is inserted. (**E**) Both screws are inserted so that no threads cross the tibiotalar joint. (**F**) The positions of the screws are checked fluoroscopically to verify correct position. (**G**) After the guide pins are removed, the screws are tightened further and the screw tip positions are checked fluoroscopically to verify that the subtalar joint has not been violated.

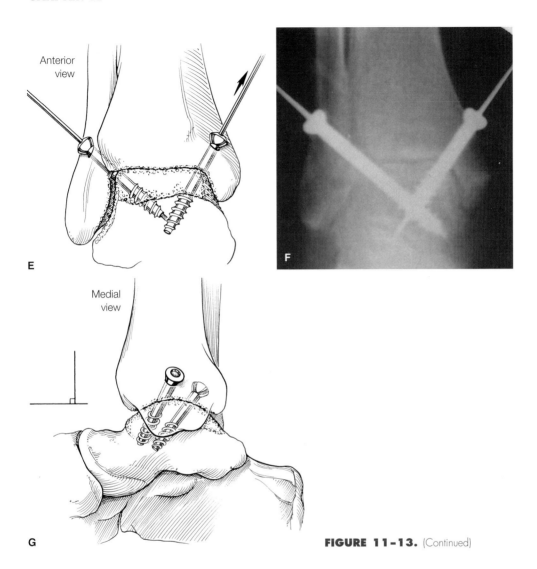

Anterior view

Medial view

E

F

G

FIGURE 11-13. (Continued)

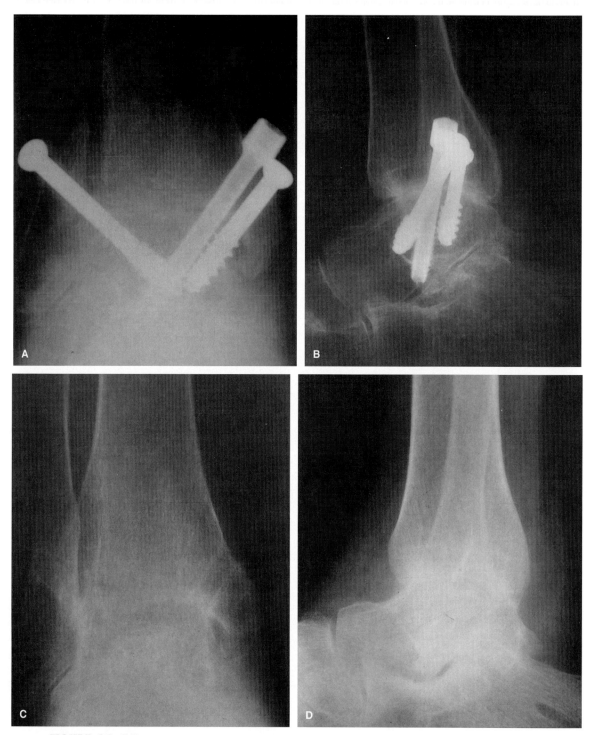

FIGURE 11–14.
A 54-year-old female with rheumatoid arthritis whose preoperative x-rays are seen in Figure 11-8. (**A**) AP x-ray 8 weeks after arthrodesis. A third screw is used medially because of the osteoporotic bone. (**B**) Lateral x-ray 8 weeks after arthrodesis. (**C**) AP x-ray with screws removed, demonstrating solid fusion. (**D**) Lateral x-ray after screws removed, showing solid fusion.

literature as 3 to 12 months.[7,17–19] In our series, the average time to union after arthroscopic arthrodesis is 9 weeks on average. This compares favorable with Myerson and Quill, who found the mean time to fusion to be 8.7 weeks.[11] They used cross-screw fixation in both methods. The rapid rate of union may be technique-dependent; as with the arthroscopic technique, there is no periosteal stripping and therefore no interruption of the local circulation. There were no complications in the 29 cases reviewed. Most of the patients were discharged on the day of surgery or stayed overnight in an outpatient facility.

Recently, a multicenter evaluation of 75 patients found that the overall fusion rate was 91%, with 84% good or excellent results.[20] The fusion rate jumped to 96% if abandoned techniques were excluded from the results. Time to fusion was 9 weeks, which, on average, is 4 weeks less than when using open fusion techniques. The morbidity is considerably less with arthroscopic arthrodesis.

CONCLUSIONS

The relatively rapid postoperative mobilization makes the arthroscopic approach particularly appealing in elderly patients and in patients with rheumatoid arthritis and other diseases who cannot tolerate a prolonged period of non-weight bearing postoperatively. Limited incisions make arthroscopic arthrodesis useful in patients with vascular, dermatologic, diabetic, autoimmune, and other medical conditions that may contraindicate a more major surgical procedure. This procedure has been successful in patients with arteriovenous malformations of the ankle and severe peripheral vascular disease. In the appropriate setting and for the appropriate indications, the arthroscopic procedure provides an attractive alternative to traditional open methods of ankle fusion.

REFERENCES

1. Ahlberg A, Henricson AS. Late results of ankle fusion. Acta Orthop Scand 1981;52:103.
2. Boobyer GN. The long-term results of ankle arthrodesis. Acta Orthop Scand 1981;52:107.
3. Charnley J. Compression arthrodesis of the ankle and shoulder. J Bone Joint Surg 1951;33B:180.
4. Johnson FW, Boseker EH. Arthrodesis of the ankle. Arch Surg 1968;97:766.
5. Morrey BF, Wiedeman GP. Complications and long-term results of ankle arthrodesis following trauma. J Bone Joint Surg 1980;62A:777.
6. Said E, Hunka L, Siller TM. Where ankle fusion stands today. J Bone Joint Surg 1978;60B:211.
7. Morgan CD, Henke JA, Bailey RW, Kaufer H. Long-term results of tibiotalar arthrodesis. J Bone Joint Surg 1985;67A:546.
8. Schneider D. Arthroscopic ankle fusion. Arth Video 1983;3.
9. Morgan DC. Arthroscopic tibiotalar arthrodesis. Jefferson Orthop J 1987;16:50.
10. Myerson MS, Allon SM. Arthroscopic ankle arthrodesis. Contemp Orthop 1989;19:21.
11. Myerson MS, Quill G. Ankle arthrodesis—a comparison of an arthroscopic and an open method of treatment. Clin Orthop 1991;268:84.
12. Ogilvie-Harris DJ, Lieberman I, Fitsialos D. Arthroscopically assisted arthrodesis for osteoarthrotic ankles. J Bone Joint Surg 1993;75A:1167.
13. Dent CM, Patil M, Fairclough JA. Arthroscopic ankle arthrodesis. J Bone Joint Surg 1993;75B:830.
14. Mann RA, Coughlin M. Surgery of the foot and ankle. St. Louis: CV Mosby, 1993:676.
15. Mazur JM, Schwartz E, Simon SR. Ankle arthrodesis: long-term follow-up with gait analysis. J Bone Joint Surg 61A:964;1979.
16. Marcus RE, Balourdas GM, Heiple KG. Ankle arthrodesis by chevron fusion with internal fixation and bone grafting. J Bone Joint Surg 65A:833;1983.
17. Campbell CJ, Rinehart WT, Kalenak A. Arthrodesis of the ankle: deep autogenous graft with maximum cancellous bone apposition. J Bone Joint Surg 1974;56A:63.
18. Scranton PE Jr. Use of internal compression in arthrodesis of the ankle. J Bone Joint Surg 1985;67A:550.
19. Holt EW, Hanson ST, Mayo KA, Sangeorzan BJ. Ankle arthrodesis using internal screw fixation. Clin Orthop 1991;268:21.
20. Mann JA, Glick JM, Morgan CT, et al. Arthroscopic ankle arthrodesis: experience with 75 cases. Presented at the annual meeting of the American Academy of Orthopaedic Surgeons, Orlando, Florida, February 1995.

BIBLIOGRAPHY

Buck P, Morrey BF, Chan EYS. The optimum position of arthrodesis of the ankle. J Bone Joint Surg 1987;69A:1052.

Mann RA, Van Manen JW, Wapner KL, et al. Ankle fusion. Clin Orthop 1991;268:49.

Maurer RC, Cimino WR, Cox CV, Satow GK. Transarticular cross-screw fixation: a technique of ankle arthrodesis. Clin Orthop 1991;268:56.

Arthroscopic Surgery: The Foot and Ankle,
by Richard D. Ferkel.
Lippincott-Raven Publishers, Philadelphia © 1996.

12

Subtalar Arthroscopy

Richard D. Ferkel

*T*he appropriate application of arthroscopic technology to various parts of the body takes time and experience, as has been demonstrated in knee and shoulder arthroscopy. Although many clinical and experimental studies concerning ankle arthroscopy have been published, few reports are available concerning the subtalar joint. With the advent of smaller arthroscopes with improved fields of vision and clarity and the development of small-joint instrumentation, arthroscopy of the subtalar joint has become more feasible.

The first report of subtalar arthroscopy was by Parisien and Vangsness in 1985.[1] They used amputation specimens to determine the feasibility of subtalar arthroscopy. Both 2.2- and 2.7-mm arthroscopes were used, and the specimens were dissected at the end of the arthroscopic examination to determine where they were looking with their instruments in various positions. Since then, other reports and presentations have followed.[2,3]

LANDMARKS

The extraarticular anatomy in this region was discussed in Chapter 5, but certain anatomic structures and landmarks are important to emphasize here (Fig. 12-1). The lateral malleolus is routinely palpable and is the key to identifying the posterior facet of the subtalar joint. The sinus tarsi is also usually palpable, although it can be filled with large amounts of adipose tissue. Inversion and eversion of the foot may be helpful in palpating the sinus tarsi. In addition, the lateral talar dome can be palpated as the anterolateral portion slides out from under the distal tibia as the ankle is taken from a dorsiflexed into a plantarflexed position.

Posterior to the lateral malleolus lie the sural nerve and peroneal tendons (Fig. 12-2). The sural nerve is usually 2 cm posterior and 2 cm inferior to the lateral malleolus. The peroneal tendons pass along the posterior surface of the distal fibula and are tightly held in the peroneal groove by the retinaculum. The lateral ankle ligaments include the anterior talofibular ligament, the calcaneofibular ligament, and the posterior talofibular ligament. The anterior talofi-

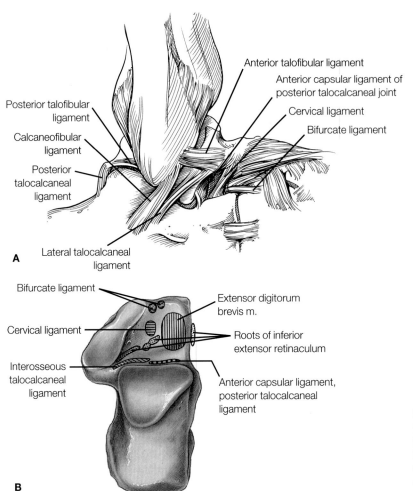

Posterior talofibular ligament

Calcaneofibular ligament

Posterior talocalcaneal ligament

Anterior talofibular ligament

Anterior capsular ligament of posterior talocalcaneal joint

Cervical ligament

Bifurcate ligament

Lateral talocalcaneal ligament

A

Bifurcate ligament

Cervical ligament

Interosseous talocalcaneal ligament

Extensor digitorum brevis m.

Roots of inferior extensor retinaculum

Anterior capsular ligament, posterior talocalcaneal ligament

B

FIGURE 12-1.

Ligaments of the subtalar joint. (**A**) Superficial lateral view of the subtalar joint with bones and ligaments. From this position, the interosseous ligament cannot be seen. (**B**) Superior view of insertion sites on the calcaneus with the talus removed.

bular ligament is a broad, thin ligament with the most inferior margin superior to the posterior facet of the subtalar joint. The calcaneofibular ligament courses deep to the peroneal tendons in an oblique fashion from the tip of the fibula toward the most posterior portion of the calcaneus. As it crosses the subtalar joint, it also stabilizes this joint, and a steep surface can be expected arthroscopically. The posterior talofibular ligament is also superior to the subtalar joint. The posterior portion of the subtalar joint is very close to the posterior ankle joint, and as the talus tapers the posterior talofibular ligament is just proximal to the posterior subtalar joint line.

Palpation of surface landmarks on the medial side of the foot begins with the articulation of the talar head and the navicular, felt as the forefoot is inverted and everted. The sustentaculum tali is palpated one

fingerbreadth beneath the tip of the medial malleolus. The posterior portion of the subtalar joint is more difficult to palpate because of its deep position and the fact that it is covered by the Achilles, the flexor hallucis longus, and the joint capsule. The os trigonum is present in 7% to 10% of people, and has a 50% incidence of bilaterality.

INTRAARTICULAR ANATOMY

The subtalar joint may be divided into anterior and posterior articulations, separated by the sinus tarsi and the tarsal canal. The anterior subtalar joint (talocalcaneal navicular joint) is formed by the anterior aspect of the talus, the posterior surface of the navicular, the anterior portion of the calcaneus, and the

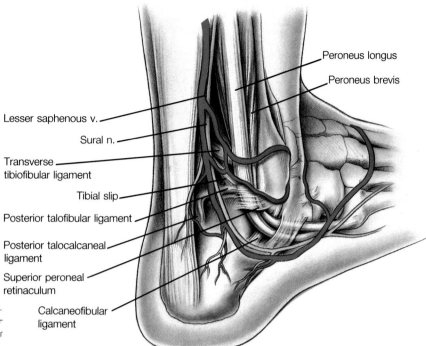

FIGURE 12-2.

Posterolateral view of the right ankle. Note the course of the lesser saphenous vein and sural nerve and their associated branches.

calcaneonavicular (spring) ligament (Figs. 12-3, 12-4). The anterior articulation is separated from the posterior articulation by the tarsal canal. The tarsal canal is formed by a sulcus in the undersurface of the talus and the superior surface of the calcaneus, and laterally the opening is termed the sinus tarsi. The borders of the tarsal canal include the anterior portion of the posterior subtalar joint capsule, which forms the posterior boundary of this canal. The ante-

rior boundary is the posterior portion of the talocalcaneal navicular joint capsule. There is a 45° angle of orientation of the long axis of the sinus tarsi to the lateral aspect of the calcaneus. According to Cahill, the tarsal canal is about 10 to 15 mm high, 3 to 5 mm wide, and 15 to 20 mm long.[4] It gives attachments to the medial root of the inferior extensor retinaculum, the cervical ligament, the ligament in the tarsal canal (interosseous talocalcaneal ligament), and fatty tissue and blood vessels (Fig. 12-5). This is discussed later in the chapter.

The posterior talocalcaneal or posterior subtalar joint is formed by the posterior calcaneus facet on the inferior surface of the talus and the corresponding posterior facet on the calcaneus (see Fig. 12-4). The posterior facet of the calcaneus is convex, the posterior facet of the inferior surface of the talus concave. This is shaped much like a saddle joint and the motion is that of a mitered hinge. Its long axis is obliquely located about 40° to the midline of the foot, and its joint capsule is reinforced laterally by the lateral talocalcaneal ligament and calcaneofibular ligament and in line with the synovium.

There is much debate over the ligamentous support of the subtalar joint. One of the first detailed

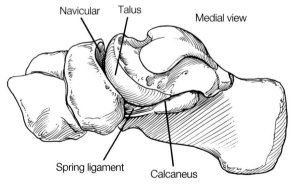

FIGURE 12-3.

Anteromedial subtalar joint and talonavicular joint, demonstrating the important location of the spring ligament.

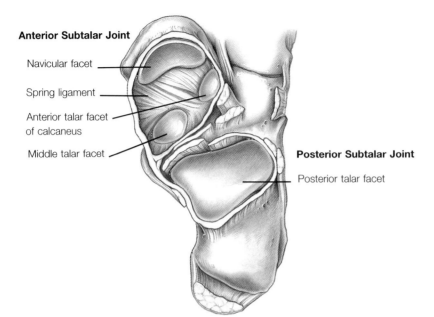

Anterior Subtalar Joint

Navicular facet

Spring ligament

Anterior talar facet
of calcaneus

Middle talar facet

Posterior Subtalar Joint

Posterior talar facet

FIGURE 12-4.

Anterior subtalar joint with talus opened away from the calcaneus.

descriptions of the anatomy of the contents of the sinus tarsi and tarsal canal was by Wood Jones in 1944.[5] Since then, several papers have discussed these ligaments. Last in 1952 determined that the cervical ligament was the strongest bond between the talus and the calcaneus.[6] Cahill described the presence of three lateral roots for the inferior extensor retinaculum and emphasized that the retinaculum consisted of two layers, one superficial and one deep to the extensor tendons.[4] In 1978 Schmidt defined five distinct ligaments within the sinus tarsi and canal.[7] Viladot and associates in 1984 divided the ligaments into peripheral or central.[8] More recently, Harper categorized the supporting structures into superficial, intermediate, and deep layers[9] (Table 12-1). Stephens and Sammarco described the stabilizing role of the lateral ligament complex around the subtalar joint.[10]

Our dissections have concurred with Harper's work, dividing the supporting structures into three layers. The superficial or peripheral layer includes (Fig. 12-6):

1. The lateral talocalcaneal ligament, which runs from the lateral tubercle of the talus to the lateral surface of the calcaneus. Its fibers are anterior and parallel to the fibers of the calcaneofibular ligament.

2. The posterior talocalcaneal ligament, directed downward and laterally from the posterolateral tubercle of the talus to the superior and medial surface of the calcaneus

3. The medial talocalcaneal ligament, originating from the medial tubercle of the talus and coursing anteriorly and inferiorly to insert on the sustentaculum tali

TABLE 12-1.
LATERAL LIGAMENTOUS SUPPORT OF THE SUBTALAR JOINT

Superficial layer

Lateral root of the inferior extensor retinaculum

Lateral talocalcaneal ligament

Calcaneofibular ligament

Posterior talocalcaneal ligament

Medial talocalcaneal ligament

Intermediate layer

Intermediate root of the inferior extensor retinaculum

Cervical ligament

Deep layer

Medial root of the inferior extensor retinaculum

Interosseous talocalcaneal ligament

(Modified from Harper MC. The lateral ligamentous support of the subtalar joint. Foot Ankle 1991;12:354.)

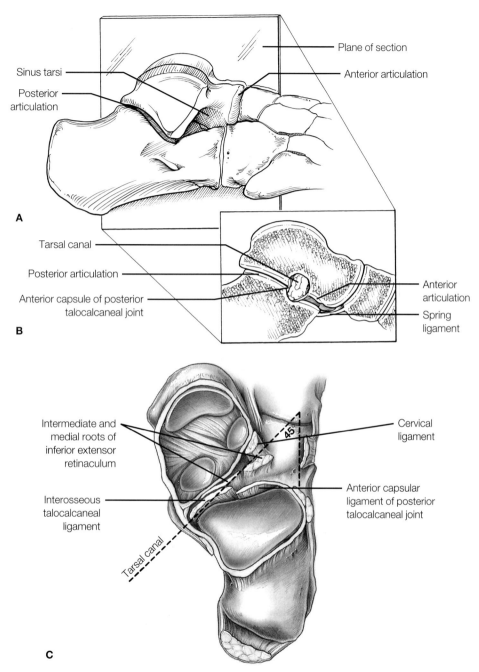

FIGURE 12-5.

Sinus tarsi. (**A**) Lateral view. The sinus tarsi and tarsal canal separate the anterior and posterior articulations of the subtalar joint. The plane of section helps to demonstrate the anatomy more clearly. (**B**) After sectioning, the tarsal canal and subtalar articulations are more clearly seen. (**C**) Axial view of the tarsal canal. Note the location of the interosseous talocalcaneal and cervical ligaments. There is a 45° angle of orientation of the long axis of the sinus tarsi to the lateral aspect of the calcaneus.

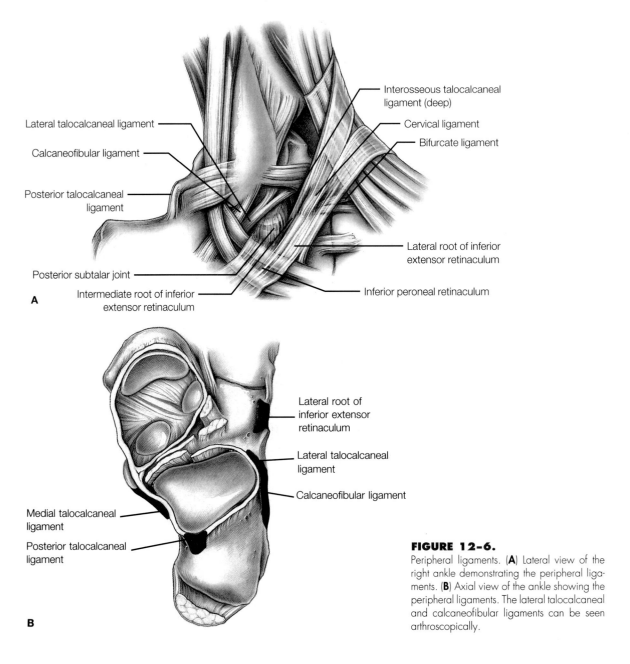

Lateral talocalcaneal ligament

Calcaneofibular ligament

Posterior talocalcaneal ligament

Posterior subtalar joint

A Intermediate root of inferior extensor retinaculum

Interosseous talocalcaneal ligament (deep)

Cervical ligament

Bifurcate ligament

Lateral root of inferior extensor retinaculum

Inferior peroneal retinaculum

Lateral root of inferior extensor retinaculum

Lateral talocalcaneal ligament

Calcaneofibular ligament

Medial talocalcaneal ligament

Posterior talocalcaneal ligament

B

FIGURE 12-6.
Peripheral ligaments. (**A**) Lateral view of the right ankle demonstrating the peripheral ligaments. (**B**) Axial view of the ankle showing the peripheral ligaments. The lateral talocalcaneal and calcaneofibular ligaments can be seen arthroscopically.

4. The lateral root of the inferior extensor retinaculum, superficial fibers that blend into the deep fascia on the lateral aspect of the foot, where they may be continuous with the inferior peroneal retinaculum

5. The calcaneofibular ligament, which runs just posterior to the lateral talocalcaneal ligament.

The intermediate layer of ligaments comprises (Fig. 12-7):

1. The intermediate root of the inferior extensor retinaculum. This root is a relatively strong, broad band inserting on the calcaneus at the floor of the tarsus sinus and canal, just posterior to the cervical ligament.

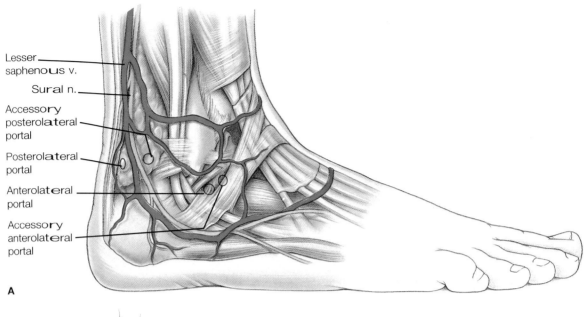

Lesser
saphenous v.

Sural n.

Accessory
posterolateral
portal

Posterolateral
portal

Anterolateral
portal

Accessory
anterolateral
portal

A

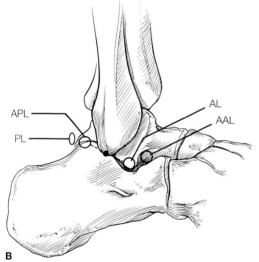

APL

PL

AL

AAL

B

FIGURE 12-8.

Subtalar portals. (**A**) The anterolateral and posterolateral subtalar portals and accessory portals are made using extreme caution to avoid injury to the neurovascular structures. (**B**) With the soft tissues removed, the location of the portals is seen in relation to the subtalar joint and fibula. (**C**) Surgical view of the location of the anterolateral portals.

are the retinacular ligaments. The medial root is a slender ligament lying deeper within the sinus tarsi, inserting into the calcaneus close to the ligament of the tarsal canal. Insertional fibers of the extensor digitorum brevis, as well as blood vessels and adipose tissue, are intermingled with the retinacular ligaments.

2. The ligament of the tarsal canal (interosseous talocalcaneal ligament) is the most important ligament uniting the talus and the calcaneus. It prevents eversion, heel valgus, and depression

of the longitudinal arch. The ligament of the canal is a broad band originating from the sulcus calcanei on the floor of the tarsal canal and runs obliquely upward and medially at 45°, inserting onto the inferior surface of the talus behind the cervical ligament.

The subtalar joint is enveloped by a thin capsule and does not communicate with other joints. The joint capsule has a posterior pouch as well as medial, lateral, and anterior capsular recesses.

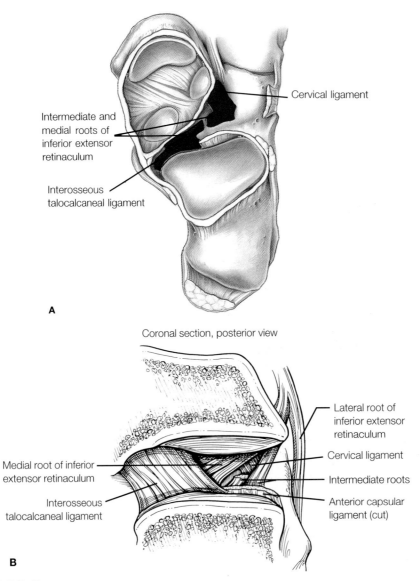

Coronal section, posterior view

FIGURE 12-7.

Deep ligaments. (**A**) Axial view of the subtalar joint demonstrating the deep ligaments. (**B**) Coronal section of the subtalar joint showing the course of the interosseous talocalcaneal ligament in relation to the cervical ligament and surrounding roots.

2. The cervical ligament, originating from the floor of the sinus tarsi and running in a superior oblique direction to insert onto the inferior aspect of the talar neck. The cervical ligament, which is thought to limit inversion, is covered superficially by the extensor digitorum brevis muscle and by the stem of the inferior extensor retinaculum. The

ligament consists of prominent fascicles intermingled with loose connective tissue and fat.

The deep layer of ligaments includes (see Fig. 12-7):

1. The medial root of the inferior extensor retinaculum. This and the intermediate root

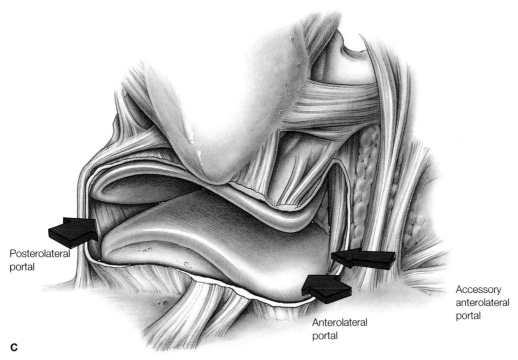

Posterolateral
portal

Accessory
anterolateral
portal

Anterolateral
portal

C

FIGURE 12-8. (Continued)

INDICATIONS FOR ARTHROSCOPY

The diagnostic indications for subtalar arthroscopy include persistent pain, swelling, stiffness, locking, or catching resistant to all conservative care. The therapeutic indications include debridement of chondromalacia, excision of osteophytes, lysis of adhesions with posttraumatic arthrofibrosis, synovectomy, removal of loose bodies, debridement and drilling of osteochondritis dissecans, fracture assessment and reduction, and arthrodesis. Other indications for subtalar arthroscopy will no doubt arise as expertise in this area increases. Patients with obvious degenerative joint disease of the tibiotalar joint who are candidates for arthrodesis sometimes also have degenerative changes of the subtalar joint. The subtalar joint can be inspected arthroscopically before tibiotalar fusion, if there is a question as to whether a tibiotalar or subtalar arthrodesis should be performed.[11]

CONTRAINDICATIONS

The absolute contraindications to subtalar arthroscopy include localized infection and advanced degenerative joint disease, particularly with deformity. Relative contraindications include severe edema and poor vascular status.

PORTALS

Two primary and two accessory portals are generally used (Figs. 12-8, 12-9). The anterolateral portal is about 2 cm anterior and 1 cm distal to the tip of the lateral malleolus. The posterolateral portal is at or 0.5 cm proximal to the tip of the fibula, and remains closer to the Achilles than the fibula to avoid injury to the peroneal tendons, sural nerve, and short (lesser) saphenous vein. The accessory anterolateral portal is usually slightly anterior and superior to the anterolateral portal. One must keep enough separation between portals to allow proper triangulation and instrumentation without crowding. The accessory anterolateral portal is best made under direct vision while looking from either the posterolateral or anterolateral portal. The accessory posterolateral portal is made lateral to the posterolateral portal, using extreme caution to avoid injury to the previously discussed structures. It is best made under direct vision and appropriate triangulation.

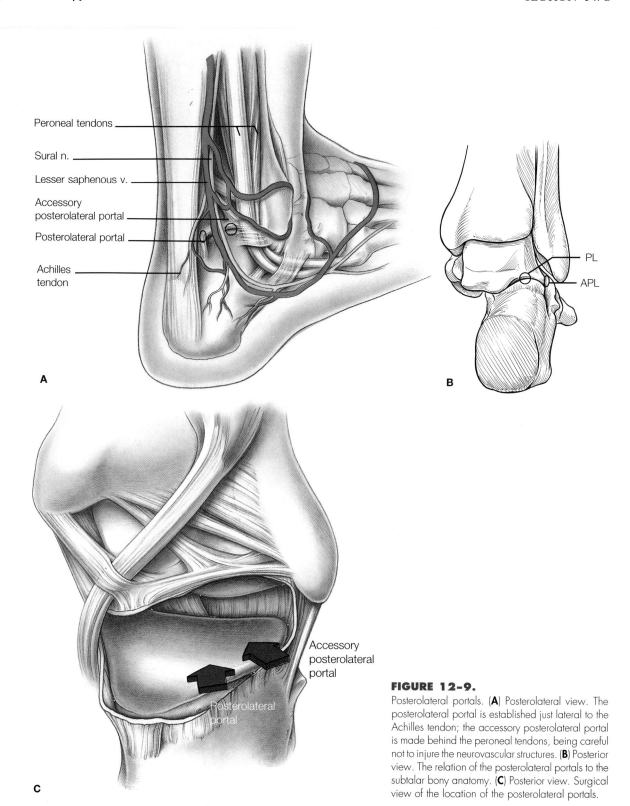

Peroneal tendons

Sural n.

Lesser saphenous v.

Accessory
posterolateral portal

Posterolateral portal

Achilles
tendon

A

PL

APL

B

Accessory
posterolateral
portal

Posterolateral
portal

C

FIGURE 12-9.

Posterolateral portals. (**A**) Posterolateral view. The
posterolateral portal is established just lateral to the
Achilles tendon; the accessory posterolateral portal
is made behind the peroneal tendons, being careful
not to injure the neurovascular structures. (**B**) Posterior
view. The relation of the posterolateral portals to the
subtalar bony anatomy. (**C**) Posterior view. Surgical
view of the location of the posterolateral portals.

INSTRUMENTATION

The instruments used for subtalar arthroscopy are similar to those used in the ankle (Table 12-2). The arthroscope generally used is a 2.7-mm 30° short arthroscope. Sometimes a 70° arthroscope is quite helpful to look around corners and to facilitate instrumentation. In joints too tight to allow a 2.7-mm arthroscope, a 1.9-mm 30° arthroscope is used (Fig. 12-10). Usually a 2.9-mm shaver-type blade can be used, but smaller 1.9- and 2-mm blades are available (Fig. 12-11).

TECHNIQUE

Subtalar arthroscopy can be performed in a similar manner to that of the ankle. The patient can be positioned in the lateral decubitus position, the supine position, or flexed 90° at the knee. Distraction can be used when appropriate, with invasive or noninvasive instrumentation. The decision to use distraction is made at the time of surgery based on the ease of visualization and the nature of the pathology approached.

Preferred Approach

Subtalar arthroscopy is generally done using general or regional anesthesia. Relaxation is critical to allow good distraction and maximum visualization; therefore, local anesthesia is not recommended.

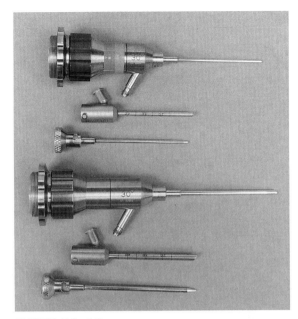

FIGURE 12-10.
1.9-mm and 2.7-mm 30° video arthroscopes are used for subtalar arthroscopy. The cannulae are 2.2 and 2.9 mm, respectively.

TABLE 12-2.
INSTRUMENTS FOR SUBTALAR ARTHROSCOPY

Needed:
- 1.9- & 2.7-mm 30° and 70° short video arthroscopes with lightweight chip cameras
- 2.0- & 2.9-mm full-radius blades, whiskers, and burrs
- 18-gauge spinal needle
- 2 19-gauge needles and 55-cc syringe with IV tubing

Otherwise include:
- Small-joint probe, small-joint grasper
- Ring curettes, pituitary
- K-wires
- Drill

The patient is positioned in a supine position with a sandbag under the buttock, and a thigh holder is positioned to flex the hip 45°. A tourniquet is applied to the thigh and used as needed. The sterile foot holder and clamp are attached to the table. Landmarks are marked with a pen and the noninvasive strap is used for distraction (Fig. 12-12). The joint is distended by inserting a 19-gauge needle into the posterolateral portal, avoiding injuries to the sural nerve and lesser saphenous vein. Care must be taken to avoid puncturing too proximally, lest the posterior aspect of the ankle joint be entered. Correct position is verified in the subtalar joint by assessing backflow.

With the joint distended through the posterolateral portal, the anterolateral portal is established as previously outlined. This portal is verified by seeing fluid come out of the needle when it is appropriately positioned anteriorly. Care must be taken to angle the needle in the anterolateral portal posteriorly and slightly superiorly to avoid entering the sinus tarsi and abrading the articular surface (Fig. 12-13).

Once the proper position of both portals has been established, a small stab incision is made, being extremely careful to avoid injuries to the neurovas-

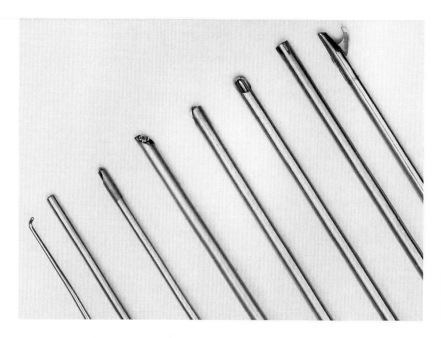

FIGURE 12-11.
Small-joint instrumentation includes probe, 2.0-mm and 2.9-mm shavers and burrs, and small-joint baskets.

cular structures. Although the posterolateral portal is more dangerous than the anterolateral, branches of the superficial peroneal nerve can be injured anteriorly as well. A 2.7-mm short 30° arthroscope with interchangeable cannula is inserted. Inflow can initially be done through the arthroscope, and joint inspection is accomplished with a small probe (Fig. 12-14). If distraction is necessary to improve visualization, invasive or noninvasive techniques are used depending on the patient's size, the pathology present, and the narrowness of the subtalar joint. Noninvasive and invasive distraction allow for manipulation of the subtalar joint. A switching stick is helpful to allow the insertion of instruments that do not go through the standard cannulae.

Intraoperative shaving, loose body removal, burring, and other procedures can be done by alternating from anterior to posterior (Fig. 12-15). Ac-

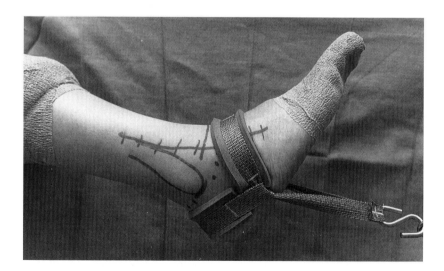

FIGURE 12-12.
Noninvasive distraction. It is important with subtalar arthroscopy to position the strap low enough to avoid interference with the anterolateral and posterolateral portals.

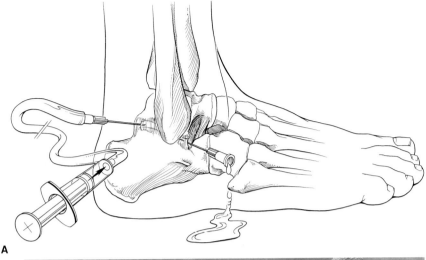

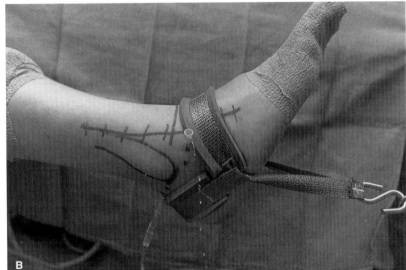

FIGURE 12-13.
Distention of the subtalar joint. (**A**) The posterolateral portal is established with a small-gauge needle and distended with saline. The anterolateral portal is then made with a second needle, and flow verifies the location of the subtalar joint anteriorly. (**B**) Locating the posterolateral and anterolateral portals by verifying good flow in a patient with soft-tissue distraction.

cessory portals are most useful when the posterior portal does not permit adequate visualization of the anterior compartment with instrumentation anterior, and vice versa. Accessory portals are also useful to provide a separate inflow to keep the capsule distended. Generally, this involves placing the arthroscope in the anterolateral portal and the shaver, grasper, or probes in the accessory anterolateral portal (Fig. 12-16). The anterior and posterior portals can be interchanged depending on the location of the pathology and are frequently used interchangeably in the case.

Diagnostic Examination

Once the portals have been established, visualization is done by means of a 13-point examination, starting from the anterior subtalar joint and going lateral and posterior. The examination is done the same way every time to ensure that no area is omitted from visualization and that pathology is not missed.

After the arthroscope is inserted through the anterolateral portal and the inflow through the posterolateral portal, the anterior portion of the posterior subtalar joint is visualized (Fig. 12-17). Initially visu-

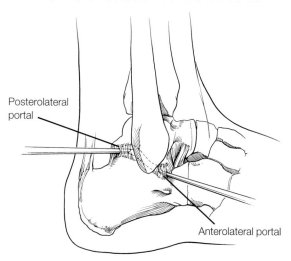

FIGURE 12–14.

While looking from the posterolateral portal, the joint can be probed through the anterolateral portal.

alized is area 1, the deep interosseous talocalcaneal ligament (1A and B). Area 2 is the more superficial portion of the interosseous talocalcaneal ligament. The interosseous talocalcaneal ligament separates the posterior subtalar joint from the sinus tarsi and anterior subtalar joint. The articulation of the anterior portion of the posterior subtalar joint is seen in areas 3A and B. Area 4 is the anterolateral corner of the joint. Area 5 is the lateral gutter, with the reflection of the lateral talocalcaneal ligament seen anterior to the calcaneofibular ligament (5A and B). The reflection of the calcaneofibular ligament is seen more posteriorly in the lateral gutter in area 6. The lateral talocalcaneal and calcaneofibular ligaments form the lateral support for the capsule and subtalar joint.

The arthroscope is then exchanged into the posterolateral portal, with inflow through the anterolateral portal. Visualization from the posterior portal of the posterior subtalar joint is done in a sequential manner, going from lateral to medial (Fig. 12-18). If the subtalar joint is distracted significantly, the interosseous talocalcaneal ligament can be seen as well as the anterior capsular ligament. More commonly, visualization starts while viewing the lateral gutter and the capsular reflections of the lateral talocalcaneal ligament and calcaneofibular ligament (areas 5 and 6). The articulation of the midportion

of the talus and calcaneus is assessed in area 7. Area 8 is the posterolateral gutter; this area is carefully assessed for synovitis and loose bodies (8A and B). The posterolateral recess and the posterior gutter are then carefully evaluated in the normal bare area where the articulation ends, and the posterior corner of the talus is assessed (areas 9 and 10). The posteromedial recess is seen in area 11. Area 12 is the most posteromedial corner of the talocalcaneal joint that can be seen arthroscopically (12A and B). Area 13 is the most posterior aspect of the talocalcaneal joint; in this region. The Stieda process or os trigonum is visualized on the talus (13A and B).

Postoperatively, the wounds are closed with 4-O nylon stitches and a compression dressing and posterior splint is applied. The splint and stitches are removed at 5 to 7 days and range of motion exercises are begun. A compressive below-the-knee stocking is also used postoperatively while swelling is resolving.

The surgery is done on an outpatient basis and the patient is discharged 1 to 2 hours after surgery.

PATHOLOGY

Subtalar arthroscopy can be used for a variety of indications, as discussed above.

For patients with chronic pain over the os trigonum that is unresponsive to conservative care, and positive x-ray and bone scan changes, subtalar arthroscopy is indicated (Fig. 12-19*A,B*). The os trigonum is best visualized from the posterolateral portal, using the accessory posterolateral portal for instrumentation and the anterolateral portal for inflow. Alternatively, a 70° arthroscope can be used from the anterolateral portal to look around the corner to see the os trigonum, and instrumentation can be done posterolaterally. The os trigonum is evaluated with a probe and also dynamically, by moving the ankle and subtalar joints. A nonunion of the os trigonum reveals significant motion at its fibrous attachment to the talus and irregularity and sometimes chondromalacia and fibrosis at its insertion (see Fig. 12-19*C,D*). Extreme caution is needed when excising the os trigonum to avoid injuring the flexor hallucis longus and neurovascular bundle, which are just medial to it. A banana knife is inserted and the fibrous attachments to the talus are released (see Fig.

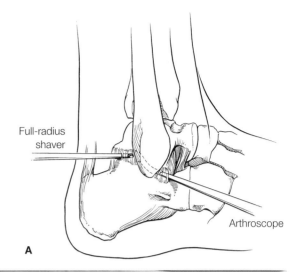

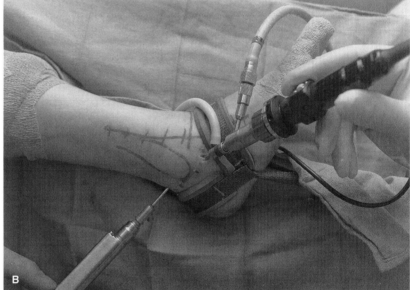

FIGURE 12-15.
Intraarticular shaving. (**A**) Using interchangeable cannulae, the arthroscope and shaver can be moved between the anterior and posterior portals. (**B**) With the two-portal technique, inflow goes through the arthroscope sheath and exits via the intraarticular shaver.

12-19*E*). A shaver and reverse-angle curette are then used to free the os trigonum to release the surrounding ligaments and capsule and "shell it out" (see Fig. 12-19*F,G*). Instruments should be used only under direct visualization. Once the fragment is loose, it is removed with a grasper (see Fig. 12-19*H,I*). Postoperatively, the patient is immobilized in a below-the-knee cast or removable cast boot for 3 to 4 weeks, followed by a rehabilitation program.

Subtalar arthroscopy can also be used to evaluate osteochondral lesions of the talocalcaneal joint (Fig. 12-20*A,B*). If the lesion is loose and nonviable, it is excised and then abraded or drilled (see Fig. 12-20*C,D*). These patients are usually kept non-weight-bearing and then are begun on range of motion and strengthening exercises.

The most common indication for subtalar arthroscopy is chronic pain in the posterior subtalar joint and sinus tarsi after a single or repeated inversion sprain of the ankle and subtalar region. The exact location of chronic postsprain pain can be difficult to determine positively because of the close proximity of the sinus tarsi, subtalar joint, and inferior aspect of

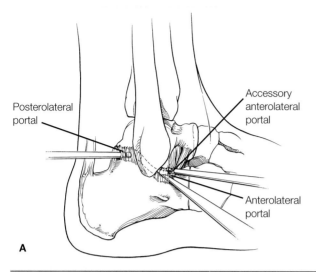

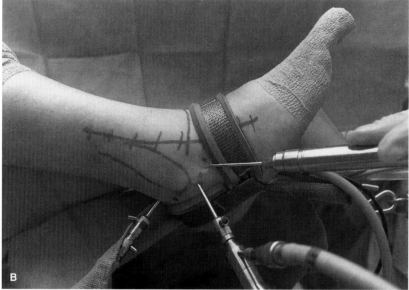

FIGURE 12-16.
Three-portal technique. (**A**) Using a separate portal for inflow gives better joint distention with the use of the shaver. (**B**) On this patient, the arthroscope is in the accessory anterolateral portal, the shaver is in the anterolateral portal, and inflow is in the posterolateral portal.

the lateral gutter of the ankle (see Fig. 12-1*A*). Selective injections can assist in determining the location of the pain and the appropriate treatment. Posterior subtalar fibrosis and scarring is amenable to arthroscopic debridement and synovectomy (Fig. 12-21).

Sinus tarsi syndrome was first described by O'Connor in 1958.[12] About 70% of the cases involve trauma, usually a significant inversion sprain of the ankle. The exact etiology is not clearly defined, but scarring and degenerative changes to the soft-tissue structures of the sinus tarsi are thought to be the most common causes of pain in this region[13–16] (see

Fig. 12-5). The presence of nerve endings in the ligamentous tissue within the sinus and tarsal canals suggest the possibility that injury to these nerves and loss of their proprioceptive function could be a factor in this condition.[17]

Clinically, these patients have pain in the lateral side of their foot, in the area of the lateral opening of the sinus tarsi, that is most severe with deep palpation, standing, and walking on uneven ground, and during rotation of the subtalar joint. The patient may also have a feeling of instability or giving way of the ankle, particularly on uneven surfaces. Injec-

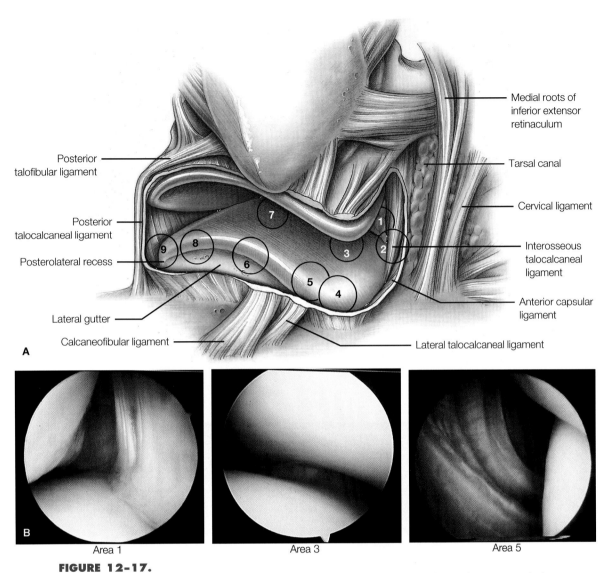

Medial roots of
inferior extensor
retinaculum

Tarsal canal

Cervical ligament

Interosseous
talocalcaneal
ligament

Anterior capsular
ligament

Lateral talocalcaneal ligament

Posterior
talofibular ligament

Posterior
talocalcaneal ligament

Posterolateral recess

Lateral gutter

Calcaneofibular ligament

A

B

Area 1

Area 3

Area 5

FIGURE 12-17.
Six-point examination of the subtalar joint (viewed from the anterolateral portal). (**A**) Lateral view. The posterior subtalar joint is examined starting at the most medial portion of the talocalcaneal joint, progressing laterally and then posteriorly. (**B**) Arthroscopic views at positions 1, 3, and 5.

tion of a local anesthetic into the sinus tarsi usually alleviates the pain and feeling of instability for several hours, but routine x-rays and stress examinations reveal no evidence of instability of the ankle or subtalar region.[18]

Because pain in the ankle and subtalar joint is hard to differentiate, patients with such complaints usually undergo arthroscopy of both areas concurrently. In patients with chronic sprain pain, the sub-

talar joint has been found to be normal, with pathology localized to the lateral gutter of the ankle.[11] If subtalar fibrosis and scarring is found, it is debrided as needed. In patients with sinus tarsi syndrome, part of the interosseous ligament, cervical ligament, and fibrofatty tissue is removed in the lateral 1 to 1.5 cm of the sinus to avoid injury to the blood supply of the talus[18] (Fig. 12-22). In these patients, a short-leg

(*text continues on page 250*)

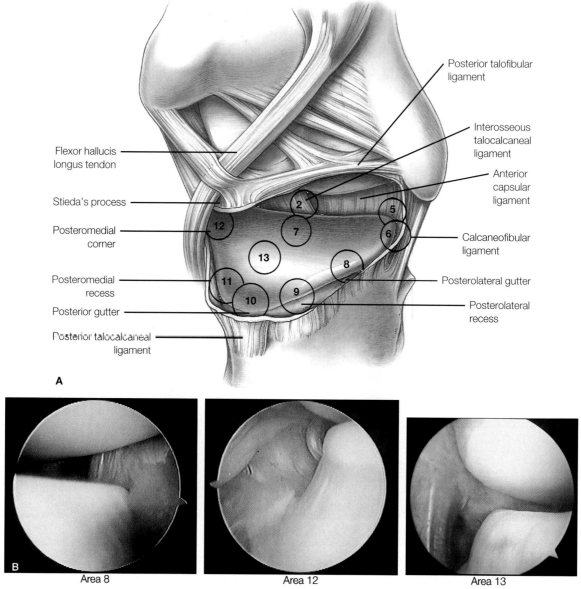

Posterior talofibular
ligament

Interosseous
talocalcaneal
ligament

Anterior
capsular
ligament

Calcaneofibular
ligament

Posterolateral gutter

Posterolateral
recess

Flexor hallucis
longus tendon

Stieda's process

Posteromedial
corner

Posteromedial
recess

Posterior gutter

Posterior talocalcaneal
ligament

A

Area 8

Area 12

Area 13

FIGURE 12-18.

Seven-point examination of the subtalar joint (viewed from the posterolateral portal). (**A**) The posterior examination starts by visualizing along the lateral gutter, going posterolaterally, then posteriorly and medially, and ending centrally. (**B**) Arthroscopic views at positions 8, 12, and 13.

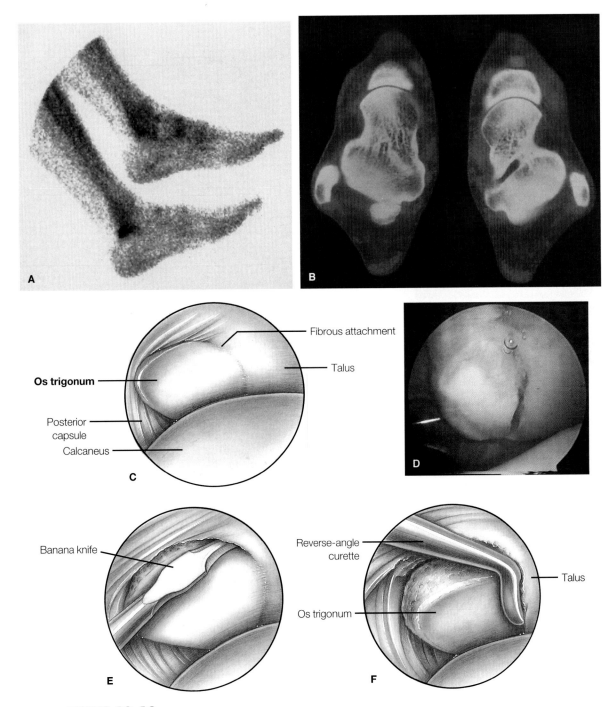

FIGURE 12-19.

Excision of os trigonum. (**A**) Bone scan demonstrates marked increased activity of the os trigonum, representing a nonunion in this area. (**B**) Axial bilateral hindfoot CT scan showing the os trigonum present on the right ankle but absent on the left. (**C**) The os trigonum has a fibrous attachment that can be well seen with subtalar arthroscopy. (**D**) In symptomatic patients, a large gap can exist between the os trigonum and posterior talus. (**E**) A banana knife is used to release the soft-tissue attachments to the os trigonum, using extreme care to avoid injuring the flexor hallucis longus and neurovascular bundle medially. (**F**) Reverse-angle curettes are useful in this area to release soft-tissue attachments to the os trigonum. (**G**) While visualizing from the anterolateral portal, the reverse-angle curette can be inserted through the posterolateral portal. (**H**) Once the os trigonum is free, it is removed with a grasper. (**I**) As the os trigonum is removed from the subtalar joint, the flexor hallucis longus is well seen.

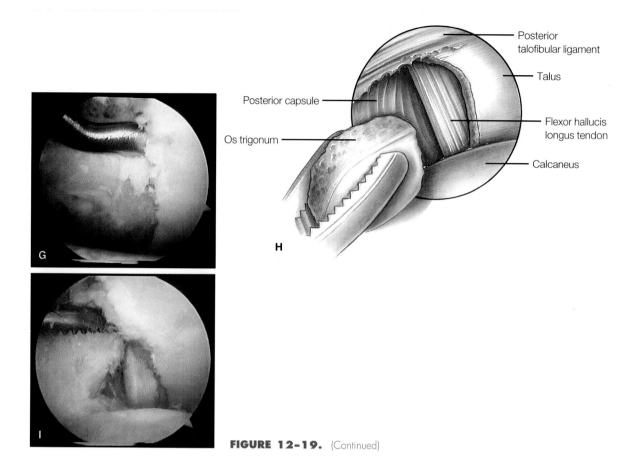

FIGURE 12-19. (Continued)

cast or removable walking boot is worn for 3 to 4 weeks, and then rehabilitation is instituted.

Arthrodesis of the subtalar joint is a newer application of subtalar arthroscopy. The indications for subtalar arthrodesis are similar to those for ankle fusion, and patients with persistent unremitting pain that does not respond to conservative methods are candidates for this procedure. Ideally, they should have degenerative changes localized only to the subtalar joint, such as after a calcaneal fracture, and the talonavicular and calcaneocuboid joints are normal. The procedure is indicated in subtalar joints that do not have significant angular or rotatory deformity, significant bone loss, or severe ankylosis.

The primary fusion is done in the posterior talocalcaneal facet, which is the largest facet in the subtalar joint. It is easily accessible and makes up most of the surface area of the subtalar joint. It is not as important to try to fuse the middle facet, although

this can be done after resecting the contents of the sinus tarsi. The anterior facet of the subtalar joint is even more difficult to reach arthroscopically and generally is not fused.

The technique for subtalar arthroscopic arthrodesis includes the use of joint distraction; Tasto has reported that inserting a lamina spreader in the sinus tarsi opens the posterior subtalar joint significantly wider, allowing easier instrumentation.[19] Two anterior portals are used for instrumentation, and the posterior portal is used for inflow. The soft tissues are debrided and removed, and the articular surfaces of the talocalcaneal joint are resected with a ring curette and shaver. A burr is used to abrade the surfaces lightly to good bleeding bone. The middle facet can be resected in a similar manner after all soft tissue has been removed from the sinus tarsi region. The foot is then put in the appropriate position (about 5° valgus) and the joint is compressed together. A small incision is made medial to the ante-

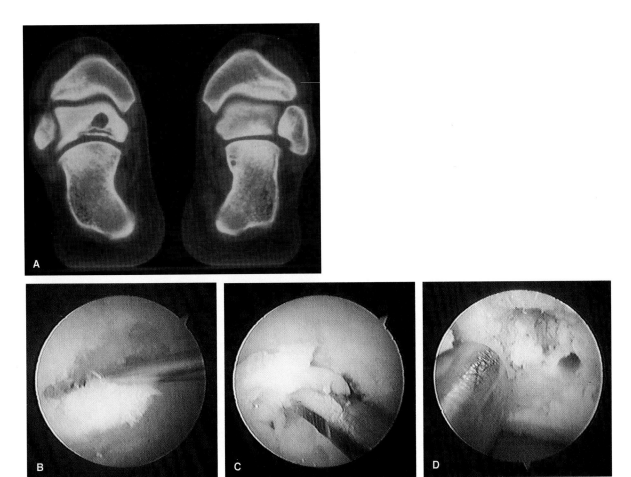

FIGURE 12-20.
Osteochondral lesion of the talus. (**A**) Bilateral hindfoot coronal CT scan demonstrating osteochondral lesion of a large portion of the articular surface of the inferior talus, with a large cyst superior to the defect. (**B**) Arthroscopic probing of the lesion. (**C**) The lesion is debrided with a banana knife. (**D**) Once the loose osteochondral lesion has been removed, drilling is accomplished through a small-joint cannula.

rior tibial tendon and the anterosuperior aspect of the talar neck is exposed. Using an anterior cruciate ligament drill guide, a ⅛" guide pin is inserted superiorly from the talar neck across the talocalcaneal joint to exit just lateral to the Achilles tendon on the inferior lateral aspect of the calcaneus. The pin is then drilled out the calcaneus until its tip is flush with the talar neck. The length of the screw is then determined, and a self-drilling, self-tapping 6.5-mm cannulated cancellous screw is inserted over the guide pin in a retrograde fashion, so that the screw head is in the calcaneus and the threads are flush with the talar neck (Fig. 12-23).

The wounds are then closed with nonabsorbable

suture and the patient is placed in a well-padded posterior splint. At 1 week, the stitches are removed and the patient is placed in a short-leg (non-weight-bearing) cast for an additional 2 weeks. A weight-bearing cast or removable cast boot is then applied for an additional month. At this point, the cast boot is continued until clinical and radiologic union has been achieved.

Recently Tasto reported on his technique of subtalar arthrodesis in nine patients.[19] His patients were placed in the lateral decubitus position and standard anterolateral and posterolateral portals were established. As previously mentioned, a small lamina spreader was inserted through the anterolateral portal into the sinus

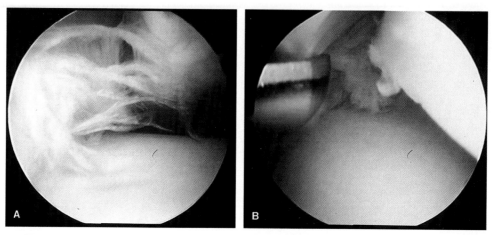

FIGURE 12-21.
Fibrosis of the subtalar joint. (**A**) Arthroscopic view of torn portions of the interosseous ligament of the left subtalar joint. (**B**) After debridement of the interosseous ligament and removal of scar tissue, the remaining joint looks clean.

tarsi to provide internal skeletal distraction. The average follow-up in Tasto's study was 17 months, and the average time to union was 10 weeks. There were no nonunions or other complications.

RESULTS

I have performed subtalar arthroscopy on 75 patients, and recently the first 50 patients were studied.[19] These patients were followed for an average of 32 months (range 16 to 51 months). In 21 patients with chronic lateral ankle pain, the subtalar joints were completely normal. The remaining 29 patients had the following diagnoses at arthroscopy: synovitis, 7; degenerative joint disease, 5; subtalar dysfunction (sinus tarsi syndrome), 5; chondromalacia, 4; os trigonum nonunion, 4; arthrofibrosis, 2; loose bodies, 1; and osteochondral lesion of the talus, 1. Overall, 86% had good or excellent results. The results were affected by the amount of degenerative change, the associated

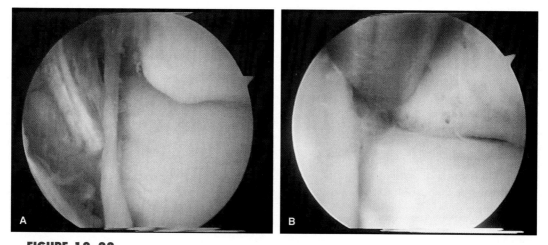

FIGURE 12-22.
Sinus tarsi syndrome. (**A**) Left subtalar joint with previous tear of the interosseous ligament and scarring along the interosseous ligament and sinus tarsi region. (**B**) Arthroscopic debridement of the sinus tarsi and interosseous ligament with the intraarticular shaver.

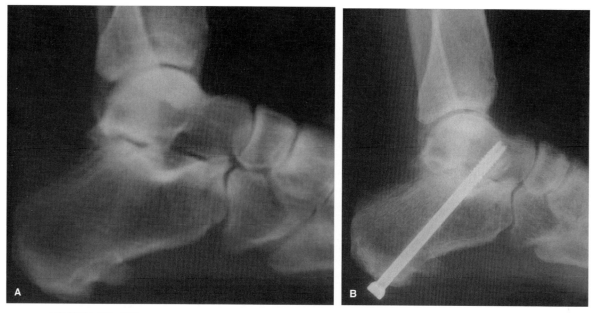

FIGURE 12-23.
Subtalar arthrodesis. (**A**) Preoperative lateral x-ray of a patient with a previous calcaneal fracture and persistent pain isolated to the subtalar joint. (**B**) Postoperative x-ray 6 months after subtalar arthrodesis, showing the posterior subtalar joint to be completely fused.

ankle pathology, and the patient's age and activity level. There were no major complications.

FUTURE

Arthroscopy of the subtalar joint is still in its early stages of development. Arthroscopy of the subtalar joint represented 14% of the arthroscopies of the foot and ankle done between 1984 and 1994 in my practice. As instrumentation improves and experience increases, this technology will expand. In the future, evaluation of subtalar dysfunction and sinus tarsi syndrome will be improved through the use of subtalar arthroscopy. In addition, arthrodesis of the subtalar, calcaneocuboid, and talonavicular joints will become more common as better techniques evolve for patients with little or no angular deformity.

REFERENCES

1. Parisien JS, Vangsness T. Arthroscopy of the subtalar joint: an experimental approach. Arthroscopy 1985;1:53.

2. Parisien JS. Arthroscopy of the subtalar joint. In Guhl J, ed. Arthroscopy of the ankle. Thorofare, NJ: Slack, 1988:133.

3. Parisien JS. Arthroscopy of the posterior subtalar joint. In Jahss MH, ed. Disorders of the foot and ankle. Philadelphia: WB Saunders, 1991:230.

4. Cahill DR. The anatomy and function of the contents of the human tarsal sinus and canal. Anat Rec 1965;153:1.

5. Wood Jones F. The talocalcaneal articulation. Lancet 1944;24:241.

6. Last RJ. Specimens from the Hunterian Collections. 7. The subtalar joint (specimens S 100 1 and 2 100 2). J Bone Joint Surg 1952;34B:116.

7. Schmidt HM. Shape and fixation of band systems in human sinus and canalis tarsi. Acta Anat 1978; 102:184.

8. Viladot A, Lorenzo JC, Salazar J, et al. The subtalar joint: embryology and morphology. Foot Ankle 1984;5:54.

9. Harper MC. The lateral ligamentous support of the subtalar joint. Foot Ankle 1991;12:354.

10. Stephens MM, Sammarco GJ. The stabilizing role of the lateral ligament complex around the ankle and subtalar joints. Foot Ankle 1992;13:130.

11. Williams MM, Ferkel RD. Subtalar arthroscopy: in-

dications, technique, and results. Arthroscopy 1994; 10:345.

12. O'Connor D. Sinus tarsi syndrome—a clinical entity. J Bone Joint Surg 1958; 40A:720.
13. Meyer JM, Lagier R. Post-traumatic sinus tarsi syndrome: an anatomical and radiological study. Acta Orthop Scand 1977; 48:121.
14. Cahill DR. The anatomy and function of the contents of the human tarsal sinus and canal. Anat Rec 1965; 153:1.
15. Regnauld B. Sinus tarsi syndrome. In Regnauld B, ed. The foot: pathology, etiology, semiology, clinical investigation, and therapy. New York: Springer-Verlag, 1986:298.
16. Vidal J, Fassio B, Buscayret C, et al. Instabilite externe de la cheville. Importance de l'articulation sour-astragalienne: nouvelle technique de reparation (Lateral ankle instability. The importance of the subtalar joint: new technique of repair). Rev Chir Orthop 1974; 60:635.
17. Clanton TO, Schon LC. Athletic injuries to the soft tissues of the foot and ankle. In Mann RA, Coughlin MJ, eds. Surgery of the foot and ankle, 6th ed. St. Louis, CV Mosby, 1993:1095.
18. Taillard W, Meyer JM, Garcia J, et al. The sinus tarsi syndrome. Int Orthop 1981; 5:117.
19. Tasto JP. Subtalar arthrodesis. Presented at Arthroscopy Association of North America, Orlando, Florida, February 1995.

BIBLIOGRAPHY

Frey C, Gasser S, Feder K. Arthroscopy of the subtalar joint. Foot Ankle 1994; 15:425.
Lawrence SJ, Botte MJ. The sural nerve in the foot and ankle: an anatomic study with clinical and surgical implications. Foot Ankle 1994; 15:490.

Arthroscopic Surgery: The Foot and Ankle,
by Richard D. Ferkel.
Lippincott-Raven Publishers, Philadelphia © 1996.

13

Great-Toe Arthroscopy

Richard D. Ferkel

*I*n the past, evaluating the small joints of the foot, including the great toe, has been difficult, except by arthrotomy. With the advent of small-joint and extra-small-joint arthroscopes and instrumentation, arthroscopy of these small joints is now possible.

The use of the arthroscope in the great-toe metatarsophalangeal (MTP) joint was described originally by Watanabe and associates, who wrote about performing arthroscopy on 22 MTP joints as well as interphalangeal joints of the foot.[1] Yovich and McIlwraith discussed the use of the arthroscope to debride osteochondral fractures in MTP joints of horses in 1986.[2] Lundeen reported on 11 great-toe arthroscopies in the podiatry literature in 1987, but no results were given.[3] Bartlett described successful arthroscopic debridement of an osteochondritis dissecans lesion of the first metatarsal head.[4] Ferkel and Van Buecken detailed the technique in the first large-scale series of cases.[5]

GROSS ANATOMY

The first MTP joint is a chondroloid joint and is a source of frequent pathology. The MTP joint of the great toe is composed of the metatarsal head and neck, the proximal phalanx, and the medial and lateral sesamoids. The sesamoid complex consists of two sesamoid bones, eight ligaments, and seven muscles[6] (Figs. 13-1 through 13-3). Most of these structures are concentrated on the plantar surface of the joint. The dorsal surface of the MTP joint is dominated by the extensor hallucis longus tendon (EHL), which lies in the dorsal midline. The extensor hallucis brevis tendon is just plantar and lateral to the EHL. The sagittal hood spreads out from the tendon sheath, encasing the ligaments to form a confluence of thickened capsular tissue extending plantarward to the collateral ligaments in the midline both medially and laterally. These capsuloligamentous structures align at the equator of the joint. These fanlike structures extend from the upper condylar region of the first metatarsal head to the base of the proximal phalanx.

(text continues on page 258)

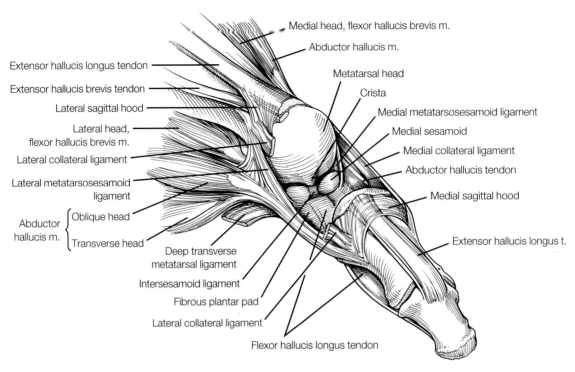

FIGURE 13-1.
Superolateral view of the bone–ligament–capsular anatomy of the metatarsophalangeal joint.

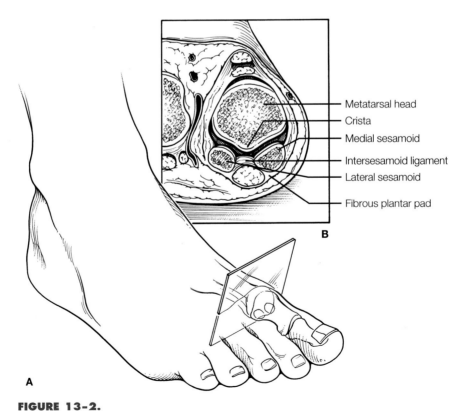

FIGURE 13-2.
Sesamoid position. (**A**) Plane of cross section to study the sesamoids. (**B**) Cross-sectional anatomy of the metatarsal head with the medial and lateral sesamoids separated by a small bony ridge, or crista.

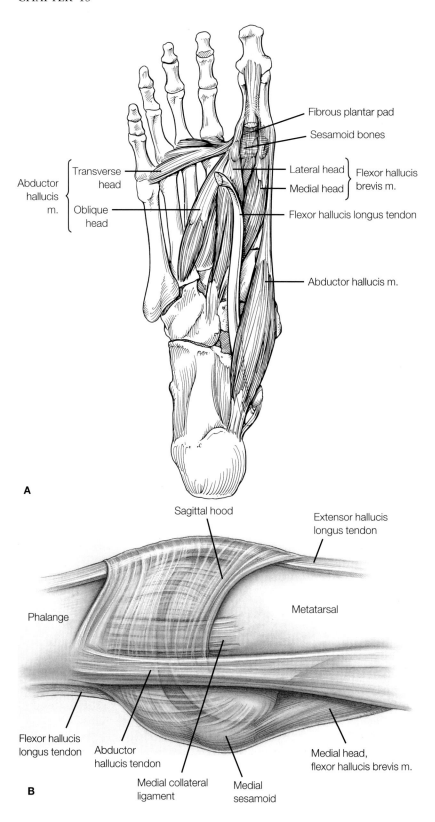

A

Fibrous plantar pad

Sesamoid bones

Abductor
hallucis
m. { Transverse head

Oblique head }

Lateral head

Medial head } Flexor hallucis brevis m.

Flexor hallucis longus tendon

Abductor hallucis m.

B

Sagittal hood

Extensor hallucis longus tendon

Phalange

Metatarsal

Flexor hallucis longus tendon

Abductor hallucis tendon

Medial collateral ligament

Medial sesamoid

Medial head, flexor hallucis brevis m.

FIGURE 13-3.
(**A**) Plantar view of the metatarsophalangeal joint with the surrounding muscles and tendons. (**B**) Medial view of the first metatarsophalangeal joint and surrounding anatomy, including the sagittal hood and the medial collateral ligament.

A small bony ridge or crista separates the two sesamoid bones as they lie in their respective grooves (see Figs. 13-1, 13-2). A dense plantar pad covers the sesamoids and anchors them to the proximal phalanx. The medial sesamoid is usually slightly more distal than the lateral one. This allows visualization more easily via the arthroscope. The sesamoids are encased by two heads of the flexor hallucis brevis tendons (see Figs. 13-1, 13-3A).

The capsuloligamentous complex of the MTP joint is the key factor contributing to its stability.[7] Minimal stability is offered by the bony architecture of the joint and long flexor and extensor tendons. The adductor and abductor hallucis tendons provide some support to the lateral and medial capsule, respectively; the short flexor and extensor tendons blend into the capsule and give strong stabilizing elements (see Figs. 13-1, 13-3A). The medial and lateral collateral ligaments provide strong support and have two components, the metatarsophalangeal and the metatarsosesamoid ligaments. The ligaments' origins are on the medial or lateral border of the metatarsal head and fan out onto the proximal phalanx and plantar plate[8] (see Fig. 13-3B). The arterial supply to the big toe is provided by the dorsal and plantar metatarsal arteries, branches of the dorsalis pedis artery (occasionally, the first plantar metatarsal artery is considered the terminal branch of the lateral plantar artery).[7] The dorsal medial vein of the big toe joins the medial arm of the dorsal venous arcade and contributes to the formation of the greater saphenous vein[9,10] (Figs. 13-4, 13-5A).

The superficial peroneal nerve provides much of the sensation to the great-toe MTP joint. It splits into a median, dorsal cutaneous branch above the ankle joint. This nerve then passes obliquely across the forefoot at the level of the first MTP joint. It has consistently been found to lie 2 to 5 mm plantar medial to the EHL. The medial plantar nerve appears between the abductor hallucis and the flexor digitorum brevis and gives off a proper digital nerve to the great toe and the three common digital nerves. This nerve innervates the medial and plantar aspect of the great toe. At the level of the MTP joint, it passes just plantar to the collateral ligament. On the lateral side of the great toe, the proper digital nerve lies beneath the transverse metatarsal ligament (see Figs. 13-4, 13-5B).

BIOMECHANICS

The importance of the great-toe MTP joint to weight bearing and gait is obvious. The great toe supports more than twice the load of the lesser toes, with the maximum force reaching 40% to 60% of body weight in normal walking.[11-13] During running and jumping, these forces are increased proportionally.[14] The instant center of motion for the first MTP joint falls within the first metatarsal head.[12] With range of motion of the MTP joint, a gliding motion occurs at the joint surface.

INDICATIONS FOR ARTHROSCOPY

The diagnostic indications for arthroscopy of the great-toe MTP joint include persistent pain, swelling, stiffness or locking, or grinding symptoms despite conservative treatment. The therapeutic indications include treatment of chondromalacia, synovitis, osteochondral lesions, osteophytes, loose bodies, arthrofibrosis, and perhaps in the future arthrodesis. The contraindications include the presence of infection, advanced degenerative joint disease, severe edema, or poor vascular status.

PORTALS

Three portals are commonly used in arthroscopy of the great-toe MTP joint: dorsomedial, dorsolateral, and medial (Figs. 13-6, 13-7). The dorsomedial portal is placed just medial to the EHL at or slightly distal to the joint line. Care must be taken when establishing this portal to avoid injury to the medial dorsal cutaneous branch of the superficial peroneal nerve. The dorsolateral portal is placed just lateral to the EHL at or just distal to the joint line. Because the proper digital nerve lies beneath the transverse metatarsal ligament, the nerve is usually not in danger with the placement of this portal. The medial portal is placed through the medial capsule, midway between the dorsal and plantar aspects of the joint. It is usually established under direct vision because of the narrowness of the space in which it lies. In addition, extreme caution must be taken to avoid injury to the surrounding neurovascular structures.

INSTRUMENTATION

Because of the small size of the great-toe MTP joint, small instrumentation is mandatory. A short 2.7- or 1.9-mm arthroscope is used with a 30° obliquity. An interchangeable cannula system is used so that the arthroscope and shaver can be shifted from one portal to another without repeated punctures into the capsule (Fig. 13-8). To prevent injury to the articular surface or the arthroscope, a small, lightweight chip camera (videoscope) is preferred. The light source is the same as for standard arthroscopic procedures, but a smaller light cord may be necessary. Because of the size of this cord, breakage is easier, and replacement cords must be available at the time of surgery.

The shaver is an important tool for MTP arthroscopy. A small-joint system is needed that uses both 2.9- and 2.0-mm full-radius blades, burrs, and whiskers. Instruments ranging in size from 1.6 to

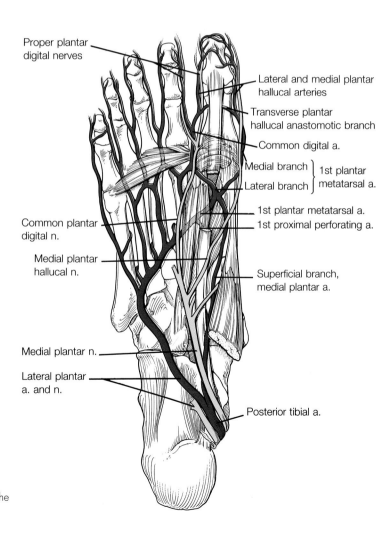

FIGURE 13-4.
Plantar view of the neurovascular supply of the great toe.

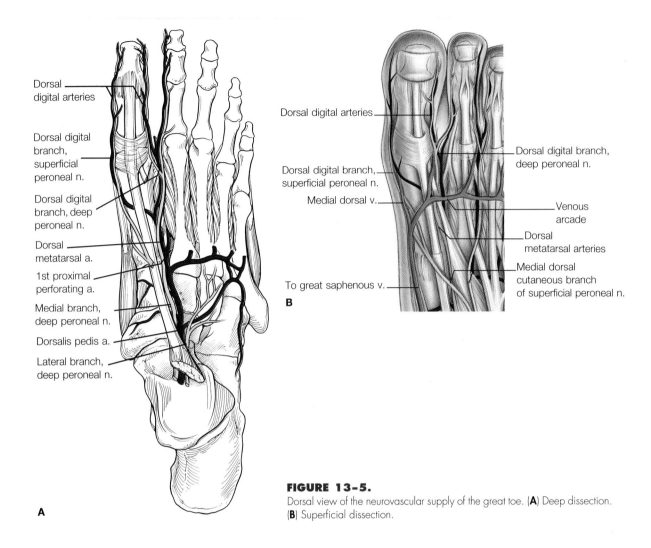

Dorsal
digital arteries

Dorsal digital
branch,
superficial
peroneal n.

Dorsal digital
branch, deep
peroneal n.

Dorsal
metatarsal a.

1st proximal
perforating a.

Medial branch,
deep peroneal n.

Dorsalis pedis a.

Lateral branch,
deep peroneal n.

Dorsal digital arteries

Dorsal digital branch,
superficial peroneal n.

Medial dorsal v.

To great saphenous v.

B

Dorsal digital branch,
deep peroneal n.

Venous
arcade

Dorsal
metatarsal arteries

Medial dorsal
cutaneous branch
of superficial peroneal n.

FIGURE 13-5.
Dorsal view of the neurovascular supply of the great toe. (**A**) Deep dissection.
(**B**) Superficial dissection.

A

2.3 mm in diameter are used. These include a probe, Freer, basket, grasper, and curette (Fig. 13-9).

DISTRACTION

The first MTP joint space is quite small, and its contours make certain aspects of it difficult to visualize. By using joint distraction, the entire joint can be examined and surgery performed without scuffing the articular surfaces. The distraction choices available include noninvasive and invasive techniques.

Noninvasive distraction can be applied either manually or from a fingertrap suspended from a pul-

ley attached to the ceiling or to a shoulder holder apparatus. Using the trap and suspension, adequate visualization can be obtained in most cases without difficulty. In a rare case (particularly in a multioperated toe) invasive distraction may be used with a mini-external fixation device. Suggested equipment for great-toe arthroscopy is listed in Table 13-1.

PREFERRED METHOD

Arthroscopy of the first MTP joint can be done under general, epidural, spinal, or local anesthesia. The patient is positioned supine with the foot pad

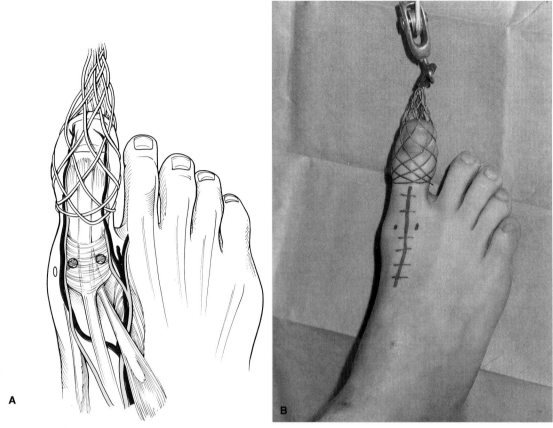

FIGURE 13-6.

Dorsal view of great-toe portals. (**A**) Note the position of the medial, dorsomedial, and dorsolateral portals to the surrounding tendons and neurovascular structures. (**B**) Dorsomedial and dorsolateral portals separated by the extensor hallucis longus tendon, with the toe suspended from a sterile device.

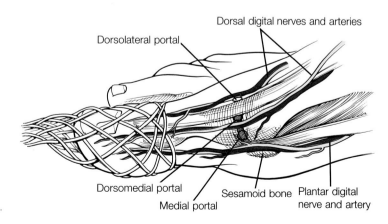

FIGURE 13-7.

Medial oblique view of great-toe portals.

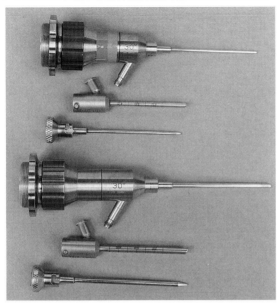

FIGURE 13-8.
Small-joint video arthroscopes. The 1.9-mm (*top*) and 2.7-mm (*bottom*) 30° oblique arthroscopes are used for great-toe arthroscopy.

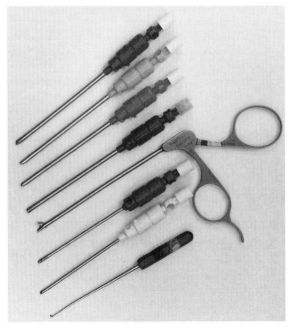

FIGURE 13-9.
Small-joint instruments (probe, basket, different-sized shaver blades) are used in great-toe arthroscopy.

TABLE 13-1.
SUGGESTED EQUIPMENT FOR GREAT-TOE ARTHROSCOPY

Tourniquet
Shoulder holder
Sterile toetrap
2.7- and 1.9-mm 30° arthroscopes
Sterile video cameras
Small-joint shaver system
2.0 full-radius and turbo whisker blades
2.9 full-radius and abrader blades
25-gauge 1.25" needles
10-cc syringe
2.0 baskets
2.0 probe
2.0 curette

Position: Supine with tourniquet; remove cassette and pad from end of table and pad opposite leg only; shoulder holder on opposite side of the table to suspend toe via trap.

removed from the operating table. A sterile toe trap is attached to the great toe and the end of the trap is suspended over a pulley by a rope, using the shoulder holder system. A counterweight is needed to elevate the foot slightly off the table. The use of a tourniquet is optional (Fig. 13-10).

After anesthesia is established, anatomic landmarks and portals are marked carefully before distending the joint. The dorsolateral portal is established first because of the absence of significant neurovascular structures in this area. A 19-gauge needle is placed in the joint just lateral to the EHL at or just distal to the joint line, and the joint is distended with normal saline. Before making the dorsolateral portal with a knife, a second 19-gauge needle is placed through the dorsomedial portal just medial to the extensor hallucis longus at or just distal to the joint line. Once adequate flow is established from one needle to the other, the dorsolateral incision is then made with a #11 blade (Fig. 13-11*A*). The incision is made only through the skin, and the soft tissues are spread bluntly with a mosquito clamp down to the capsule. A 2.9- or 2.0-mm cannula is then advanced into the joint using a blunt-tipped obturator.

The appropriate arthroscope is then inserted to inspect the joint (see Fig. 13-11*B,C*). Both 2.7-mm 30° oblique and 1.9-mm 30° oblique arthroscopes

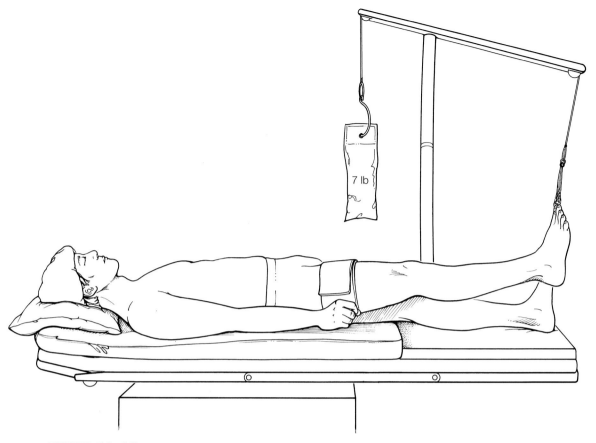

FIGURE 13-10.
Great-toe arthroscopy setup. The traction device is hung from the opposite side of the table to suspend the toe with the sterile trap.

have been used successfully. The larger scope gives improved picture clarity and allows greater fluid inflow via the cannula. The 1.9-mm 30° arthroscope allows easier maneuverability in tight joints without damaging the articular cartilage. Recent advances in arthroscope technology have provided the 1.9-mm arthroscope with an excellent picture quality not available in the past.

The dorsomedial portal is established just medial to the EHL, using the needle first. Extreme caution must be taken to spread the tissues to avoid injury to the dorsomedial branch of the superficial peroneal nerve, which lies just plantar to this portal. The straight medial portal is best established under direct vision by needle placement midway between the dorsal and plantar surfaces of the joint (see Fig. 13-11*D*). Because this portal is used to visualize both

the dorsal aspect of the joint and the sesamoids, placement is critical. Caution should be exercised to avoid injury to the medial proper plantar digital nerve.

The arthroscope and instruments are switched through the three portals to allow optimal visualization of the entire joint and to manage the intraarticular pathology (see Fig. 13-11*E*). Initially inflow is done through the side port on the arthroscopic cannula, using a 50-cc syringe and intravenous extension tubing. However, for efficiency, a high-flow system should be set up using 3-liter bags of lactated Ringer's solution attached to the cannula. The best flow is obtained when all three portals are used and inflow is directly made through a third cannula instead of the arthroscope sheath (see Fig. 13-11*F*).

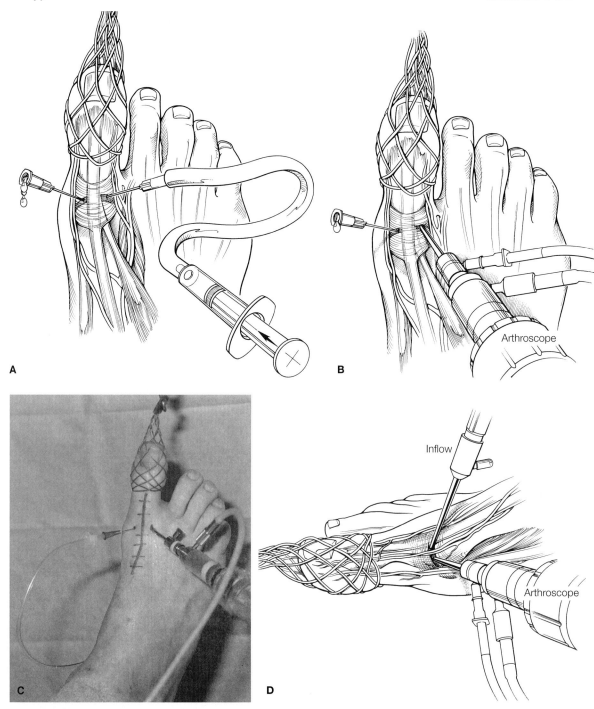

FIGURE 13-11.

Preferred method for great-toe arthroscopy. (**A**) The joint is distended from the dorsolateral portal and flow is verified with a needle through the dorsomedial. (**B**) The arthroscope is inserted through the dorsolateral portal to perform the diagnostic examination. (**C**) During the diagnostic examination, inflow is done through the arthroscope sheath and outflow through the dorsomedial portal. (**D**) The medial and plantar structures are best seen through the medial portal, especially the sesamoids. (**E**) Two-portal technique, with the shaver dorsolaterally and the arthroscope dorsomedially. (**F**) Inflowing through a third separate arthroscopic portal (three-portal technique) provides maximum joint distention and helps avoid the problem of joint-space collapse while using motorized instrumentation.

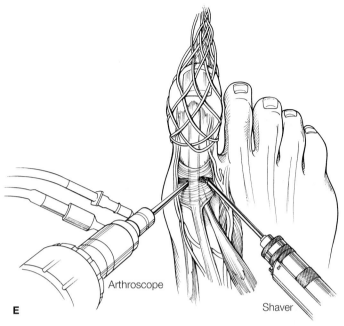

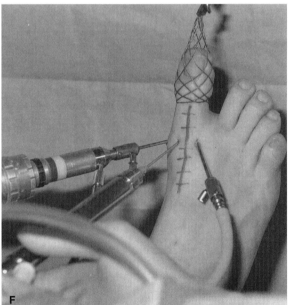

FIGURE 13-11. (Continued)

ARTHROSCOPIC ANATOMY

A systematic sequential examination of the MTP joint, starting lateral and progressing medially, is then performed by rotating the arthroscope and instruments through the three portals. A 13-point examination has been developed through the dorsolateral portal that includes the:

1. Lateral gutter
2. Lateral corner of the metatarsal head
3. Central portion of the metatarsal

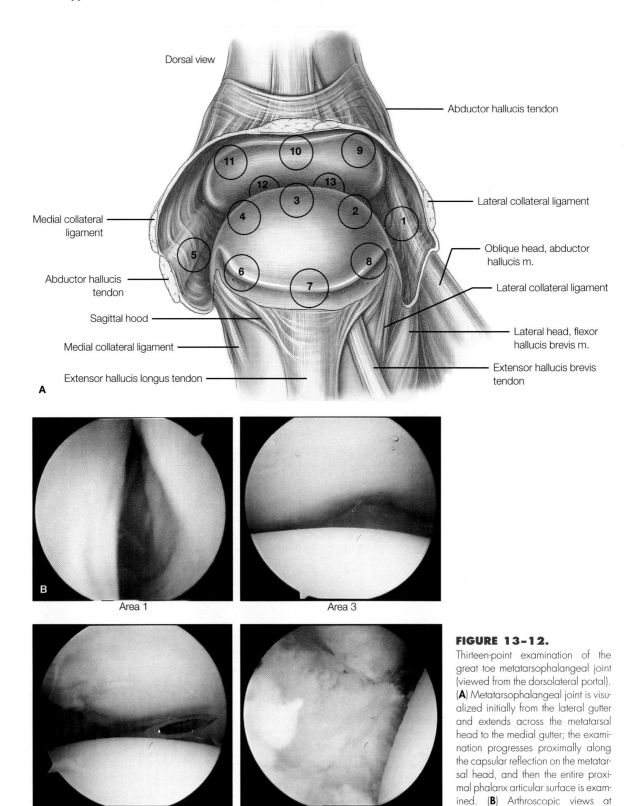

Dorsal view

Abductor hallucis tendon

Lateral collateral ligament

Medial collateral ligament

Oblique head, abductor hallucis m.

Lateral collateral ligament

Abductor hallucis tendon

Sagittal hood

Medial collateral ligament

Extensor hallucis longus tendon

Lateral head, flexor hallucis brevis m.

Extensor hallucis brevis tendon

A

B

Area 1

Area 3

Area 4

Area 5

FIGURE 13-12.

Thirteen-point examination of the great toe metatarsophalangeal joint (viewed from the dorsolateral portal). (**A**) Metatarsophalangeal joint is visualized initially from the lateral gutter and extends across the metatarsal head to the medial gutter; the examination progresses proximally along the capsular reflection on the metatarsal head, and then the entire proximal phalanx articular surface is examined. (**B**) Arthroscopic views at positions 1, 3, 4, and 5.

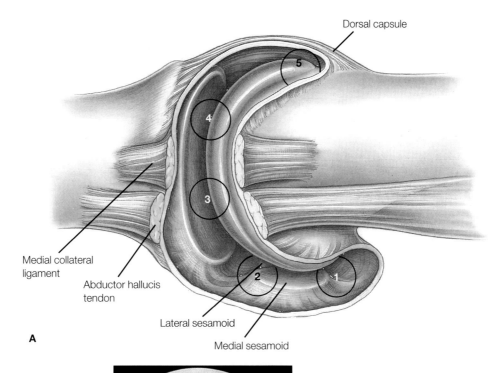

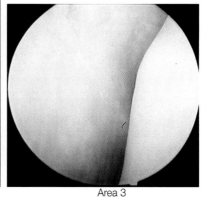

FIGURE 13-13.
Five-point medial examination of the great toe metatarsophalangeal joint (viewed from the medial portal, sagittal head removed). (**A**) The articulation of the metatarsal head with the sesamoids is visualized, and then the arthroscope is brought more centrally and superiorly to visualize the metatarsophalangeal joint. (**B**) Arthroscopic views at positions 2 and 3.

Area 2

Area 3

4. Medial corner of the metatarsal head
5. Medial gutter
6. Medial capsular reflection
7. Central bare area
8. Lateral capsular reflection
9. Medial portion of the proximal phalanx
10. Central portion of the proximal phalanx
11. Lateral portion of the proximal phalanx
12. Medial sesamoid
13. Lateral sesamoid (Fig. 13-12).

Certain portions of the joint may be better visualized through the dorsomedial or straight medial portals, particularly the plantar surfaces, including the sesamoids (through the straight medial portal).

The examination through the medial portal (five points) includes the posterior plantar capsule, the medial and lateral sesamoids, the central metatarsal head, the superior metatarsal head, and the dorsal capsular structures (Fig. 13-13).

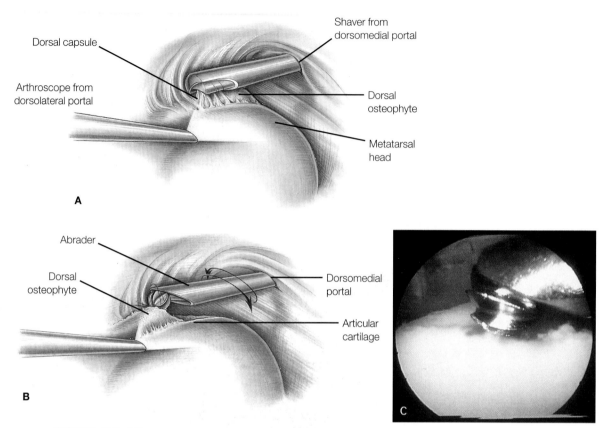

FIGURE 13-14.

Excision of dorsal osteophyte. (**A**) While looking from the dorsolateral portal, the shaver lifts the soft tissue off the osteophyte from the dorsomedial portal (viewed proximally from within metatarsophalangeal joint). (**B**) A small-joint abrader then removes enough osteophyte to permit adequate metatarsophalangeal joint dorsiflexion. (**C**) Arthroscopic view of osteophyte removal with a motorized burr. (**D**) Preoperative x-ray of a 19-year-old ballet dancer with pain over the dorsal aspect of the great toe metatarsophalangeal joint. (**E**) Postoperative x-ray at 1 week demonstrates adequate excision of the osteophyte and metatarsal head.

If a pathologic lesion is identified, a small-joint arthroplasty system and small-joint instruments are used (see Fig. 13-11*D*). The wounds are closed with one 4-0 nylon stitch and a bulky compressive foot dressing is applied for the first 4 days. This dressing can then be removed and a light dressing applied, using a wood-soled shoe until the swelling and pain are diminished. Stitches are usually removed in 7 to 10 days. The patient is started on range of motion and strengthening activities as soon as they are comfortable. As soon as swelling and pain are diminished in the MTP joint, a stiff-soled walking shoe may be substituted for the wooden postop shoe.

PATHOLOGY

Arthroscopy of the great toe can be used in several pathologic conditions, as mentioned above. The most common indication is treatment of degenerative joint disease of the MTP joint, including chondromalacia and dorsal osteophytes. Arthroscopic cheilectomy is indicated with mild to moderate dorsal osteophytes and only mild limitation of motion. With larger osteophyte formation and significant reduction in joint motion, a conventional cheilectomy is preferred.

Arthroscopic cheilectomy is performed using all three of the above-mentioned portals. Inflow is usually through the straight medial portal, visualization from the dorsolateral portal. The shaver is used from the dorsomedial portal to lift the soft tissue off the dorsal osteophyte dorsally and proximally (Fig. 13-14*A*). The small-joint burr is then inserted and the osteophyte is removed in its entirety from distal to proximal and medial to lateral. A small amount of the dorsal articular surface is also removed to help increase the postoperative range of motion (see Fig. 13-14*B,C*). After surgery, the patient is placed in a wood-soled shoe and is allowed to be partially weight-bearing with crutches.

One week postoperatively, the stitches are removed and a postoperative x-ray is performed and compared with the preoperative one (see Fig. 13-14*D,E*). The patient is placed in a light dressing, begins range of motion and strengthening exercises, and is encouraged to wear a flexible shoe 2 weeks postoperatively.

Great-toe arthroscopy is also useful in the evaluation and treatment of osteochondral lesions of the metatarsal head and proximal phalanx. Usually this lesion can be seen on plain x-rays, but sometimes only an MRI or CT scan will demonstrate its presence (Fig. 13-15*A–C*). At surgery, the lesion is evaluated and, if loose, is excised (see Fig. 13-15*D*). The exposed bone is then abraded with a small-joint abrader to a bleeding surface to stimulate the formation of new fibrocartilage (see Fig. 13-15*E,F*). Follow-up x-rays are done to monitor subsequent healing (see Fig. 13-15*G*).

Postoperatively, a compression dressing is used for 1 week, and then a light dressing is applied after the stitches are removed. The patient starts gentle range of motion and strengthening exercises 1 week postoperatively, but a wood-soled shoe is worn for 1 month to protect the MTP joint.

Arthroscopy of the great toe is also useful for

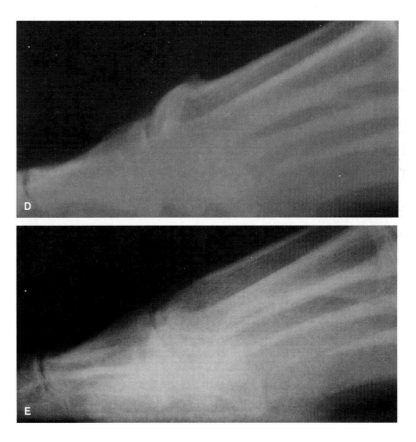

FIGURE 13-14. (Continued)

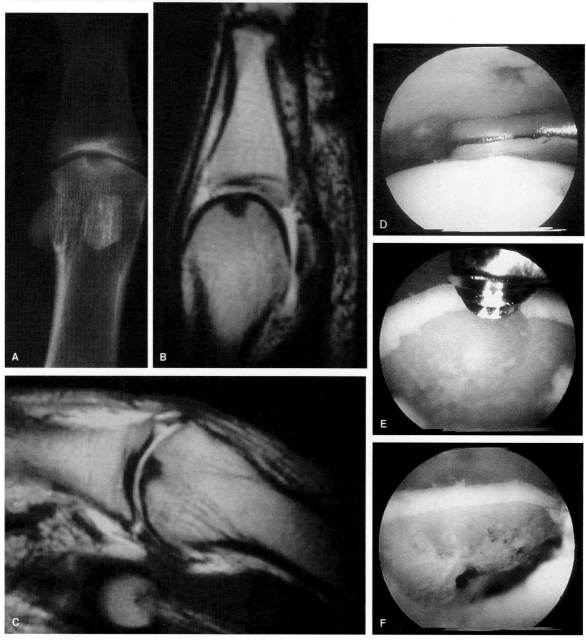

FIGURE 13–15.

Osteochondral lesion of the metatarsal head in a 35-year-old professional basketball player. (**A**) Preoperative antero-posterior x-ray demonstrates a cystic lesion on the central portion of the articular surface of the metatarsal head. (**B,C**) Preoperative gadolinium MRI scan of the first metatarsophalangeal joint (T1-weighted image). (**B**) Axial scan demonstrating a 4- to 5-mm low-signal-intensity subchondral lesion at the midportion of the first metatarsal head. The overlying articular cartilage appears intact because the lesion does not fill with gadolinium. (**C**) Sagittal MRI showing a low-signal-intensity osteochondral lesion of the metatarsal head. Although gadolinium did not leak into the lesion, arthroscopy found a flap tear of articular cartilage in this location. (**D**) Excision of the lesion using a small ring curette. (**E**) Abrasion arthroplasty performed with a small joint burr. (**F**) After abrading the osteochondral lesion of the metatarsal head, the tourniquet should be released and bleeding assessed. (**G**) Follow-up x-ray at 10 months demonstrates the osteochondral lesion to be healing, with minimal lucency now apparent.

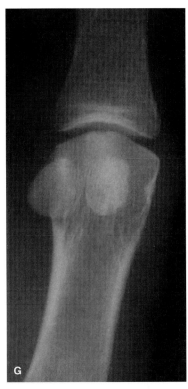

FIGURE 13-15. (Continued)

joint disease (5), arthrofibrosis (4), synovitis (3), osteophytes (3), osteochondral lesions of the metatarsal head (3), loose bodies (2), and chondromalacia (2). Results were graded as good, fair, and poor based on a rating system and our goal in surgery, which was to relieve pain and swelling, increase motion, and improve function. The overall results were 73% good, 13.5% fair, and 13.5% poor.

Many of the patients in the study had had previous surgery (41%), which made the surgery more difficult; however, most of these patients still noted improvement in their pain and limitations. Although improvement of range of motion was hard to correlate with ultimate results, overall patients improved an average of 7° in dorsiflexion and 6° in plantarflexion where they had a preoperative limitation. No complications were seen in this study, and all patients were done as outpatients.

The 3 patients rated fair and the 3 rated poor all had significant degenerative joint disease in their toes; the latter patients subsequently went on to have toe arthrodeses because of persistent pain.

FUTURE

Arthroscopy of smaller joints such as the great toe and lesser toes is still in its infancy. As instrumentation improves and experience increases, this technology will expand. In the future, arthrodesis of the great-toe joint appears feasible in certain isolated cases. In addition, we have done lesser-toe arthroscopy on patients with Freiberg's infarction of the second and third MTP joints with some success. Although technically difficult, it may be possible in the future also to perform simple bunionectomies arthroscopically. At present, arthroscopy of the great-toe MTP joint is not a common procedure: in my practice, between 1984 and 1994, only 4% (22/541) of all arthroscopies of the foot and ankle involved the great toe.

other conditions, including debridement of synovitis (especially gout), removal of loose bodies, and excision of scar tissue from the arthrofibrotic joint. This latter situation is usually created from a previous bunionectomy or fracture, with resultant joint stiffness and pain.

CLINICAL RESULTS

In my practice, 22 patients have had arthroscopy of the great MTP joint. There were 7 male and 15 female patients, with the right side operated on 14 times and the left side 8 times. The age of the patients at surgery ranged from 18 to 70 years (average 40 years). The average length of follow-up was 54 months (range 13 to 70 months), and 9 patients had previous open surgery. The time period from initial patient complaints of great-toe pain to surgery was 37 months. The primary postoperative diagnosis included degenerative

REFERENCES

1. Watanabe M, Ito K, Fuji S. Equipment and procedures of small-joint arthroscopy. In Watanabe M, ed.

Arthroscopy of small joints. New York: Igaku-Shoin, 1986:3.

2. Yovich JV, McIlwraith CW. Arthroscopic surgery for osteochondral fractures of the proximal phalanx, the metacarpophalangeal and metatarsophalangeal joints in horses. J Am Vet Med Assoc 1986;188:273.

3. Lundeen RO. Arthroscopic approaches to the joints of the foot. J Am Podiatr Med Assoc 1987;77:451.

4. Bartlett DH. Arthroscopic management of osteochondritis dissecans of the first metatarsal head. Arthroscopy 1988;4:51.

5. Ferkel RD, Van Buecken K. Great toe arthroscopy: indications, technique and results. Presented at Arthroscopy Association of North America, San Diego, April 1991.

6. Alvarez R, Haddad RJ, Gould N, Trevino S. The simple bunion: anatomy at the metatarsophalangeal joint of the great toe. Foot Ankle 1984;4:229.

7. Sarrafian SK. Anatomy of the foot and ankle, 2d ed. Philadelphia: JB Lippincott, 1993.

8. Clanton TO, Butler JE, Eggert A. Injuries to the metatarsophalangeal joints in athletes. Foot Ankle 1986;7:162.

9. Gilbert A. Composite tissue transfers from the foot: anatomic basis and surgical technique. In Symposium on microsurgery 14. St. Louis: CV Mosby, 1976:230.

10. Poirier P, Charpy A. Traite d'anatomie humaine, vol II. Paris: Masson, 1902:839.

11. Johnson KA, Buck PG. Total replacement of the first metatarsophalangeal joint. Foot Ankle 1981;1:307.

12. Sammarco GJ. Biomechanics of the foot. In Frankel VH, Nordin M, eds. Biomechanics of the skeletal system. Philadelphia: Lea & Febiger, 1980:193.

13. Stokes IAF, Hutton WC, Stott JRR. Forces under the hallux valgus foot before and after surgery. Clin Orthop 1979;142:64.

14. Nigg BM. Biomechanical aspects of running. In Nigg BM, ed. Biomechanics of running shoes. Champaign, IL: Human Kinetics, 1986:1.

BIBLIOGRAPHY

Acton RK. Surgical anatomy of the foot. J Bone Joint Surg 1967;49A:555.

Hamilton WG. Surgical anatomy of the foot and ankle. CIBA Clin Symp 37, 1985.

Jahss MH. The sesamoids of the hallux. Clin Orthop 1981;157:88.

Joyce JJ, Harty M. Surgical anatomy and exposure of the foot and ankle. In Wilson JC Jr, ed. American Academy of Orthopaedic Surgeons Instructional Course Lectures, XIX. St. Louis: CV Mosby, 1970:1.

Kelikian H, Kelikian AS. Correlative anatomy of the ankle joint. In Kelikian H, Kelikian AS, eds. Disorders of the ankle. Philadelphia: WB Saunders, 1985:1.

Mankey MG, Mann RA. Biomechanics of the first metatarsophalangeal joint. Sem Arthroplasty 1992;3:2.

Shereff MJ, Bejjani FJ, Kummer FJ. Kinematics of the first metatarsophalangeal joint. J Bone Joint Surg 1986;68A:392.

Arthroscopic Surgery: The Foot and Ankle,
by Richard D. Ferkel.
Lippincott-Raven Publishers, Philadelphia © 1996.

14

Foot and Ankle Rehabilitation

Melanie Reid and Richard D. Ferkel

Although much has been written about the rehabilitation of joints such as the knee and the shoulder, very little has been published regarding the functional rehabilitation of the foot and ankle. The purpose of this chapter is to present current concepts regarding rehabilitation to full function after an injury or surgery to the foot and ankle.

In the past, the full rehabilitation of this complex was often considered unnecessary because the foot was viewed as a static structure. Recently, however, the foot has gained increased respect and is now considered a keystone in maintaining bipedal posture and mobility. Roger Mann correctly defines the foot as "a dynamic mechanism functioning as an integral part of the locomotor system."[1]

As surgical techniques have advanced, it has become possible to salvage larger recovery potentials from an injured limb.[2,3] Consequently, rehabilitation has needed to keep pace, as improper or inadequate postoperative rehabilitation can seriously impair the recovery to maximum function.[4-9]

Function is defined by structure. An architect designs a structure to fulfill a functional purpose. Similarly, studying the foot's structure may lead to clues about its function. Once the purpose has been defined, then rehabilitation techniques may aim to restore as much function as possible.

Techniques sometimes change rapidly to stay in vogue with current trends. In the discussion that follows, we have tried to maintain perspective on the techniques used to treat an injured foot. The goal of the rehabilitation process is to restore the extremity to its maximum functional potential.

STRUCTURE AND FUNCTION

The anatomy of the foot and ankle has been well documented and was discussed in Chapter 5 (Fig. 14-1).

The talocrural joint (or ankle) is a modified hinge joint, working on a transverse axis to provide dorsiflexion and plantarflexion movements.[10-12] It unites the leg to the foot complex and is composed of three main bones—

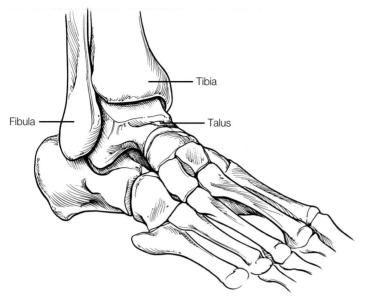

FIGURE 14-1.
Oblique drawing of the foot and ankle.

the tibia, fibula, and talus—firmly bound by strong ligaments. Included are the medial and lateral collateral ligaments, which assist by inhibiting unwanted inversion and eversion during weight bearing (WB) onto the joint (Fig. 14-2).

The foot complex is composed of much smaller bony elements, also bound by an integrated ligamentous system. Most proximal are the talus and calcaneus, also known as the hindfoot. The cuboid and navicular, articulating with the three cuneiforms,

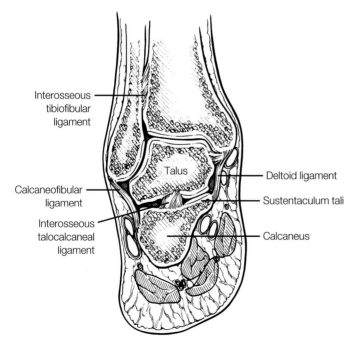

FIGURE 14-2.
Coronal cross section (anterior view) of the foot and ankle with the surrounding stabilizing ligaments.

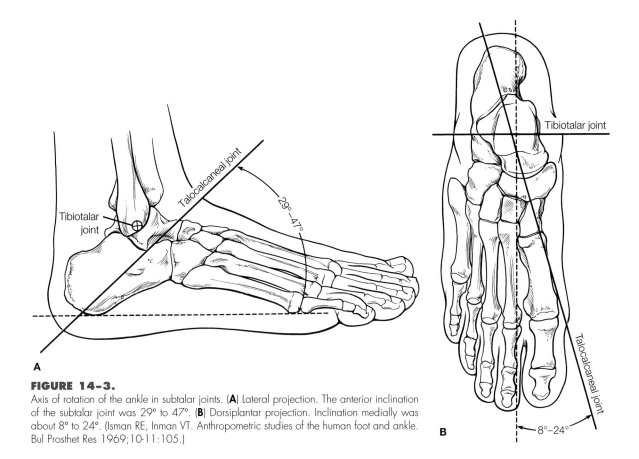

FIGURE 14–3.
Axis of rotation of the ankle in subtalar joints. (**A**) Lateral projection. The anterior inclination of the subtalar joint was 29° to 47°. (**B**) Dorsiplantar projection. Inclination medially was about 8° to 24°. (Isman RE, Inman VT. Anthropometric studies of the human foot and ankle. Bul Prosthet Res 1969;10-11:105.)

make up the midtarsal region. The five metatarsals, followed by the proximal and distal phalanges, are components of the forefoot.[13]

The vital subtalar joint is enclosed in the foot complex.[14] It is chiefly composed of the talus articulating with the calcaneus. The anterior talocalcaneal articulation is continuous with the talonavicular articulation, thus forming the foot's largest synovial joint. It moves around a triplanar oblique axis to provide the whole foot with pronation and supination in both WB and non-weight-bearing (NWB) positions[15] (Fig. 14-3). The movements that combine to produce pronation and supination are shown in Table 14-1. This joint is especially important in providing and accommodating the foot in normal gait patterns.

TABLE 14–1.
WEIGHT-BEARING AND NON-WEIGHT-BEARING POSITION OF THE FOOT

	CALCANEUS POSITION	FOREFOOT POSITION	ANKLE POSITION	TALUS POSITION
NWB supination	Inversion	Adduction	Plantar flexion	—
WB supination	Inversion	Adduction	Plantar flexion	Abduction
NWB pronation	Eversion	Abduction	Dorsiflexion	—
WB pronation	Eversion	Abduction	Dorsiflexion	Adduction

Reviewing the foot's role in locomotion provides a better understanding of its function[16] (Fig. 14-4). During walking, the foot is vital in the initial contact, midstance, and push-off phases. In initial contact, the heel hits the ground with a force 25% more than body weight. Electromyographic activity has been reported only in the anterior tibial muscles in this phase. Most of the impact appears to be absorbed during simultaneous subtalar pronation and tibial internal rotation.

In midstance, the body weight is transferred over the foot to prepare for push-off. Force-plate recordings substantiate that 50% to 60% of the body weight is placed on the foot at this stage. Muscular activity is high in the intrinsic foot muscles and posterior tibial muscles while the calcaneus begins to invert. It is accompanied by forefoot adduction, which initiates supination. This supination creates some rigidity to allow for weight transfers.[1,17,18]

In push-off, the foot load again exceeds 25% of the supported body weight on the other foot, as weight is transferred over. Muscular activity continues in the foot intrinsics and posterior tibial muscles to allow for pro-gressive supination of the forefoot. Toe extension in preparation for toe-off increases the plantar aponeurosis tension to assist in continued elevation of the medial longitudinal arch and supination (Table 14-2).

The functions of the foot complex may be divided into two main areas: stability and mobility. For stability, the foot is the static base of support for posture and also acts as a rigid lever to assist in push-off. Mobility, however, is dynamic and is demonstrated in three ways: dynamic shock absorption is magnified by the foot's flexible transmission and dispersion abilities; dynamic proprioceptive stability is noted while accommodating to uneven surfaces during WB;[19] and gait control is maintained, especially deceleration at initial contact.[10,11]

REHABILITATION MODALITIES

Again, the main goal of rehabilitation is to restore maximum functional potential.[20-22] The goals are the same after surgery or an acute injury, and whether the patient is an elite athlete or a sedentary

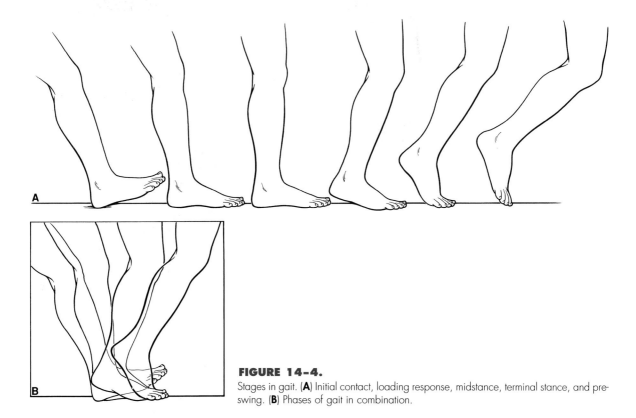

FIGURE 14-4.
Stages in gait. (**A**) Initial contact, loading response, midstance, terminal stance, and pre-swing. (**B**) Phases of gait in combination.

TABLE 14-2.
SUMMARY

	FORCE	+ EMG ACTIVITY	FOOT POSITION
Initial contact	25% excess of body weight	Anterior tibial	Pronation tibial Internal rotation
Midstance	50–60%	Intrinsic foot Posterior tibial	Supination
Push off	25% excess of body weight	Intrinsic foot Posterior tibial Toe extended	Supination

grandparent; however, age and lifestyle differences influence the expected maximum potentials.[23]

Electrical Stimulation Devices

Electrical stimulation devices (Fig. 14-5) offer variable wave forms, frequencies, and intensities.[24–26] Benefits from each device have not always been proven, but they provide some symptomatic relief.

Ice

Ice, an often-used modality, can influence the circulatory response in an acutely injured joint.[27] Its vasoconstrictive properties are used to alleviate acute swelling and effusion, and its anesthetic property is exceptionally beneficial.[28]

Massage

There are various styles of massage or soft-tissue manipulation, each with a particular goal. Effleurage massages are light, using a circular technique to encourage more efficient circulation. Myofascial release techniques aim to influence proper soft-tissue matrix alignment mechanically in healing tissue. It can be more aggressive and forceful than effleurage.

Joint Mobilization

There are various techniques and approaches (Fig. 14-6), but all have similar goals. The two purposes of joint mobilization are to restore accessory joint movement, aiding the return of the active movement range and minimizing muscle atrophy and the formation of scar tissue; and to improve circulation to the joint by augmenting physiologic healing.[11,29–31]

Heat

Heat can be presented in numerous forms. The standard hydroculator is commonly used. The effects of ultrasound have not been thoroughly documented in recent literature, but its thermal properties continue to benefit the injured joint.[27] Both ultrasound and electrical stimulation can be used to help transfer certain medications across the skin's porous surface. Phonophoresis (the cutaneous transmission of medication using ultrasound energy) and iontophoresis (the electrical dispersion of ions across a permeable membrane [skin]) can provide symptomatic relief when used within the correct parameters.[24,25,32]

Exercises

Therapeutic exercises offer an advantage over other passive modalities.[23,33–35] Exercises can involve active participation by the patient to help retrain the in-

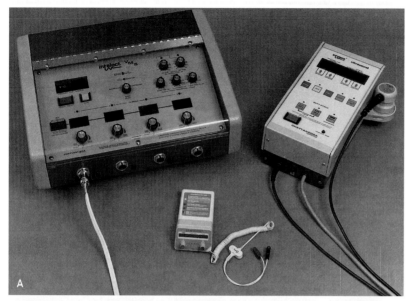

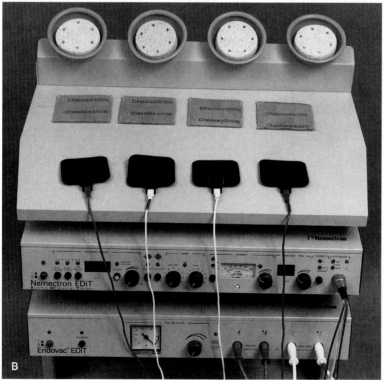

FIGURE 14-5.

Rehabilitation modalities. (**A**) The VMS Electrical Stimulation device, used for pain, swelling, and muscle reeducation (*left*); Phoresor plantarphoresis, used to deliver medication for pain control (*center*); ultrasound, used with aquatic gel or with a medication for phonophoresis (*right*). (**B**) Interferential stimulation unit used for pain and swelling management.

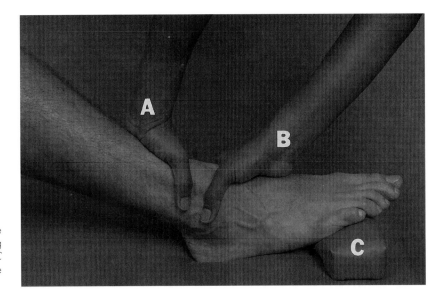

FIGURE 14-6.
A posterior glide of the talus on the tibia and fibula. *A* is the stabilizing force. *B* is the mobilizing force. *C* is used to help position and rest the foot.

jured limb and gain full function. Such active participation can contribute to improved carryover and patient compliance with a home program once formal rehabilitation is completed.

There are four main types of exercises.

Passive Exercises

Passive exercises involve no voluntary muscle contraction by the patient. They are used to increase range of motion within the joint, to stress healing ligamentous structures gently to avoid excessive scar formation, and to facilitate mild nutritional changes in the cartilage by improving circulation with increased range of motion.

Active-Assisted Exercises

Active-assisted exercises initiate voluntary muscle contraction to begin the reeducation process. If a painful arc is present in the available range of motion, the assistance given can allow the patient to maintain an improved physiologic range of motion instead of being completely limited by a painful end range.

Active Exercises

Active exercises involve full patient participation. They are usually started once full pain-free passive range of motion has been obtained. Active exercises can train eccentric and concentric muscle contractions. Eccentric contractions load an elongating muscle; concentric contractions load a shortening muscle. Eccentric training is essential to return a patient to any stop-and-go sport that involves rapid deceleration and quick changes in direction (eg, football, racquetball, tennis). Concentric training, although important, does not form the major part of normal activity.

Resistive Exercises

Resistive exercises retrain strength and power by progressively increasing the weight and the rate of movement throughout the available range.[36] These exercises can be used to develop selective hypertrophy within a muscle group. Muscle fiber tension is progressively trained by slowing the rate of contraction while increasing the resistance.

Passive and active-assisted exercises are commonly used when a joint is acute and rigid. Figures 14-7 and 14-8 demonstrate exercises used to improve mobility and flexibility in the injured joint.

Active and resistive exercises may be subdivided further into the following four categories:

Isometric Exercises

Isometric exercises involve voluntary muscle contraction without stretching or increasing joint range of motion. The compressive joint forces ob-

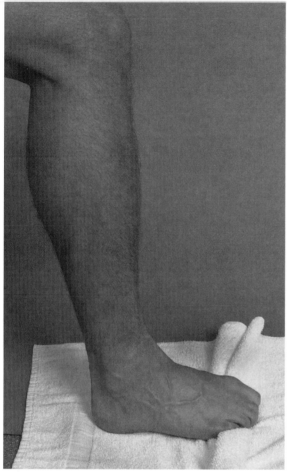

FIGURE 14-7.
Active toe flexion while "curling" a towel.

tained here are vital to improve nutrition to an immobilized joint. These exercises can develop more muscle tension than some resistive exercises, but they strengthen the muscles only at a given range. Multiangle isometrics are commonly used to avoid retraining only at one particular range, but these may be used only after the joint can safely accept stressing range of motion.

Isotonic Exercises

Isotonic exercises can initiate aerobic conditioning, as they can use faster muscle contraction rates by training voluntary muscle recruitment efficiency.

Eccentric and concentric muscle retraining can be used with these exercises.

Isokinetic Exercises

In isokinetic exercises, maximum resistance is maintained throughout the range to ensure that full work is completed at all angles of the range.[8,37,38] Various equipment is available; Cybex, Orthotron, KinCom, Biodex, and Lido offer software packages to allow biofeedback and to improve patient compliance. They also allow the patient to use various modes of exercise within a workout to meet his or her needs.

Plyometric Exercises

Plyometric exercises involve an eccentric contraction followed by an immediate concentric contraction. This motion is used when jumping through an obstacle course of varying heights and distances. Such drills can help retrain athletes in rapid deceleration followed by immediate acceleration; this is needed in most sports involving rapid changes of direction. (Isometric exercises tend to be more static; the others tend to be more dynamic.)

Plyometrics have been used by coaches and trainers in retraining injured athletes.[9,38] They are being used more commonly in the traditional rehabilitation setting, as athletes are increasingly expecting to return to preinjury levels of performance. Weekend athletes sometimes have expectations of recovery similar to those of seasoned athletes (Fig. 14-9).

Functionally, the foot and ankle complex requires both stability and mobility components in the rehabilitation process to return to maximum function.[39] Traditional rehabilitation has not always emphasized dynamic stability or proprioception retraining, and much has been written about the chronic ankle instability resulting from insufficient joint proprioception.[40,41] The normally functioning foot's ability to accommodate uneven surfaces and to maintain balance with the external forces bearing down on it is unique; the development of rehabilitation exercises using various equipment emphasizes this important component (Fig. 14-10). Dynamic stability is vital to regain maximum functional potential for both activities of daily living and high-

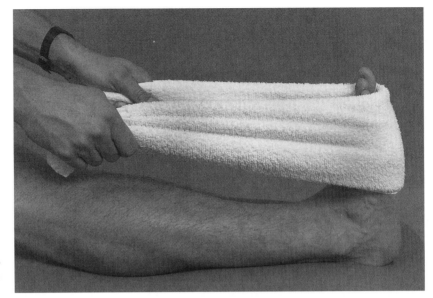

FIGURE 14-8.
Passive ankle dorsiflexion in a non-weight-bearing position, using a towel to assist.

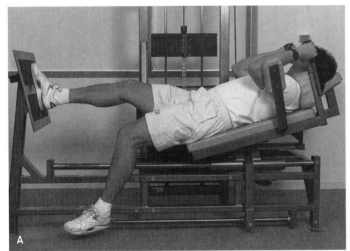

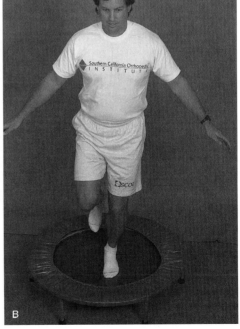

FIGURE 14-9.
(**A**) Unilateral leg-press exercise in a safe, partial weight-bearing position. (**B**) Unilateral trampoline balance drills to encourage increased weight-bearing balance and to initiate proprioception training.

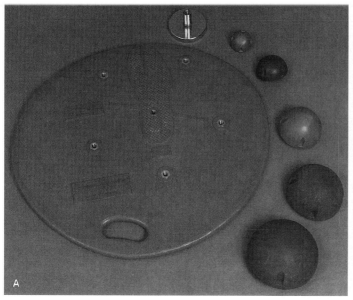

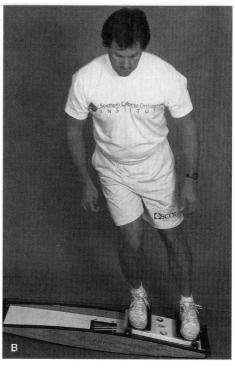

FIGURE 14–10.

(**A**) A BAPS board with its assorted sizes of balls and weights. (**B**) A Fitter encourages medial/lateral ankle and knee training and is especially useful in preparing skiers to return to their sport.

intensity sports, which require a combination of various muscle contractions, various speeds of muscle contractions, and rapid changes in movement or direction.

PHASES OF REHABILITATION

There are four basic phases of rehabilitation (some authors subdivide them, but they remain broad in this text). Phase I, the acute or symptomatic phase, is the immediate postoperative or postinjury phase; the goals are to control and alleviate the acute symptoms of trauma. In phase II, acute symptoms are controlled enough to allow rehabilitation techniques involving more active patient participation. In phase III, low symptom reactivity allows progression to full normal activity levels. Aggressive techniques may be used to ensure full patient participation in returning to normal strength and endurance. Strength should be trained statically and dynamically. The main task in phase IV is to facilitate normal subconscious coordination, proprioception, and agility, vital for athletes in all activities.[42]

The time frames for each phase vary depending on the surgical procedure, the pathology involved, and the patient's healing abilities. Advancement to a higher phase may be discontinued if symptoms recur, but may gradually proceed once they are controlled.

Phase I

Phase I goals are to decrease acute symptoms, such as swelling and pain, and to initiate safe cardiovascular training to promote overall conditioning. Passive modalities such as electrical stimulation, ice, and gentle passive motion exercises may help to minimize soft-tissue dysfunction, such as contractures. The effects of immobilization have been reported by many; joint stiffness and muscle atrophy are common results.[4,5] NWB exercises that allow safe motion while promoting circulation and healing are also encouraged in this phase. Isometric strengthening exercises may be tolerated provided symptoms of acute distress are not activated.

Cardiovascular training should be initiated here, but often this is delayed until later phases. The current interest in fitness has led to the development of cardiovascular alternatives to traditional jogging. Cybex's upper-body ergometer allows safe cardiovascular training without involving any active effort from the feet (Fig. 14-11). A pool is an ideal NWB environment in which to initiate range of motion in the acutely injured joint[43–45] (Fig. 14-12).

Phase II

The goals here are to maintain symptom control, to initiate active strengthening, to initiate proprioceptive training, and to continue cardiovascular training. Phase I techniques can be continued here as needed. Passive modalities should be decreased as much as possible to promote more active patient participation.

Active-assisted range on the involved joints can

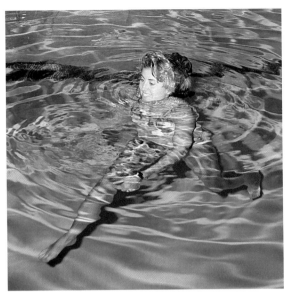

FIGURE 14-12.
Non-weight-bearing lower-extremity exercises in the pool are an effective means of rehabilitation while remaining non-weight-bearing.

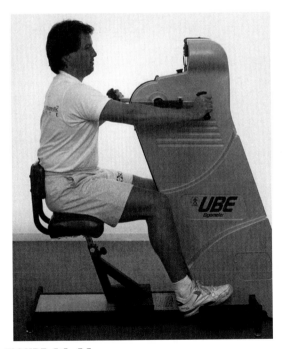

FIGURE 14-11.
An upper-body cardiovascular exerciser is an excellent way to train or maintain cardiovascular capacity while allowing the ankle to rest safely.

progress to active range exercises. Active motions of inversion, eversion, pronation, and supination should be started, as these are foot motions needed in the normal walking pattern. Joint mobilization techniques to the talocrural and subtalar joints may be indicated if the range is restricted, thus preventing the required motions. This passive technique should be terminated once full available range has been obtained.

Once simple, active exercises are achieved, gentle NWB proprioception exercises may begin on devices such as the BAPS board.[46] Early and safe training of balance and coordination may prevent the rapid deterioration of such spontaneous and vital protective reactions. The lack of proprioception in the foot is often blamed for common recurrent chronic injuries, and an early retraining program may help decrease the frequency of such injuries.[47,48]

Cardiovascular training can continue from phase I until WB is permitted on the injured foot. A stationary bicycle (upright or recumbent) can be used initially before progressing to WB activities such as walking. A pool can be a safe NWB environment in which to train for cardiovascular endurance.

Phase III

The goals in this phase are to increase active strengthening; to continue progressive proprioception and coordination training, especially in WB positions; and to continue WB cardiovascular training. Active resistive exercises should be aggressive to cause muscle hypertrophy and development without evoking any acute symptoms of increased swelling or pain or decreased range of motion. Various techniques are available, including manual techniques such as proprioceptive neuromuscular facilitation and numerous isokinetic and isotonic modalities. A pulley-type machine allows eccentric strengthening by teaching muscle control, which is vital in daily activities such as walking (decelerating at heelstrike) and in sports involving quick directional changes.

Proprioception training at this stage should be in WB positions to duplicate normal activities of daily living. A BAPS board or a balance board of any type allows progression into both bilateral and unilateral standing positions (Fig. 14-13), and also allows progressive resistive training. Supination, pronation, inversion, and eversion can be specifically trained on such a device. A Fitter or Skier's Edge (see Fig. 14-10*B*) may also allow WB proprioceptive training. WB on the foot should be fully normal before progressing to aggressive WB strengthening exercises.

Cardiovascular training may continue in WB activities using the treadmill, Stairmaster, or rowing or skiing machines. Instructing the patient to monitor his or her target heart rate and working intensity may promote active patient participation.

Phase IV

The goal in this phase is to return the patient to his or her preinjury or presurgery level of function in the desired sport and involves the creative use of rehabilitation techniques.[49-52] In this phase, many therapists and trainers assess the athlete's level of performance, based on his or her physical abilities and the demands of the sport, and then develop specific drills to assist the athlete in his or her weakest areas. Good accessory joint motion is needed in all available joints, as well as flexible lower extremity muscles, especially the gastrocsoleus, hip flexor, and adductor groups. The medial longitudinal arch should be able to support adequate body weight without deformation. Subtalar positioning is vital for the above and may need to be corrected with orthotics to permit full, normal static WB on the foot.[12,53]

Agility and coordination drills that involve repetitive, quick multidirectional changes in movement are most effective at this stage.[36,38,42] Simple equipment, such as trampolines and sport cord, can be used, along with imagination in simulating troublesome movements. Interval training and cross-training are often used.

Sometimes the patient's abilities may not permit a safe return to the sport. Orthotic devices, braces, and taping techniques are available for assistance.[54-59] The effects of bracing on decreasing the frequency of reinjury are controversial; the decision to use bracing is usually left to the surgeon, the patient, or the rehabilitation therapist (Fig. 14-14).

SUMMARY

Many physiologic and psychological factors are involved in rehabilitation and must be taken into account.[39,51,60] Rehabilitation goals should be realistic, and communication about these goals with the patient, physician, therapist, and trainer can help ensure a high success rate. Open communication is vital in providing satisfaction to all those involved in a lengthy rehabilitation process. The more traumatic an injury is to a patient, the more important it is to take all these human aspects into account. Returning the patient to maximum previous function (Fig. 14-15) remains the ultimate goal of a complete and thorough program.

SAMPLE PROGRAMS

Sample rehabilitation progressions using the above methods are described in the following.

Example 1

This patient underwent arthroscopic internal fixation of a displaced medial malleolar fracture. The patient is immobilized 4 weeks in a cast with limited

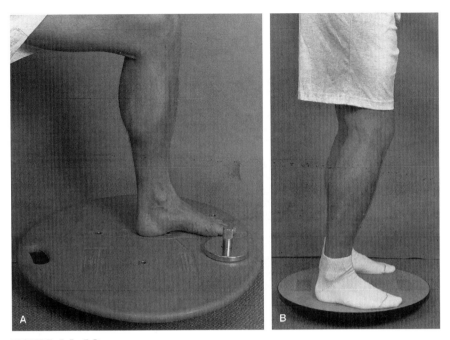

FIGURE 14-13.
(**A**) A BAPS exercise in sitting allows strengthening while avoiding joint compression. (**B**) A standing balance exercise on a simple balance board. Exercises may be progressed to unilateral ones later.

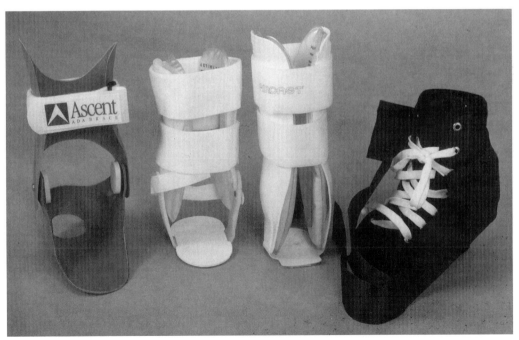

FIGURE 14-14.
Protective ankle braces (*left to right*): ADA brace, active ankle brace, aircast, lace-up brace.

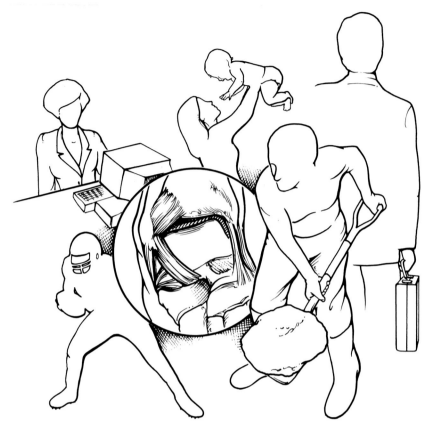

FIGURE 14-15.
The goal of rehabilitation is to return the injured person to all pre-injury activities.

WB in weeks 3 and 4. At 4 weeks, the patient is placed in a cast-brace and starts full WB and physiotherapy.

Weeks 0 to 4

- Patient is NWB.

Weeks 4 to 6

- Modalities to decrease pain and swelling
- Passive range of motion in NWB positions to stretch dorsiflexion and plantarflexion directions
- Gentle active exercises for the foot intrinsic muscles in NWB positions
- UBE for cardiovascular endurance
- Gait training with cast-brace and crutches
- Pool therapy to accomplish any of the above goals.

Weeks 6 to 8

- Gradually decrease the use of modalities
- Gait training to increase WB with brace, without assistive devices depending on stability of the injury and tissue healing capabilities
- BAPS exercises in sitting to initiate balance and proprioception; no inversion and eversion
- General lower extremity strengthening
- Pool therapy to accomplish any of the above goals if needed.

Weeks 8 to 10

- Joint mobilization if passive range of motion is not completely obtained
- Stationary bicycling with or without brace; progress to treadmill
- Stretching in WB positions (standing)
- Trampoline balance drills to improve WB and proprioception

- BAPS drills in standing, in all directions
- Continue lower extremity strengthening.

Weeks 10 to 12

- Emphasize full WB and proprioception
- Trampoline drills
- BAPS and Fitter drills
- Stairmaster
- Running activities
- Return to previous activity level.

Example 2

The patient had chronic sprain pain after a basketball injury and underwent arthroscopic debridement for anterolateral impingement of the ankle. Postoperatively he was immobilized in a posterior splint for 5 days and then was placed in a compression stocking and short-leg walking boot. Therapy is initiated 1 to 2 weeks postoperatively.

Weeks 1 and 2

- Modalities to decrease pain and swelling
- Passive range of motion to increase dorsiflexion and plantarflexion
- Active exercises to foot intrinsics
- General lower extremity strengthening
- BAPS exercises in NWB positions; dorsiflexion and plantarflexion only
- Gait training to increase WB status gradually
- Pool therapy to accomplish any of the above goals.

Weeks 2 to 4

- Decrease use of modalities
- Should have full range of motion; joint mobilization to restore accessory motion
- General lower extremity strengthening
- Active stretching in WB position (standing)
- Trampoline balance drills to increase WB on the injured limb
- BAPS drills sitting, progressing to standing, to include inversion and eversion stresses
- Stationary or recumbent bicycling

- Pool therapy to accomplish any of the above goals if needed.

Weeks 4 to 6

- Continue with aggressive lower extremity strengthening, concentric and eccentric
- Unilateral trampoline and BAPS drills
- Agility drills with random changes in direction to emphasize medial/lateral stresses; use of Fitter
- Initiate running drills.

Weeks 6 to 8

- Stretching before and after exercises
- Aggressive lower extremity strengthening, concentric and eccentric
- Plyometric exercises with jumping and reaching functional drills
- Agility drills incorporated into plyometric work with an emphasis on quick medial/lateral changes in direction
- Running or jogging for cardiovascular endurance
- Gradual return to sport.

REFERENCES

1. Mann R, Inman VT. Structure and function. In DuVries HL, ed. Surgery of the foot. St. Louis: CV Mosby, 1965:1.
2. Ferkel RD, Fischer SP. Progress in ankle arthroscopy. Clin Orthop 1989;240:210.
3. Ferkel RD, Scranton PE Jr. Current concepts review: arthroscopy of the ankle and foot. J Bone Joint Surg 1993;75A:1233.
4. Finsen V, Benum P. Osteopenia after ankle fractures: the influence of early weight bearing and muscle activity. Clin Orthop 1989;245:261.
5. Freeman MAR, Dean MRE, Hanham IWF. The etiology and prevention of functional instability of the foot. J Bone Joint Surg 1965;47B:678.
6. Garrick JG. The frequency of injury, mechanism of injury, and epidemiology of ankle sprains. Am J Sports Med 1977;5:241.
7. Cass JR, Morrey BF. Ankle instability: current concepts, diagnosis, and treatment. Mayo Clin Proc 1984;59:165.

8. Davies GJ. A compendium of isokinetics in clinical usage and rehabilitation techniques. Onalaska, WI: S & S Publishers, 1987.

9. Chu D. Plyometrics. Livermore, CA: Bittersweet Publishing Co, 1989.

10. Norkin CC. Joint structure and function. Philadelphia: FA Davis, 1983.

11. Corrigan B. Practical orthopaedic medicine. Cambridge, England: Butterworth & Company, 1983.

12. Donatelli RA, ed. The biomechanics of the foot and ankle. Philadelphia: FA Davis, 1990.

13. Grant JCB. Grant's atlas of anatomy, 7th ed. Baltimore: Williams & Wilkins, 1978.

14. Perry J. Anatomy and biomechanics of the hindfoot. Clin Orthop 1983;177:9.

15. Root ML, Orien WP, Weed JN. Clinical biomechanics, vol 2: Normal and abnormal function of the foot. Los Angeles: Clinical Biomechanics Corp., 1977.

16. Nordin M, Frankel VH, eds. Basic biomechanics of the musculoskeletal system. Malvern, PA: Lea & Febiger, 1989.

17. Donatelli R. Normal biomechanics of the foot and ankle. J Orthop Sports Phys Ther 1985;7:91.

18. Vaughan CL, ed. Biomechanics of sport. Boca Raton, FL: CRC Press, 1989.

19. Chusid JG. Correlative neuroanatomy and functional neurology. Los Altos, CA: Lange Medical Publications, 1982.

20. Pitman CA. Rehabilitative exercises following ankle injuries. Orthopedics 1990;13:723.

21. Long JP. Rehabilitation and return to activity after sports injuries. Primary Care 1984;11:137.

22. Hickson RC, Marone JR. Exercise and inhibition of glucocorticoid-induced muscle atrophy. Exer Sports Sci Rev 1993;21:135.

23. DeLisa JA. Rehabilitation medicine. Philadelphia: JB Lippincott, 1988.

24. Snyder-Mackler L. Clinical electrophysiology: electrotherapy and electrophysiologic testing. Baltimore: Williams & Wilkins, 1989.

25. Nelson RM, Currier DP. Clinical electrotherapy. East Norwalk, CT: Appleton-Century-Crofts, 1987.

26. Knight K. Electrical muscle stimulation during immobilization. Phys Sports Med 1980;8:147.

27. Micholvitz SL, ed. Thermal agents in rehabilitation. Philadelphia: FA Davis, 1990.

28. Wilkerson GB. Treatment of the inversion ankle sprain through synchronous application of focal compression and cold. Athletic Training 1991;26:220.

29. Loitz BJ, Frank CB. Biology and mechanics of ligament and ligament healing. Exer Sports Sci Rev 1993;21:33.

30. Paris SV, Patla C. E1 course notes: extremity dysfunction and manipulation. Atlanta: Institute of Graduate Health Sciences, 1988.

31. Maitland GD. Peripheral manipulation, 3rd ed. London: Butterworth-Heinemann, 1991.

32. Kloth L. Electrophoresis in the management of acute soft tissue trauma. Stimulus 1983;8:3.

33. Atha J. Strengthening muscle. Exer Sports Sci Rev 1981;9:1.

34. Berger RA. Applied exercise physiology. Philadelphia: Lea & Febiger, 1982.

35. deLateur BJ. Therapeutic exercise to develop strength and endurance. In Kottke FJ, Stillwell GK, Lehmann JF, Krusen JF, eds. Handbook of physical medicine and rehabilitation, 3rd ed. Philadelphia: WB Saunders, 1982.

36. DeLorme TL, Watkins AL. Techniques of progressive resistance exercise. Arch Phys Med Rehabil 1948;29:263.

37. Ivy JL, Withers RT, Brose G, et al. Isokinetic contractile properties of the quadriceps with relation to fiber type. Eur J Appl Physiol 1981;47:247.

38. Albert M. Eccentric muscle training in sports and orthopedics. New York: Churchill Livingstone, 1991.

39. Andrews JR, Harrelson GL, eds. Physical rehabilitation of the injured athlete. Philadelphia: WB Saunders, 1991.

40. DeMaio M, Paine R, Drez D Jr. Chronic lateral ankle instability—Inversion sprains: Part I. Orthopedics 1992;15:87.

41. Brunt D, Andersen JC, Huntsman B, et al. Postural responses to lateral perturbation in healthy subjects and ankle sprain patients. Med Sci Sports Exer 1992;24:171.

42. Kottke FJ. From reflex to skill: the training of coordination. Arch Phys Med Rehabil 1980;61:551.

43. Gall SL. Swim fins—adding splash to the laps. Phys Sportsmed 1990;18:91.

44. Bergel R. Aquatic therapy—exercises in water. American Back Society Symposium.

45. Duffield MH. Exercise in water. Baltimore: Williams & Wilkins, 1976.

46. Lattanza L, Gray GW, Kantner RM. Closed versus open kinematic chain measurements of subtalar joint eversion: implications for clinical practice. J Orthop Sports Phys Ther 1988;9:310.

47. Rebman LW. Ankle injuries: clinical observations. J Orthop Sports Phys Ther 1986;8:153.

48. Molnar ME. Rehabilitation of the injured ankle. Clin Podiatr Med Surg 1989;6:657.

49. Clancy WG Jr. Specific rehabilitation for the injured recreational runner. In AAOS Instructional Course Lectures, vol 38, 1988:483.

50. Oviatt R, Hemba G. Oregon State: sandblasting through the PAC. National Strength and Conditioning Association Journal 1991;13:40.

51. Sammarco GJ. Conditioning and rehabilitation of the athlete's foot and ankle. In Jahss MH, ed. Disorders of the foot and ankle. Philadelphia: WB Saunders, 1991:2797.

52. Hoover RL. Rehabilitation: a functional protocol. J School Health 1977;4:238.

53. Tiberio D. Evaluation of functional ankle dorsiflexion using subtalar neutral position—a clinical report. Physical Therapy 1987;67:955.

54. Novick A, Kelley DL. Position and movement changes of the foot with orthotic intervention during the loading response of gait. J Orthop Sports Phys Ther 1990;11:301.

55. Kimura KF, Nawoczenski DA, Epler M, Owen MG. Effect of the AirStirrup in controlling ankle inversion stress. J Orthop Sports Phys Ther 1987;9:190.

56. Lane SE. Severe ankle sprains. Treatment with an ankle-foot orthosis. Phys Sportsmed 1990;18:43.

57. Bullard RH, Dawson J, Arenson DJ. Taping the athletic ankle. J Am Podiatr Med Assoc 1979; 69:727.

58. Myburgh KH, Vaughan CL, Isaacs SK. The effects of ankle guards and taping on joint motion before, during, and after a squash match. Am J Sports Med 1984;12:441.

59. Wilkerson GB. Comparative biomechanical effects of the standard method of ankle taping and a taping method designed to enhance subtalar stability. Am J Sports Med 1991;19:588.

60. Coakley J. Sport and socialization. Exer Sports Sci Rev 1993;21:169.

Arthroscopic Surgery: The Foot and Ankle,
by Richard D. Ferkel.
Lippincott-Raven Publishers, Philadelphia © 1996.

15

Complications in Ankle and Foot Arthroscopy

Richard D. Ferkel

Arthroscopy of the ankle and foot has progressed significantly since Burman first tried to perform arthroscopy on the ankle in 1931.[1] As equipment and instrumentation have advanced, especially over the last 10 years, newer techniques have been developed. As the number of arthroscopic procedures has increased and more demanding procedures have been developed, the opportunity for significant complications has also increased.

HISTORY

In Small's 1988 prospective study in which 21 surgeons participated, the overall complication rate for all arthroscopy was 1.7%, and the complication rate for ankle arthroscopy was 0.7%.[2] Guhl in 1988 reported on 131 cases with 13 complications for a rate of about 10%.[3] In 1989 Martin and associates[4] reported a long-term follow-up on a series of 101 ankles with a 15% complication rate; Barber and colleagues[5] reported an incidence of 17% in 53 cases. Ferkel and Guhl reported on complications in the first 518 cases with an overall rate of 9.8%; the most common complication was neurologic.[6] These rates of 10% to 17% are significant, and emphasize the extreme caution that must be used in performing arthroscopy of the ankle and foot.

TYPES OF COMPLICATIONS

Various complications can be associated with arthroscopic surgery of the ankle and foot (Fig. 15-1, Table 15-1): systemic, preoperative, and procedure-related.[7] Systemic complications include those related to illness, the stress of injury, anesthesia, and surgery. Atelectasis, pulmonary embolus, myocardial infarction and other cardiopulmonary events, loss of limb, and even loss of life are all potential systemic complications. Preoperative complications include lack of preoperative planning, failure to obtain appropriate preoperative studies, and operating for the wrong

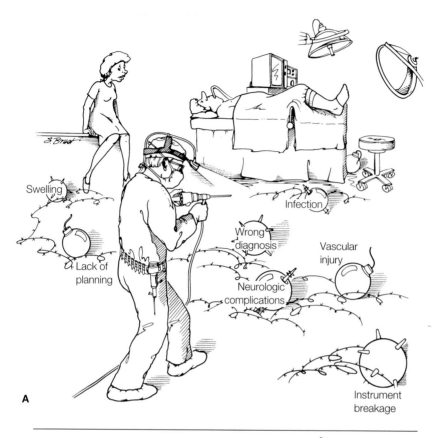

A

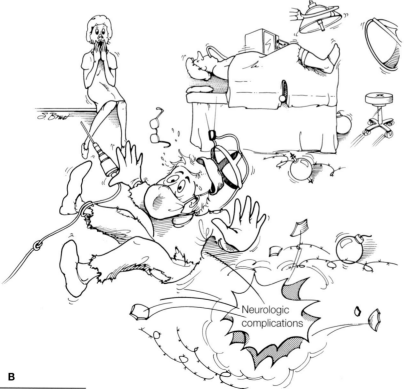

B

FIGURE 15-1.
Arthroscopy complications. (**A**) Doing ankle arthroscopy is like walking through a minefield: the arthroscopic surgeon must maneuver carefully to avoid a complication (explosion). (**B**) Poor technique can lead to the most common complication in ankle arthroscopy, which is neurologic.

TABLE 15-1.
COMPLICATIONS OF FOOT
AND ANKLE ANTHROSCOPY

- Operating on wrong extremity
- Missed diagnosis
- Tourniquet complications
- Neurovascular injury
- Tendon injury
- Ligament injury
- Wound complications
- Infection
- Articular cartilage damage
- Compartment ischemia/compartment syndrome
- Hemarthrosis
- Postoperative effusion
- Reflex sympathetic dystrophy
- Fluid management complications
- Distraction-related complications
- Postoperative stress fracture
- Instrument breakage
- Thrombophlebitis and pulmonary embolism

diagnosis. Most complications in the ankle and foot are procedure-related.

Neurovascular Injury

Neurovascular structures can be injured by incorrect portal placement, careless distraction pin placement, prolonged or inappropriate distraction, or excessive tourniquet use. The most common complication in ankle and foot arthroscopy is neurologic. This usually involves a temporary paresthesia of the superficial nerves, but occasionally can be associated with permanent paresthesia or paresis. Neuromas can also form from injury to the nerve during surgery. The anteromedial portal can be associated with injury to the greater saphenous vein or saphenous nerve. The anterocentral portal is not recommended because of potential injury to the dorsalis pedis artery and deep peroneal nerve (Fig. 15-2).

The anterolateral portal is associated with significant risk to the superficial peroneal nerve. Injury to this nerve is the most common neurologic complication. Variations in the superficial nerve were described in Chapter 5. Preoperatively, it is critical to try to identify the nerve and its branches and mark them to avoid injury. However, in some patients,

particularly those who are obese, the nerve may not be seen either directly or through transillumination.

Nerve damage may be minimized by vertically incising only the skin with the knife blade, followed by careful spreading of the subcutaneous tissues with the hemostat before penetrating the capsule. Repeated passage of instruments through the portal site without the use of a protective cannula can increase the risk of neurovascular injury. An interchangeable cannula system is helpful to avoid repetitive soft-tissue injury.

The posterolateral portal is routinely used and places the lesser saphenous vein and sural nerve at risk. Caution must be exercised when making this portal, as with all others, to minimize complications. The posteromedial portal is never used because of significant potential injury to the posterior tibial nerve and vessels (Fig. 15-3).

If paresthesia or pain develops after arthroscopy, its site and extent should be carefully documented. The patient should be informed about the problem and followed carefully. A positive Tinel's sign that develops over the portal site may be due to nerve contusion or neurapraxia, or to neuroma formation (Fig. 15-4). Rarely is additional surgery necessary to correct these problems.

Vascular injury can occur at the portal sites or through the use of the invasive pin distractor. The use of the anterocentral portal can be associated with injury to the dorsalis pedis artery or deep peroneal nerve (Fig. 15-5). Placing the anterocentral portal through the extensor tendons helps prevent this complication. The noninvasive distraction strap may compress the neurovascular structures, but this complication is rare.

Tourniquet

The pneumatic tourniquet facilitates arthroscopic surgery by providing improved visibility and a bloodless field. The complications associated with its use are well documented, including paresthesias, paresis, thigh pain, and perhaps thrombophlebitis. Sherman and colleagues, in a study on knee arthroscopy complications, showed there was no increase in complications with tourniquet use unless the tourniquet time exceeded 60 minutes.[8] Problems related

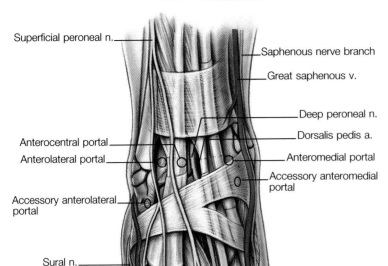

FIGURE 15-2.
Anterior view of arthroscopic portals. Caution is necessary to avoid injury to the neurovascular structures.

to the use of the tourniquet can be minimized by proper application, adequate padding, low tourniquet pressures, and reduction of tourniquet time.

Tendon Injuries

Numerous tendons traverse the ankle and foot, and they can be injured by careless portal placement or distraction pin insertion. Use of the trans-Achilles portal has been abandoned because of the increased potential for injury and possible rupture that can occur with instrumentation of the Achilles tendon. When invasive distraction is required, a blunt-tipped cannula should be inserted through the subcutaneous skin down to the tibia and calcaneus to avoid winding tendons or neurovascular structures when the pins are inserted. The flexor hallucis longus and posterior neurovascular structures can also be injured if

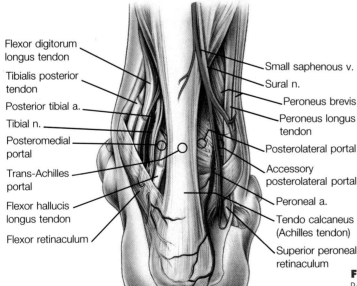

FIGURE 15-3.
Posterior arthroscopic portals. Only the posterolateral portal should be used, with care taken to avoid injury to the sural nerve and small saphenous vein.

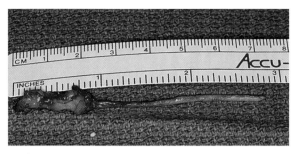

FIGURE 15-4.
Neuroma of the sural nerve excised after prolonged symptoms.

extreme caution is not used when removing a painful os trigonum via subtalar arthroscopy (see Chap. 12).

Ligament Injuries

Injury to the ligamentous structures of the ankle and foot can occur through improper portal placement, excessive debridement, and inappropriate distraction techniques. The use of accessory anteromedial and anterolateral portals can lead to injury of the deltoid or the anterior talofibular ligament. Injudicious use of the shaver and burrs can lead to injury to the ligamentous structures as well. Ankle distraction techniques also place the ligaments at risk; this risk

can be minimized by the use of appropriate distraction forces for no more than 1 to 1.5 hours. In addition, periodic relaxation of the distraction is helpful. Because of the viscoelastic property of ligaments, adequate distraction can be maintained with less force after the first half-hour of the procedure. When general anesthesia is used, the patient should be paralyzed to facilitate distraction while minimizing distraction forces. Also, the use of small pins with invasive distraction can prevent ligament injury by permitting pin bending before ligament failure.

Articular Cartilage Injury

Due to the narrow confines and shape of the joints in the ankle and foot, articular cartilage injury is more likely to occur. Great care should be exercised to avoid superficial gouges, nicks, or scuffing. Injury to articular cartilage may also occur during the introduction of the arthroscope or accessory instruments into the joint. Sharp trochars should never be used, and small-gauge needles help to set the appropriate position of the portals to avoid articular cartilage injury.

Transmalleolar portals can also lead to small defects in the articular cartilage. In rare cases, cysts can develop in the underlying bone after drilling. The

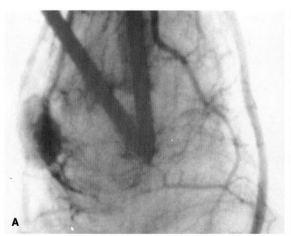
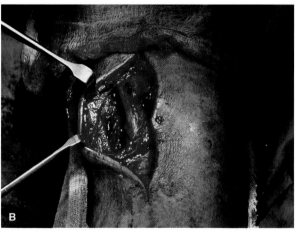

FIGURE 15-5.
Aneurysm formation. (**A**) Lateral arteriogram of a patient who underwent ankle arthroscopic arthrodesis with pin fixation. Note the aneurysm of the dorsalis pedis artery just above the joint line. (**B**) Intraoperative picture demonstrating aneurysm before resection. Aneurysm was formed by injury to the dorsalis pedis artery while using the anterocentral portal.

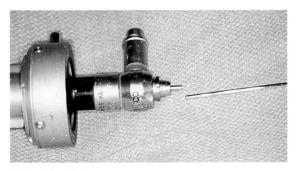

FIGURE 15-6.
This 2.5-mm arthroscope broke at the proximal end secondary to the long, heavy lever arm of the attached camera and eyepiece.

gery and prevent complications. However, these small-joint instruments are more fragile, bending and breaking more easily than larger instruments (Fig. 15-6). Greater care is required in their handling, both during surgery and while cleaning them. Before surgery all instruments should be inspected by the surgeon for loose or missing parts, fatigue damage, or other evidence of impending failure. Whenever appropriate, instruments should be replaced to prevent intraoperative breakage. Instruments should never be forced into the joint or into any tight or hard-to-reach areas.

If an instrument does break within the joint, inflow and outflow should be stopped immediately, and the arthroscope position should be fixed on the broken instrument (Fig. 15-7*A*). Small-joint graspers should be immediately introduced and the broken piece removed (see Fig. 15-7*B*). In some cases, the small fragments may migrate into the medial, anteromedial, or anterolateral recesses, or to the posterior recess of the ankle, making their retrieval much more difficult (Fig. 15-8). A small-joint suction magnet such as the Golden Retriever (Instrument Makar, Okemos, Mich.) may prove invaluable to retrieve a broken fragment. If the broken instrument cannot be found within a reasonable amount of time, a plain x-ray or fluoroscopy should be used to locate it. Preferably, nonmagnetic arthroscopic instruments should not be used because of the difficulty in retrieval. Motorized instruments such as burrs or shavers can inadvertently destroy the tip of the arthroscope or break off fragments of other metallic

articular surfaces can also be damaged by insertion of pins or screws into the subtalar joint during ankle arthrodesis, or by the placement of staples for arthroscopic ligament reconstruction. These injuries are totally avoidable, and the use of the fluoroscope is helpful to prevent these complications.

The use of small-joint arthroscopes and instrumentation and the advent of improved distraction devices have reduced the incidence of articular cartilage damage during arthroscopy.

Instrument Breakage

Due to the unique shape of the joints and the limited joint space in the ankle and foot, small-joint instrumentation is strongly recommended to facilitate sur-

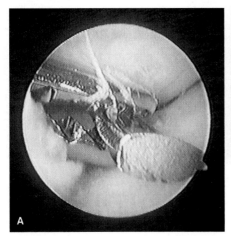

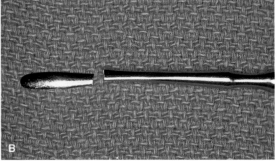

FIGURE 15-7.
Broken Freer. (**A**) Arthroscopic view showing the use of a grasper to remove the broken Freer tip. (**B**) A fatigue fracture occurred at the neck of the Freer, causing it to fail.

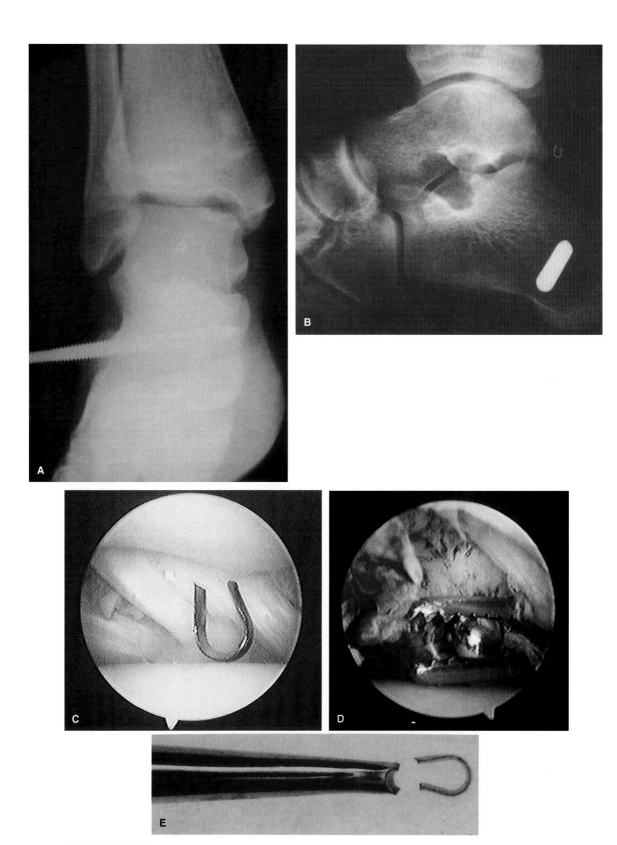

FIGURE 15-8.
Broken ring curette. (**A**) AP x-ray demonstrating a broken 3.5-mm ring curette tip inside the ankle. (**B**) Lateral intraoperative x-ray showing the ring curette tip to be in the posterior recess, just above the subtalar joint. (**C**) Arthroscopic view demonstrating broken ring curette tip floating along the posterior ankle ligaments. (**D**) The grasper is inserted and the broken ring curette tip is carefully removed. (**E**) The ring curette broke at its base due to fatigue. This curette must be carefully inspected before use for wear; if there are any questions, it should be discarded.

instruments, resulting in debris within the joint. Small-joint baskets and graspers that are designed to break at the handle and not at the tip should be used (Fig. 15-9).

Fluid Management Complications

Problems with fluid management can be divided into difficulty in joint distention, visualization, and extravasation. The key to adequate joint distention and visualization is the use of separate inflow and outflow portals. This is usually accomplished by gravity inflow, using 3-liter bags of fluid at maximal elevation. Capsular collapse and bleeding increase with excessive leakage of fluid or diminished inflow pressure.

An imbalance of too much inflow and not enough outflow can lead to fluid extravasation. Usually the amount of extravasation is mild in the ankle and foot and rapidly reabsorbs at the end of the procedure. However, complications can occur if the extravasation becomes significant into compartments of the tibia or foot. When this occurs, the procedure should be stopped to prevent serious problems.

As the quality of arthroscopic pumps and cannulae have improved, they have become increasingly popular in arthroscopy of all joints. Extreme caution

must be taken when using a pump system for ankle and foot arthroscopy. Extensive extravasation and increased pressures can develop rapidly in the operative extremity, and the potential for complication remains high (Fig. 15-10). This is particularly true when the surgeon does not pay meticulous attention to pump pressures, or the pump cannula slips into the subcutaneous space without being noticed by the surgeon.

Compartment Ischemia

Ischemia of the compartments of the distal tibia, distal fibula, and foot can lead to serious complications. This ischemia usually results from prolonged tourniquet use or excessive fluid extravasation. As previously mentioned, compartment pressures can rise significantly with the use of an arthroscopic fluid pump. In most instances, compartment pressures will rapidly decrease to normal after completion of the case and deflation of the tourniquet. However, when there is cause for concern about ischemia to any compartment, the extremity should be closely monitored and, if there is any question, pressure readings taken.

Wound Complications

Hematomas, seromas, skin slough and necrosis, and sinus tract formation are all potential wound complications associated with arthroscopic surgery of the ankle and foot. The potential for these problems may be higher than with other joints because of the lack of subcutaneous tissue, as well as the dependent nature of the ankle and foot. To decrease wound complications, patients are instructed to wash their ankle and foot with an antiseptic scrub brush the morning of surgery. At the time of surgery, a Betadine scrub is done. In addition, strict adherence to appropriate technique is mandatory to avoid wound problems. Wound problems can be minimized with proper portal placement and avoidance of closely spaced portals; the use of cannulae to facilitate instrument passage; suturing of the portals; and the use of a postoperative compression dressing and splinting.

Delayed wound healing can be associated with

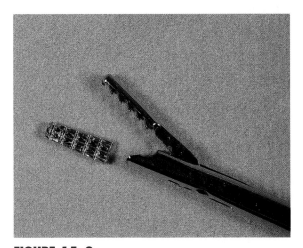

FIGURE 15-9.
Broken grasper. This grasper broke at its tip while trying to remove too large a loose body.

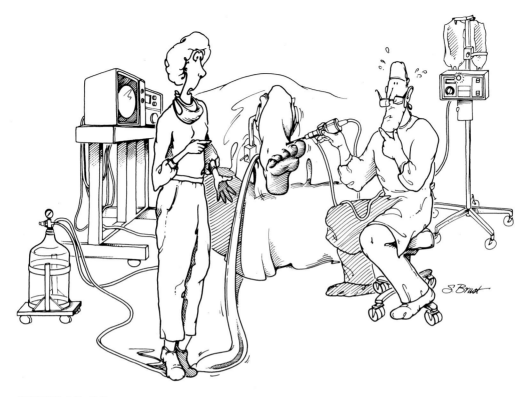

FIGURE 15-10.
Great care must be taken when using an arthroscopic pump to ensure that inflow and outflow are working correctly and that fluid extravasation is not occurring into the compartments of the distal leg and foot.

the use of invasive distractor pins. This complication is more likely to occur at the calcaneal pin site because of the lack of subcutaneous tissue there (Fig. 15-11).

If a skin problem develops, it will usually heal with appropriate care. Sinus tract formation may be more difficult to eradicate; in the case of persistent drainage, the fluid should be cultured, appropriate antibiotics administered, and the joint immobilized. If the tract still does not heal, the patient should be returned to the operating room, the sinus tract excised, the wound sutured, and the joint immobilized.

Infection

Infections following arthroscopy of the ankle and foot can be divided into superficial and deep. Ferkel, Heath, and Guhl found eight superficial infections

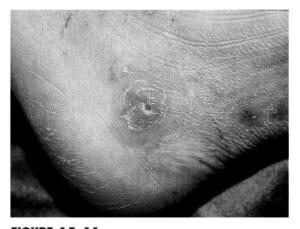

FIGURE 15-11.
Pin tract infection over the lateral calcaneus after use of invasive distraction during ankle arthroscopy. This healed with antibiotics and local wound care.

in the first 612 cases reported.[9] These superficial wound infections appeared to be related to the absence of a cannula for instrumentation, the use of Steri-Strips to close the wounds, and early mobilization of the joint following surgery. In this same series, the two deep wound infections that occurred appeared to correlate with the lack of preoperative antibiotics. The current treatment protocol includes the use of prophylactic antibiotics for 24 hours, combined with suturing of all portals and immobilization of the operated joint in a posterior splint for 5 to 7 days. With this treatment regimen, the incidence of wound problems, including infection, has been minimal.

A joint-space infection should be confirmed by joint aspiration, synovial fluid analysis, appropriate cultures, and blood tests. A septic joint should be treated by irrigation and debridement of the joint with insertion of suction drains or irrigation tubes, in conjunction with appropriate antibiotics and joint immobilization.

Postoperative Swelling

Significant postoperative effusions of the ankle and foot are rare and are usually related to bleeding or synovitis. Before removal of the arthroscope, the tourniquet should be released when appropriate and all bleeding stopped. If a bleeder cannot be found, then a drain should be inserted and removed 24 to 48 hours postoperatively. Bleeding may be aggravated by the use of aspirin or other nonsteroidal anti-inflammatory medication preoperatively; these should always be stopped at least 7 days before the procedure. Any recurrent effusion should be aspirated, with the appropriate synovial fluid analysis and cultures taken.

Thrombophlebitis and Pulmonary Embolism

Thrombophlebitis and pulmonary embolism can occur after any surgery, particularly of the extremities. If the patient has a history of previous vascular problems, consultation with a vascular specialist will assist in determining the appropriate prophylaxis after sur-

gery. In addition, tourniquet use should be avoided if possible in patients with a history of previous thrombophlebitis or pulmonary embolism. If either problem develops in the postoperative period, appropriate diagnostic studies and treatment are indicated immediately.

Reflex Sympathetic Dystrophy

Reflex sympathetic dystrophy (RSD) can develop as a result of any type of trauma, including arthroscopic surgery. The diagnosis and treatment of RSD can be difficult. A three-phase bone scan may assist in the diagnosis of this problem in the ankle and foot but is not diagnostic of the problem (Fig. 15-12). Treatment protocols vary and are controversial. Patients with RSD should be managed with a team approach consisting of the orthopedic surgeon, a pain specialist, and a physiotherapist.

Postoperative Stress Fractures

Stress fractures of the distal tibia, talus, or calcaneus can occur with the use of invasive pin distraction or transmalleolar portals. This problem can be mini-

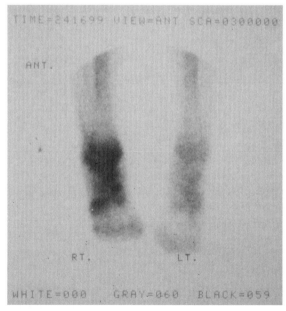

FIGURE 15-12.
Three-phase bone scan demonstrating significantly increased activity on the static as well as perfusion images, consistent with reflex sympathetic dystrophy.

mized by the use of unicortical distraction pins, correct pin placement, and postoperative protection of the extremity for 3 to 4 weeks. Postoperative stress fracture secondary to transmalleolar drilling is possible but has not been reported.

When patients have pain for more than 3 weeks at a pin insertion site, x-rays should be obtained to rule out a stress fracture. Early stress fractures may not show up initially on x-rays, and persistent pain at these sites should be treated with a removable cast boot for at least 4 weeks. Follow-up x-rays should be taken at that time. If there is evidence of periosteal healing and the patient has no pain, then increased weight bearing and activities can slowly be instituted without protection (Figs. 15-13, 15-14).

If a significant fracture of the tibia occurs, it should be treated appropriately. When $^3/_{16}''$ threaded Steinmann pins are used for distraction, the patient must not engage in running or jumping sports or similar work activities for 8 to 12 weeks. When smaller pins are used, this time may be reduced to 4 to 6 weeks.

RESULTS

Complications have recently been analyzed in the first 612 cases at the Southern California Orthopedic Institute.[9] The primary and secondary diagnoses and procedures were listed in Chapter 1.

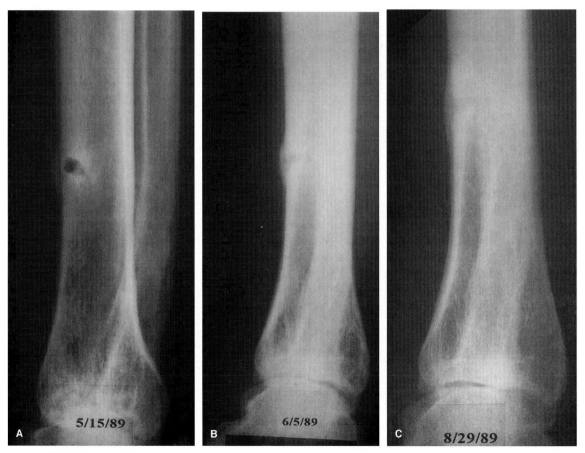

FIGURE 15-13.
Stress fracture of the anterior distal tibia. (**A**) Stress fracture has occurred because pin was placed too anteriorly. (**B**) Three weeks later, the fracture is healing. (**C**) Two and a half months later, the fracture is well healed, with good callus formation.

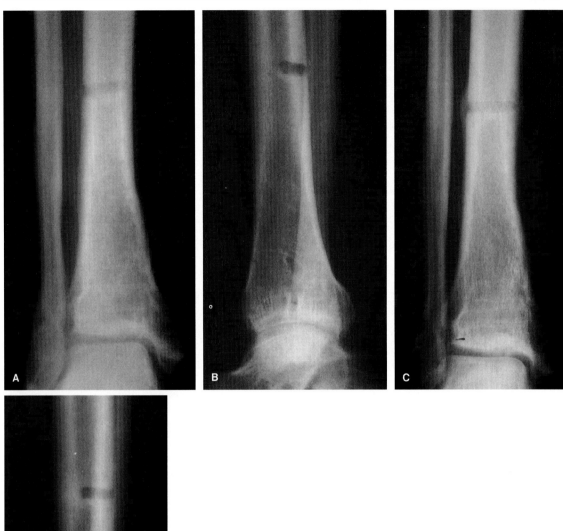

FIGURE 15-14.

Stress fracture of the posterior tibia. (**A**) AP x-ray demonstrating bicortical insertion of the distal tibial pin for invasive distraction. (**B**) Lateral x-ray shows fracture of the posterior cortex due to pin placement too posteriorly. (**C**) AP x-ray 2 months later shows good callus formation with healing of the stress fracture laterally. (**D**) Lateral x-ray 2 months later demonstrates healing of the posterior tibial stress fracture.

TABLE 15-2.
COMPLICATIONS

MAY BE PREVENTABLE	POSSIBLY PREVENTABLE	UNPREVENTABLE
Neurologic problems	Effusions	Cardiovascular problems
Hemarthrosis	Adhesions	Reflex sympathetic dystrophy
Instrument breakage	Infections	
Ecchymosis		
Wound healing problems		
Stress fracture		

The overall incidence of complications was 9%. The most common complication was neurologic (49% of all complications). The nerves primarily involved included the superficial peroneal nerve (56%; 15/27), the sural nerve (22%; 6/27), the saphenous nerve (18%; 5/27), and the deep peroneal nerve (4%; 1/27). Other complications included superficial and deep infection, distractor pin site fracture or pain, instrument failure, subsequent surgery, and a few miscellaneous problems.

Complications can be divided into preventable, possibly preventable, and unpreventable ones (Table 15-2).

TABLE 15-3.
TIPS TO AVOID COMPLICATIONS

1. Patient selection
2. Careful preoperative evaluation, including the skin, nerve, and vascular status
3. Careful physical examination and radiologic evaluation, including stress x-rays, CT scan, and MRI where applicable
4. Thorough knowledge of ankle and foot anatomy
5. Practice with sawbones or cadavers
6. Meticulous use of distraction
7. Careful portal placement
8. Use of interchangeable cannulae for arthroscope and instrumentation
9. Appropriate small-joint instrumentation
10. Perioperative antibiotics
11. Limited operative time and tourniquet use
12. Availability of magnetic retriever
13. Use of skin stitches in wounds
14. Brief postoperative immobilization
15. Appropriate rehabilitation

Overall, complications can be avoided by careful preoperative planning, meticulous surgical technique, the use of suitable small-joint instrumentation, and appropriate postoperative care. The surgeon must have a thorough understanding of the intra- and extraarticular anatomy of the ankle and foot. In addition, practicing on sawbones or cadavers can help the surgeon gain experience with small-joint instrumentation and surgical procedures. Tips to avoid complications are listed in Table 15-3.

CONCLUSIONS

Arthroscopy of the ankle and foot is associated with a significant incidence of complications. Although most of these complications are minor and resolve quickly, permanent sequelae can develop. As experience increases and techniques and instrumentation are further refined, it is to be hoped that the complication rate will decrease.

REFERENCES

1. Burman MS. Arthroscopy, a direct visualization of joints: an experimental cadaver study. J Bone Joint Surg 1931;13A:669.
2. Small NC. Complications in arthroscopic surgery performed by experienced arthroscopists. Arthroscopy 1988;4:215.
3. Guhl JF. Ankle arthroscopy. Thorofare, NJ: Slack, 1988.

4. Martin DF, Baker CL, Curl WW, et al. Operative ankle arthroscopy—long-term follow-up. Am J Sports Med 1989;17:16.

5. Barber FA, Click J, Britt BT. Complications of ankle arthroscopy. Foot Ankle 1990;10:263.

6. Ferkel RD, Guhl J, Van Buecken K, et al. Complications in 518 ankle arthroscopies. Orthop Trans 1992–1993;16:726.

7. Ferkel RD, Small HN. Complications of arthroscopy of the foot and ankle. In Mizell M, ed. Complications in foot and ankle surgery (in press).

8. Sherman OH, Fox JM, Snyder SJ, et al. Arthroscopy—"no problem surgery." An analysis of complications in 2640 cases. J Bone Joint Surg 1986;68A:256.

9. Ferkel RD, Heath DD, Guhl JF. Neurological complications of ankle arthroscopy: a review of 612 cases. Arthroscopy 1993;9:352.

Arthroscopic Surgery: The Foot and Ankle,
by Richard D. Ferkel.
Lippincott-Raven Publishers, Philadelphia © 1996.

16

Future Developments

The future of foot and ankle arthroscopy is exciting, as better equipment and more innovative ideas are developed. This chapter deals with newer technology that can be applied in arthroscopy of the foot and ankle. Some of the technologies discussed in this chapter use the principles of both arthroscopy and endoscopy to visualize not only joints but also the spaces or compartments in the foot and ankle. The first section deals with laser energy and the second discusses the use of endoscopic techniques. The following technologies and techniques are described in this chapter because their efficacy and results have not been fully demonstrated in large-scale studies.

A. *Laser Energy*
Richard D. Ferkel

LASER PRINCIPLES

The word *laser* is an acronym for light amplification by stimulated emission of radiation. It is beyond the scope of this section to discuss laser physics; excellent references on this subject are available elsewhere.[1,2] The surgical laser is an instrument that cuts, coagulates, and vaporizes. In contrast to a scalpel, which uses a mechanical force to cut tissue, a laser delivers energy (photons) in the form of an intense, coherent, collimated, single-frequency beam of light that creates a thermal effect when it is absorbed by the target material (Fig. 16-1). This heat can cause coagulation, vaporization, and cutting (actually a narrow line of vaporization). When light is transmitted onto any material, the material can reflect, transmit, scatter, or absorb it. The optical properties of a material determine the effectiveness of a given laser by controlling the interaction between the laser light and the material.[3] Laser light must be absorbed by a cell to provide energy for a photochemical

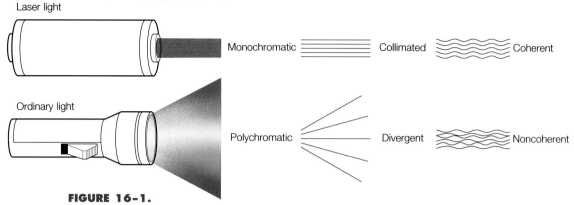

FIGURE 16-1.

Laser light characteristics. Unlike ordinary light, laser light is monochromatic, collimated, and coherent.

or photobiologic reaction: if it is not absorbed, no reaction occurs. What happens when a laser beam strikes tissue depends on the wavelength, intensity, energy, and duration of the laser irradiation and the type, color, size, and composition of the tissue.[4]

All lasers have three basic physical components (Fig. 16-2):[5] a *lasing medium,* an excitable material that can be a gas, a liquid, or a solid; an *excitation source,* which pumps high electric energy into the medium; and a *resonator,* a chamber that consists of two parallel mirrors, one of which is totally reflective and one partially reflective, to allow energy amplification and egress of the laser light. A laser beam is the product of the excitation of electrons. The electrons may rest in their ground (or lower energy level state) in a solid, liquid, or gas phase. The excitation source pumps energy into the lasing me-

dium, causing atoms in the medium to reach a higher energy state. When these atoms drop from a higher energy state to a lower energy level, they release energy in the form of protons. When enough atoms emit photons, the combined energy of these photons produces a light beam strong enough to penetrate the partially reflective mirror. This high-frequency light beam is the laser beam.

The wavelength or frequency of the emitted photons is a function of the difference between the two energy levels, and differs from one atom molecule to another.[5] The primary difference between lasers is the specific wavelength at which they emit light. Lasers currently used in orthopedics function in the infrared portion of the electromagnetic spectrum, except the Excimer (Fig. 16-3; Table 16-1).[6] Different lasers penetrate variable distances through

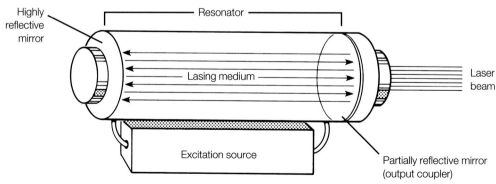

FIGURE 16-2.

Laser device. All lasers have three basic physical components: lasing medium, excitation source, and resonator. The laser beam emanates from the chamber after excitation of the crystal or gas in the chamber.

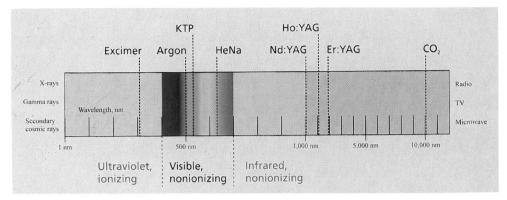

FIGURE 16–3.

Electromagnetic radiation spectrum. Various wavelengths of laser energy extend from the shorter wavelengths (*left*) in the ultraviolet area to the longer waves (*right*) in the infrared region along a perpetual line. The visible wavelengths occupy only a small portion of the spectrum. (Courtesy of John Dougherty, CMI)

TABLE 16-1.

TYPE OF LASER AND WAVELENGTH

TYPE OF LASER	WAVELENGTH (NM)	
CO_2	10,600	
Hydrogen fluoride	2,950	
ER:YAG	2,940	Infrared
Ho:YAG	2,100	
Nd:YAG	1,320	
	1,064	
Gallium arsenide	904	
Ruby	694 (red)	
Helium–neon	632 (red)	
Tunable dye	628 (red)	
	577 (yellow)	
Gold	628 (red)	Visible
Copper	578 (yellow)	
	511 (green)	
Frequency-doubled Nd:YAG	532 (green)	
Argon	515 (green)	
	488 (blue)	
Excimer		
XeF	351	
KrF	248	Ultraviolet
ArF	193	

1 nm = 10^{-9} m.
(Adapted with permission from Vangsness CT Jr., Ghaderi B, Saadatmanesh V. Lasers in arthroscopic surgery. In Parisien JS, ed. Current techniques in arthroscopy. Philadelphia: Current Medicine, 1994:1.)

tissues, depending on the absorption coefficient of the tissue and the power of the laser, and produce different tissue effects.

Laser energy may be reflected, scattered, transmitted, or absorbed by the tissue (Fig. 16-4). Effects such as cutting or ablation of tissue occur when the laser energy is absorbed by the tissues. The thermal effect has five zones: normal tissue, coagulation and

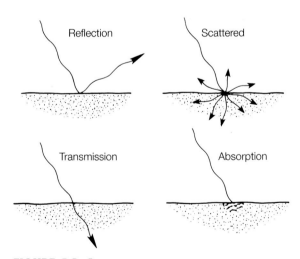

FIGURE 16-4.

When laser light strikes an object, it can be reflected, scattered, transmitted, or absorbed, or any combination of these effects. Only when laser light energy is absorbed by tissue is it transformed into effective thermal energy to produce a photothermal effect.

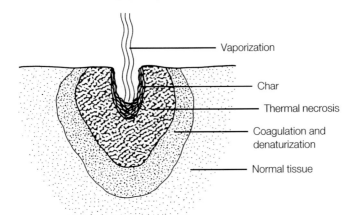

Vaporization

Char

Thermal necrosis

Coagulation and denaturization

Normal tissue

FIGURE 16–5.
The thermal effects of laser energy on tissue.

denaturation of protein, thermal necrosis, char formation, and ablation (Fig. 16-5). Coagulation occurs between 60° and 65°C. Denaturation of protein occurs between 65° and 90°C. Dehydration and shrinkage occur between 90° and 100°C. Boiling and vaporization occur at 100°C, carbonization at about 300°C.[6,7]

Laser light can be delivered in either a continuous or a pulsed beam. It can also be delivered with a free beam or by fiber. The amount of laser energy delivered to tissues can be described by different measurements (Table 16-2). The most accurate measurement is energy density, because this provides the total irradiation imparted to an exact surface area of the tissue, critical information for tissue ablation.

In the 1980s, the first clinical studies using laser-assisted arthroscopic surgery were performed using a free-beam carbon-dioxide (CO_2) laser delivered into the target tissues with the use of a wide-diameter trochar.[8–13] However, surgery of the musculoskeletal system has presented unique difficulties for the use of laser energy. The curved joint surfaces make straight

alignment of the light beam difficult. The tissues of the musculoskeletal system are fibrous and denser than other tissues of the body, giving them different light-absorption characteristics.[14] Most studies done with lasers in orthopedics have involved arthroscopic procedures, primarily in the knee. However, as experience has been gained, lasers have also been used in the shoulder, wrist, elbow, ankle, and spine.

TYPES OF LASERS

CO_2 Laser

Much of the medical laser surgery throughout the world today uses the CO_2 laser. It has the longest history of use (since 1961), and its wavelength (10.6 μm) is very efficiently absorbed by water-laden tissue. The CO_2 laser beam theoretically is ideal for operating on tissues with high water content, but it cannot be transmitted by fiber-optics. The CO_2 laser is a noncontact laser, making it ideal for the "no-touch" technique or access to tight spaces. Because CO_2 laser energy is absorbed by water, it cannot be used in an aqueous medium for arthroscopy; thus, gas insufflation of the joint is required.

Several problems are associated with the use of the CO_2 laser in ankle arthroscopy. For instance, unintended tissue can be ablated by the laser. A more common problem is the potential for gas under pressure to escape from the confines of the ankle joint,

TABLE 16–2.
ENERGY MEASUREMENTS

Joules	$=$ Watts per second
Power density	$= \dfrac{\text{Watts}}{\text{CM}^2}$
Energy density	$= \dfrac{\text{Joules}}{\text{CM}^2 \text{ (spot size)}}$

and vaporize tissue. Because of its relatively low tissue-absorption coefficient, the energy penetrates deeply in the tissue, producing unnecessary collateral damage. Therefore, a specialized tissue contact tip must be used rather than allowing free-beam application. Unlike the noncontact CO_2 and holmium:YAG lasers, which use a free beam and no-touch technique, the neodymium:YAG laser's contact hot-tip is fragile and may break with pressure.

Miller, O'Brien, and their colleagues found the neodymium:YAG laser to be a safe and efficient arthroscopic tool for performing meniscectomies, and found it to have advantages over the current instrumentation.[7,19] The neodymium:YAG laser permits fiber-optic delivery, allows easier access to confined spaces, and allows the use of conventional arthroscopic portals, techniques, and fluid environment.

Excimer Laser

Excimer lasers, introduced in the late 1980s, are pulsed gas lasers that emit ultraviolet wavelength energy. This laser can cut precisely, as well as ablate bone and cartilage. The beam is delivered through a flexible quartz optical fiber in a fluid medium. It has been called a "cold laser" because it causes photoablation of tissue with little or no thermal damage. This laser can remove layers of tissue from cartilage surfaces as the lased surface seems to melt away.[20] Raunest and Lohnert reported on the use of the 308-nanometer Excimer laser on 70 patients with chondral lesions of the knee.[21] After 6 months of follow-up, the clinical results showed the laser group had a significant reduction in pain and minimal reactive synovitis, but no differences were noted between the groups in terms of functional impairment and disability.

The disadvantages of the Excimer laser include its inherently low power and therefore slow cutting effect, large size, and high cost; the lasing medium gas is toxic. In addition, wavelengths below 0.320 μm may be mutagenic, although this has not been proven. Glossop and colleagues found no evidence of harmful effects on chondrocyte metabolism.[20]

INDICATIONS

As more experience is gained with the use of lasers and as technology advances, numerous indications for their use may evolve. In the foot and ankle, indications may include treatment of soft-tissue problems such as anterolateral impingement, nonspecific synovitis, adhesions, fibroarthrosis, and capsulitis. Lasers may also be useful in the treatment of chondromalacia and chondral defects, including osteochondritis dissecans, as well as removal of loose bodies, osteophytes, and possibly ankle arthrodesis. In the future, lasers also appear to have potential use for similar indications in the subtalar joint, the retrocalcaneal bursa, and the metatarsophalangeal joint of the first toe.

PREFERRED TECHNIQUE

Currently, the holmium:YAG laser has several advantages over the others described. It operates well in a fluid environment and uses a small-diameter fiber-optic cable protected in a metal sheath for laser-beam delivery. The durability of the delivery system permits the handpiece to be used both as an arthroscopic probe and as a laser-delivery tool. Probes are available at 0°, 15°, 30°, and 70° beam angles (Fig. 16-7). Because the handpieces are both curved and side-firing, they allow the entire ankle joint to be reached from the anterior portals (Fig. 16-8).

AAOS POSITION

The American Academy of Orthopaedic Surgeons' advisory statement was made in May 1992 and revised in July 1993: "Clinical studies reported in orthopaedic literature have not established the benefit provided by lasers when compared to other systems now in use. As further clinical research in laser applications becomes available, the Academy encourages investigators to pay special attention to those areas where the techniques can be shown to be effective additions to orthopaedic care."[22]

The current AAOS position states, "The Academy endorses a scientific approach toward the use of lasers in orthopaedic surgery and encourages further clinical and biologic study on the potential benefits and hazards of this technology. It is the individual surgeon's responsibility to become familiar with each laser's FDA clearance status, as well as the basic science and biological effects of laser techniques if he or she intends to incorporate them into clinical practice. It is also the physi-

creating subcutaneous emphysema and metastasis of gas to distant sites. To prevent these complications, a pneumatic tourniquet is used, along with low gas pressures.

Smith has developed a technique called "gas bubble" in which standard saline is used for diagnostic arthroscopy.[15,16] During the surgical aspects of the arthroscopy, the CO_2 laser is triangulated to within 3 mm of the target and a microenvironment of gas is created by bubbling the gas through the laser into the area of the target interface. With this macroenvironment of saline and microenvironment of gas, a gas bubble is created that allows the laser to work efficiently with minimal gas volume and pressure.

Despite the modifications of the CO_2 technique, most orthopedic surgeons have found the CO_2 laser cumbersome and somewhat difficult to use for arthroscopy because of the awkward articulated arms of mirrors required for beam delivery.

Holmium:YAG Laser

It became apparent that a wavelength that could be transmitted via fiber-optics and through a fluid medium was required. Lasers with these characteristics include the neodymium:YAG (Nd:YAG), the holmium:YAG (Ho:YAG), the KTP, the Excimer, and possibly the erbium:YAG. The holmium:YAG laser, a midinfrared wavelength laser, has a wavelength of 2.1 μm. The laser energy is created by stimulating a YAG crystal (yttrium, aluminum, garnet crystal with small concentrations of holmium, thallium, and chromium). Although absorbed by water, it will traverse short distances in fluid and can be used in a saline medium to vaporize biologic tissues efficiently. The holmium laser's delivery device is typically a plastic sheath surrounding a 400-μm fiber-optic cable with a metal handpiece. The small tip of the handpiece is used in a contact or near-contact mode, permitting cutting and manipulation of the target tissue with a single instrument. It is ideal for access to tight spaces in foot and ankle arthroscopy. The holmium laser can vaporize, cut, coagulate, smooth, and sculpt tissues by focusing and defocusing the beam. The holmium laser is a pulsed laser (350 μm) used at pulse rates from 1 to 20 hertz. When amplified to 15 to 30 watts of power, it produces 0.5 to 3 joules of energy per pulse. Each pulse acts independently, and the cooling effects between pulses in a fluid medium greatly limit the tissue damage[17] (Fig. 16-6).

The holmium laser's uses in the ankle include synovectomy, soft-tissue release, chondral ablation, and joint debridement.[18] It has curved handpieces or side-firing handpieces that allow the entire ankle joint, medial and lateral gutters, and most of the tibiotalar surface to be reached from anterior portals. The holmium laser allows the use of standard portals and instrumentation, permits distention with conventional fluids and fiber-optic delivery, minimizes scuffing of chondral surfaces, allows good access to tight places, and provides good hemostasis. It has minimal depth of penetration in target tissues and produces minimal thermal damage. It may also stimulate cell reproduction, which may be helpful in treating osteochondritic lesions of the foot and ankle, although this application remains unproven.

Neodymium:YAG Laser

The neodymium:YAG laser's wavelength of 1.06 μm is created by doping the YAG crystal with a small amount of neodymium. This laser beam can pass through water and is diffusely absorbed by tissue protein. The neodymium:YAG laser can cut, coagulate, excise,

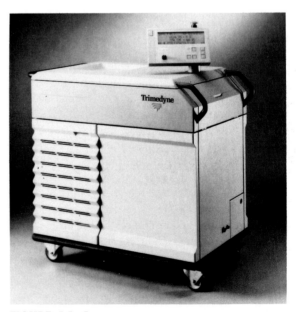

FIGURE 16-6.

Holmium:YAG laser. (Courtesy of Trimedyne, Inc.)

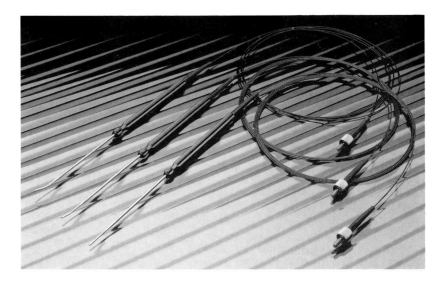

FIGURE 16-7.

Delivery systems used in arthroscopic surgery with a Holmium:YAG laser. Note the size and curvature of the different tips. (Courtesy of Coherent Medical Group.)

cian's responsibility to be sensitive to cost containment issues."[22]

As Goodfellow wrote in *The Journal of Bone and Joint Surgery* in 1992, "Until we have good outcome studies that show laser arthroscopy offers greater advantages to patients over conventional (and less expensive) techniques, those of us not actively engaged in the study of the technique or evaluating the efficacy of it should refrain from using it."[23]

FUTURE

In the future, laser technology will continue to develop and new applications for its use will be attempted. Sophisticated research is needed to reveal the effects on cell function and articular cartilage durability, and the cumulative effects of laser radiation. Although the future is exciting, caution must be exercised in using

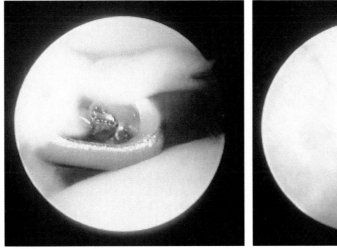

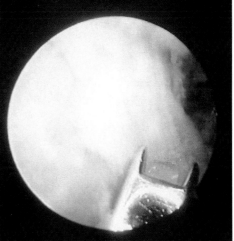

FIGURE 16-8.

Use of the Holmium:YAG laser in the ankle. (**A**) Side-firing delivery tip used to remove soft-tissue impingement. (**B**) Straight-tip device used to remove scar tissue in a patient with arthrofibrosis.

the technology indiscriminately without proper training and safe indications.

REFERENCES

1. Sherk HH. Lasers in orthopedics. Philadelphia: JB Lippincott, 1990.
2. Absten GT, Joffe SN. Lasers in medicine: an introductory guide. London: Chapman and Hall, 1989.
3. Sherk HH. Current concepts review: the use of lasers in orthopaedic procedures. J Bone Joint Surg 1993;75A:768.
4. Abelow SP. Use of lasers in orthopedic surgery: current concepts. Orthopedics 1993;16:551.
5. Miller DV, O'Brien SJ, Fealy SV, Givney MA, Kelly AM. Arthroscopic laser surgery. In Scott WN, ed. The knee. St. Louis: Mosby Yearbook, 1994:515.
6. Vangsness CT Jr., Ghaderi B, Saadatmanesh V. Lasers in arthroscopic surgery. In Parisien JS, ed. Current techniques in arthroscopy. Philadelphia: Current Medicine, 1994:1.
7. Miller DV, O'Brien SJ, Arnoczky SS, et al. The use of the contact Nd:YAG laser in arthroscopic surgery: effects on articular cartilage and meniscal tissue. Arthroscopy 1989;5:245.
8. Whipple TL, Caspari RB, Meyer JF. Arthroscopic laser meniscectomy in a gas medium. Arthroscopy 1985;1:2.
9. Whipple TL, Caspari RB, Meyer JF. Laser subtotal meniscectomy in rabbits. Lasers Surg Med 1984; 3:297.
10. Whipple TL, Caspari RB. Laser energy in arthroscopic meniscectomy. Orthopedics 1983;6:1165.
11. Philandrianos G. Carbon dioxide laser in arthroscopic surgery of the knee. Presse Med 1985;14:2103.
12. Smith JB, Nance TA. Arthroscopic laser surgery. Presented at the annual meeting of the Arthroscopy Association of North America, Coronado, California, 1983.
13. Smith JB, Nance TA. Laser energy in arthroscopic surgery. In Parisien JS, ed. Orthopedic surgery. New York: McGraw-Hill, 1988:44.
14. Miller DV, O'Brien SJ, Zarins B, et al. The optical properties of the human meniscus. Am Soc Laser Med Surg Abstracts 1991;3(Suppl):51.
15. Smith C, Dillingham M, Fanton G. The use of laser in ankle arthroscopy. In Guhl JF, ed. Foot and ankle arthroscopy. Thorofare, NJ: Slack, 1993:189.
16. Smith CF, Johansen EL, Vangsness CT, et al. Gas bubble technique in arthroscopic surgery. Sem Orthop 1992;7:86.
17. Dillingham MF, Price JM, Fanton GS. Holmium laser surgery. Orthopedics 1993;16:563.
18. Fanton GS, Dillingham MF. Arthroscopic meniscectomy using the Holmium:YAG laser—a double-blind study. Presented at the annual meeting of the Arthroscopy Association of North America, Orlando, Florida, 1990.
19. O'Brien SJ, Fealy S, Miller DV. Nd:YAG contact laser arthroscopy. Sem Orthop 1992;7:117.
20. Glossop N, Jackson R, Randle J, Reed S. The Excimer laser in arthroscopic surgery. Sem Orthop 1992;7:125.
21. Raunest J, Lohnert J. Arthroscopic cartilage debridement by Excimer laser in chondromalacia of the knee joint—a prospective randomized clinical study. Arch Orthop Trauma Surg 1990;109:155.
22. American Academy of Orthopaedic Surgeons Advisory Statement on Lasers in Orthopaedic Surgery. May 1992; revised July 1993.
23. Goodfellow JW. Current concepts review: uses and abuses of arthroscopy: a symposium. J Bone Joint Surg 1992;74A:1563.

BIBLIOGRAPHY

Black J, Sherk HH, Meller M, et al. Wavelength selection in laser arthroscopy. Sem Orthop 1992;7:72.
Garrick JG, Kadell N. The CO_2 laser in arthroscopy: potential problems and solutions. Arthroscopy 1991; 7:129.
Whipple T. The future of lasers in orthopaedic surgery. Sem Orthop 1992;7:131.

B. *Endoscopic Procedures for the Retrocalcaneal Bursa, Plantar Fascia, and Achilles Tendon*

Timothy Zimmer
Richard D. Ferkel

The first two procedures discussed in this section are considered experimental, and only a limited number of cases have been done.

ENDOSCOPIC RETROCALCANEAL DECOMPRESSION

Posterior heel pain associated with inflammation of the retrocalcaneal bursa, the secondary prominence of the posterior superior aspect of the posterior tuberosity of the calcaneus, is a common complaint. By design, the heel counter of the shoe strikes the area with considerable pressure. This causes pain and inflammation, which generally can be treated successfully with nonoperative techniques. When symptoms persist and are recalcitrant to a nonsurgical approach, surgical intervention is indicated. A single- or double-incision approach has been described, with excision of the bursa and sufficient bone stock from the posterior superior aspect of the posterior tuberosity of the calcaneus to reduce the prominent tissue profile. This procedure is ultimately successful in most cases, but is also associated with significant morbidity, as pain and heel-cord tightness may persist for 8 to 16 weeks. An endoscopic approach could potentially decrease surgical morbidity and allow faster recovery.

Anatomy

The medial and lateral borders of the Achilles tendon are palpable even in overweight patients. The insertion of the Achilles tendon on the calcaneus can also often be felt. The sural nerve passes from the posterior aspect of the calf across the musculotendinous junction of the Achilles tendon and lies about 2 cm posterior and 2 cm inferior to the lateral malleolus. Therefore, the sural nerve should not be in jeopardy when approaching the retrocalcaneal area endoscopically. The medial calcaneal nerve branching from the posterior tibial nerve and the lateral calcaneal nerve branching from the sural nerve lie closer to the surgical site, and care must be exercised to avoid injuring these structures. The Achilles tendon starts as a cylindrical structure and progressively becomes more elliptical, finally fanning out to a broad insertion across the calcaneus at about the middle of the posterior tuberosity of the os calcis.

Indications/Contraindications

Indications for endoscopic retrocalcaneal decompression include a Haglund deformity ("pump bump") and retrocalcaneal bursitis refractory to non-surgical treatment. Calcium deposits within the Achilles tendon cannot be treated arthroscopically.

Portals

Medial and lateral portals are used for resection of the retrocalcaneal bursa and are placed at the medial and lateral margins of the Achilles tendon at the level of the retrocalcaneal bursa (Fig. 16-9A). Medial and lateral accessory portals can be used along with a trans-Achilles portal, but laceration of the Achilles tendon should be avoided (see Fig. 16-9B).

Instrumentation

A 2.7-mm arthroscope with different lens angles allows entire visualization of the area. A small shaver/debrider set is also necessary, along with appropriate baskets and punches. The short length of the telescope and shaver systems facilitates instrument maneuverability (see Chap. 3).

Technique

General or regional anesthesia is necessary, and a tourniquet is needed to avoid excessive bleeding and loss of exposure. The patient is positioned prone on the operating table with the affected foot over the end of the table to allow manipulation of the ankle into dorsiflexion and plantarflexion. Also, positioning the patient distally on the table allows intraoperative fluoroscopy to evaluate bony resection.

Initially the bursa and fat are removed. The Achilles is then lifted off the calcaneus and the superior calcaneal angle is removed with a motorized burr (Fig. 16-10). The bone resection should extend distally to the insertion of the Achilles tendon without cutting or detaching it. It is important not to leave a ridge of bone at the inferior edge of the Achilles insertion on the calcaneus (Fig. 16-11). An arthroscopic pump is unnecessary; pumps may cause sufficient local extravasation to interfere with visualization.

At the completion of the procedure, single stitches are placed in each portal and a compression dressing is applied with a splint.

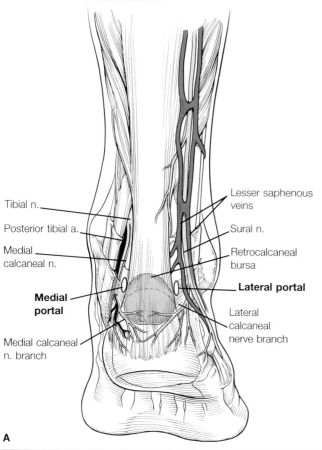

Tibial n.

Posterior tibial a.

Medial calcaneal n.

Medial portal

Medial calcaneal n. branch

Lesser saphenous veins

Sural n.

Retrocalcaneal bursa

Lateral portal

Lateral calcaneal nerve branch

A

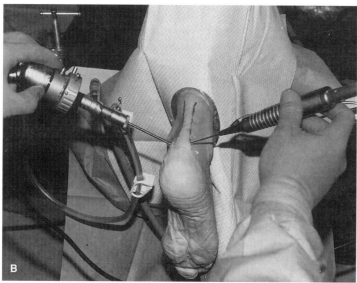

B

FIGURE 16-9.

Resection of the retrocalcaneal bursa. (**A**) Medial and lateral portals are situated at the margins of the Achilles tendon to allow access to the retrocalcaneal bursa. (**B**) With the patient prone, the arthroscope is inserted medially, the shaver laterally.

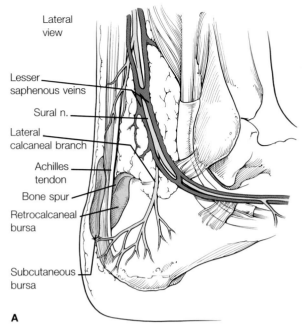

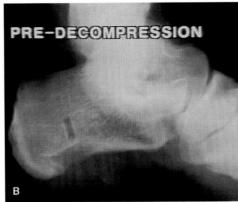

FIGURE 16-10.
(**A**) Anatomy of the retrocalcaneal and subcutaneous bursae. Note the location of the neurovascular structures.
(**B**) Preoperative lateral x-ray before decompression.

ACHILLES DECOMPRESSION

Open procedures for Achilles pathology can create significant inflammation and scarring during the healing process. An inflamed Achilles tendon tends to contract, restricting ankle motion. Achilles tendinitis and peritendinitis can recur repeatedly and often fail to respond to a nonoperative treatment plan. An endoscopic approach reduces surgical morbidity.

Anatomy

The musculotendinous junction of the triceps surae marks the superior level of the Achilles tendon. The tendon becomes cylindrical, elliptical, and finally rather thin and wide as it inserts on the os calcis. Near the musculotendinous junction, the sural nerve crosses the Achilles tendon proximally, progressing distally along the posterolateral leg and eventually passing 2 cm posterior and 2 cm inferior to the lateral malleolus. The lateral calcaneal nerve branches off the sural nerve 2 to 4 cm below the musculotendi-

nous junction. The medial calcaneal nerve branches off the posterior tibial nerve and takes a relatively direct course to the inferior aspect of the heel (see Fig. 16-9). Significant fat deposition is present deep to the Achilles, separating the tendon from the deep compartment of the leg; this becomes thicker distally. There is no true synovial sheath around the Achilles tendon, and it is covered by the peritenon alone.

Indications/Contraindications

Indications for endoscopic partial tenotomy or tendon lengthening include recurring Achilles tendinitis or peritendinitis that does not respond to stretching, splint, and anti-inflammatory treatment. Contraindications include the presence of advanced mucoid degeneration of the tendon, which should be resected. Also, poor circulation or local infection is a contraindication to the procedure.

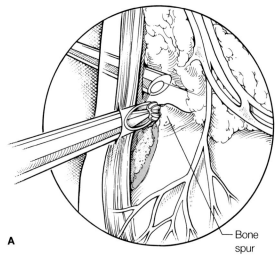

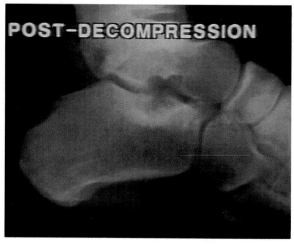

FIGURE 16-11.
Excision of Haglund deformity. **(A)** While visualizing from the medial portal, a burr is inserted laterally to remove the superior angle of the calcaneus. **(B)** Postoperative lateral x-ray demonstrating excision of the Haglund deformity.

Portals

Portals about the posteromedial aspect of the tendon are safe. One should be placed about 1.5 cm from the tendon insertion on the os calcis, and another about 1.5 cm distal to the musculotendinous junction (Fig. 16-12). A third portal can be placed midway between the other two if working distance is prohibitive (Fig. 16-13).

Instrumentation

Instrumentation is essentially the same as that for endoscopic plantar release.

Technique

The patient is positioned prone on the operating table with either general or regional anesthesia to allow use of a thigh tourniquet. The portals are es-

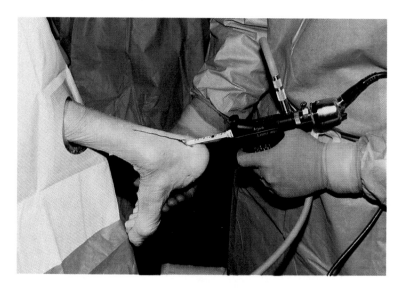

FIGURE 16-12.
Use of the inferior portal, medial aspect of the Achilles tendon, to release peritenon.

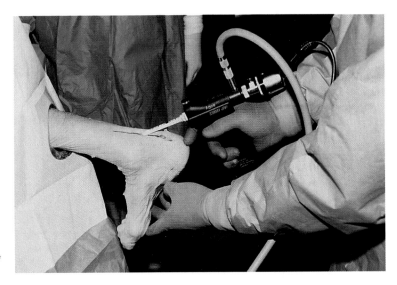

FIGURE 16-13.
Intermediate portal, medial aspect of the Achilles tendon.

tablished, spreading the subcutaneous tissue with a hemostat to protect the superficial sensory nerve branches. An arthroscopic sleeve or an endoscopic device is inserted into the sheath of the Achilles tendon. An arthroscopic pump can be used to ex-

pand this space slightly. Working between portals, the peritenon sheath can be released longitudinally, either with a retrograde knife (as is commonly done with the transverse carpal ligament) or with a punch or basket forceps (Fig. 16-14). The sheath should be released completely to the subcutaneous tissue and deep to the tendon. Care should be taken not to damage the tendon while cutting the sheath. The portals are closed with a single skin suture and a sterile compressive dressing and posterior splint are applied with the foot in neutral and slight dorsiflexion position.

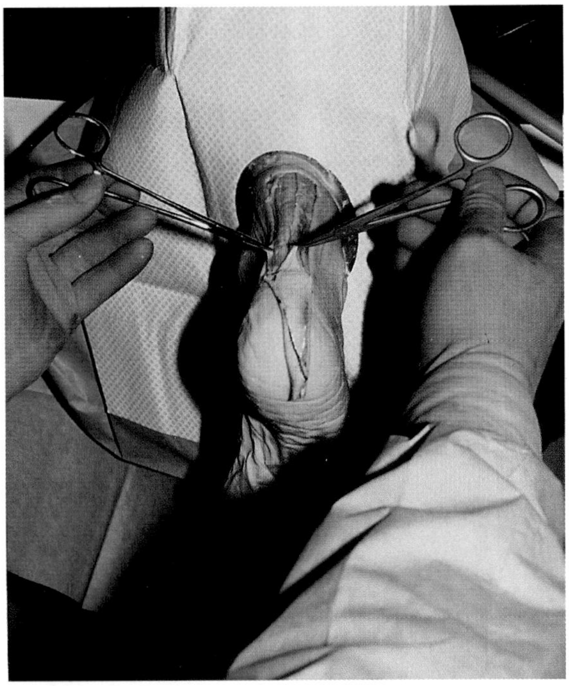

ACHILLES TENDON REPAIR

Achilles tendon repair has been reported using percutaneous sutures and was popularized by Ma.[1,2] Using these principles, endoscopy and repair of Achilles tendon ruptures can be performed. Although the authors have no experience with this technique, it has been reported by Nagai and others in Japan.[3]

ENDOSCOPIC PLANTAR FASCIAL RELEASE

Plantar heel pain is one of the most common conditions seen by the orthopedic surgeon. Most patients respond well to a course of nonoperative treatment,

FIGURE 16-14.
Cadaveric dissection after complete endoscopic release of the Achilles peritenon.

but sometimes patients fail nonoperative care and surgical intervention is indicated.

Although the terms *plantar fasciitis* and *heel pain syndrome* are used most commonly, there are many causes of heel pain.[4–7] In this section, the heel pain is isolated to the proximal origin of the plantar fascia. The onset of the pain is insidious. The pain is worse in the morning, after prolonged sitting, and after prolonged activity.

Physical examination reveals well-localized pain in the medial calcaneal tuberosity and occasionally in the central portion of the plantar fascia. The examiner must look for the various causes of heel pain, and appropriate diagnostic tests should be done.

With conservative treatment, 80% to 90% of patients with plantar fasciitis improve.[8,9] Various procedures have been advocated to treat plantar fasciitis. Plantar fasciotomy, with or without excision of the heel spurs, is the most common procedure reported for the treatment of plantar fasciitis.[10–12] Debate exists as to how much plantar fascia to release. Complete release results in loss of the windlass mechanism and loss of the longitudinal arch. In addition, most authors agree that it is unnecessary to remove the heel spur at the time of surgery.

Open plantar fascial release, either partial or complete, requires considerable soft-tissue dissection. Depending on the location of the incision and the amount of dissection, the plantar medial aspect of the heel may be left anesthetic from injury to the medial calcaneal nerve as it branches from the posterior tibial nerve. The nerve is quite small at this level and may be difficult to visualize. Open procedures may require 6 to 9 months to heel, and postoperatively, casting is done for 4 to 6 weeks. Because of high patient morbidity, an endoscopic procedure has been suggested.[13–16]

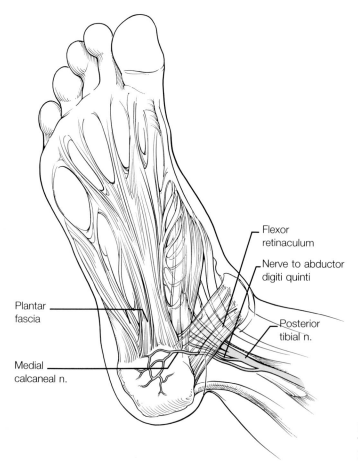

FIGURE 16–15.
The medial side of the foot, showing the flexor retinaculum, plantar fascia, and neurovascular bundle.

Anatomy

The plantar fascia can be palpated in the longitudinal arch and traced proximally to its origin on the os calcis. The plantar fascia lies superficial to the intrinsic muscles of the foot and has three portions—medial, central, and lateral. The medial flexor tendons and the neurovascular bundle are deep to this level (Fig. 16-15).

Indications/Contraindications

The indications for plantar fascia release are at least 6 to 9 months of conservative treatment without relief. Nerve entrapment should be ruled out with electrodiagnostic testing and all other causes of heel pain excluded before surgery. This procedure is contraindicated in patients with atypical heel pain, abnormal electrodiagnostic testing in the foot and ankle, and a dysvascular foot.

Portals and Instrumentation

The portals for the endoscopic plantar fascia release depend on the instrumentation available. Currently, both single- and double-portal techniques are used. The same instrumentation and arthroscopes (endoscopes) used for carpal tunnel release can also be used for plantar fascia release. The arthroscope used for this procedure is similar to the standard ones used in the knee and shoulder and measures 4.0 mm with a 30° inclination of view. The difference between the two arthroscopes is that the inclination of view in the former arthroscope looks up toward the cord instead of away from the cord, and the length of the arthroscope is 100 mm, compared with the 157-mm length of a regular arthroscope. In addition, instrumentation specific for endoscopic plantar fascia release has been developed (Fig. 16-16). The single-incision technique uses the 3M device called the Inside Job, which requires a single portal placed plantar medially. Careful portal placement will protect the medial calcaneal nerve.

The two-portal technique uses medial and lateral portals. The medial portal is made by extending a line distally near the posterior aspect of the medial malleolus, which generally will intersect the medial

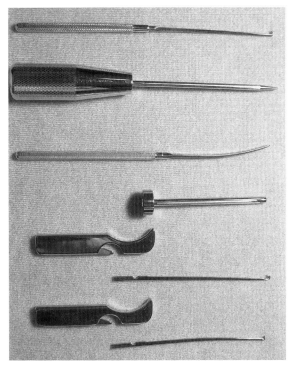

FIGURE 16–16.
Endoscopic plantar fascia release instrumentation includes a fascial probe (*top*), blunt obturator, fascial elevator, slotted cannula, and hook and triangular blades.

origin of the plantar fascia at the calcaneal tuberosity (Fig. 16-17*A,B*). Dissection superficial to the fascia allows a blunt cannula to be placed transversely across the heel to establish the lateral portal (see Fig. 16-17*C*).

Technique

The patient is placed supine on the operating table. Ankle block, regional, or general anesthesia can be used. An ankle tourniquet will improve visual clarity. For the single-portal technique, the posteromedial portal is created and the Inside Job device is placed just superficial (plantar) to the plantar fascia distal to its insertion on the inferior aspect of the os calcis (Fig. 16-18). Moving the device deeper allows visualization of the fascial insertion. The retrograde blade is deployed on the device, and three to five passes will complete release of the plantar fascia. Re-

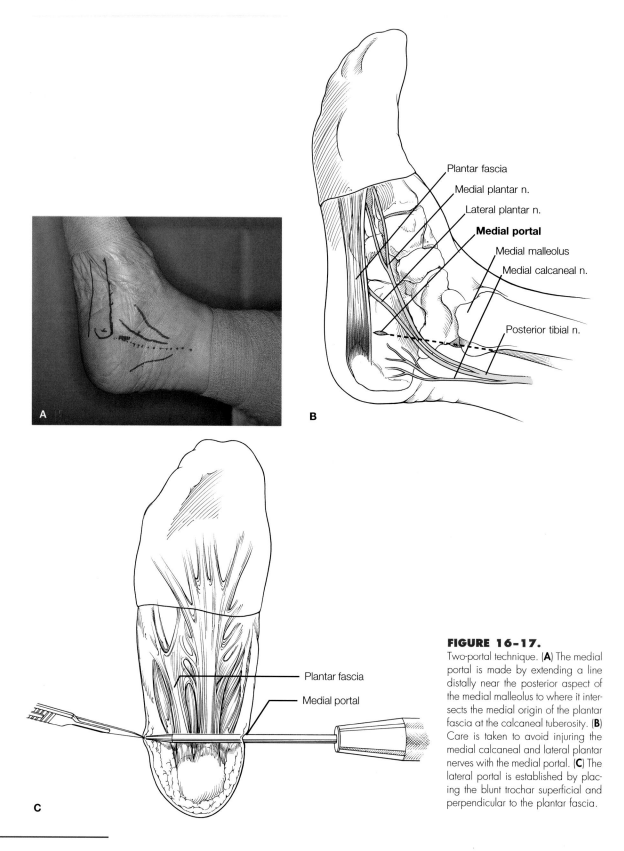

Plantar fascia

Medial plantar n.

Lateral plantar n.

Medial portal

Medial malleolus

Medial calcaneal n.

Posterior tibial n.

Plantar fascia

Medial portal

FIGURE 16–17.

Two-portal technique. (**A**) The medial portal is made by extending a line distally near the posterior aspect of the medial malleolus to where it intersects the medial origin of the plantar fascia at the calcaneal tuberosity. (**B**) Care is taken to avoid injuring the medial calcaneal and lateral plantar nerves with the medial portal. (**C**) The lateral portal is established by placing the blunt trochar superficial and perpendicular to the plantar fascia.

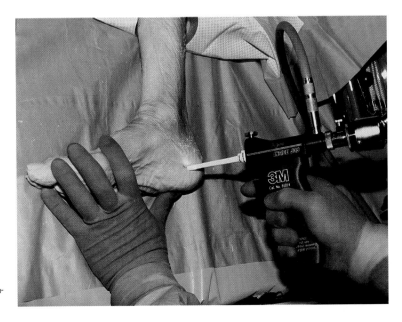

FIGURE 16-18.
Use of the single medial portal with endoscopic device.

lease is complete when the intrinsic muscles are visualized just deep to the insertion of the plantar fascia. Holding the ankle in dorsiflexion with the toes extended places the plantar fascia under tension, which helps to separate the ends of the fascia when cut (Fig. 16-19).

The two-portal technique involves making a vertical medial incision through the skin only.

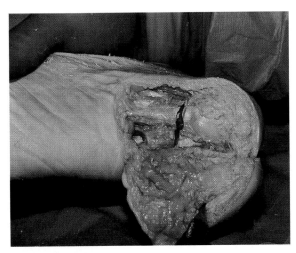

FIGURE 16-19.
Cadaveric dissection after complete release of plantar fascia endoscopically.

Blunt dissection with a hemostat is done to the level of the medial edge of the plantar fascia to avoid injuring the calcaneal nerve branch, which generally is located posteriorly. A Freer elevator is then used to lift the soft tissues away from the plantar surface of the fascia in a transverse direction. A blunt trochar is then placed through the channel and presses against the lateral skin. A bursa exists in this area, which allows a trochar to pass quite easily over to the lateral side of the foot. A second vertical incision is made over the trochar and a slotted cannula is inserted over the trochar, through the lateral portal, and the endoscope is placed laterally (Fig. 16-20). A cotton swab is passed across the cannula to remove fluid and debris from the visual field. A probe is inserted through the medial portal to determine the length of the entire plantar fascia. The medial third to half of the plantar fascia is measured, and a mark is placed on the probe and the endoscopic knives to prevent extending the incision too far laterally. The ankle and foot (including the toes) are then dorsiflexed to place tension on the plantar fascia. This also allows the flexor digitorum brevis muscle to bulge slightly when the fascia is completely released. A triangular knife blade is inserted through the medial portal and an incision is made at the lateral border of the fasciotomy (Fig. 16-21). A

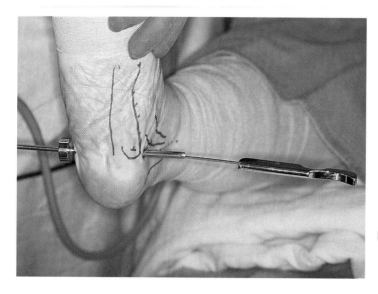

FIGURE 16-20.
Double-incision technique with the arthroscope lateral through the slotted cannula and the knife inserted through the medial portal.

hook knife is then inserted and the plantar fascia is released from lateral to medial (Fig. 16-22). Several passes may be necessary to cut the entire depth of the plantar fascia, but the underlying muscles should not be injured. The arthroscope is then passed medially and deep within the plantar fascia incision to visualize part of the deep fascia of the abductor hallucis muscle. The triangular blade is then passed several millimeters in the medial inci-

sion, and a cut is performed upward to release the portion of the deep fascia of the abductor. As there is some danger of injuring the lateral plantar nerve during this maneuver, the knife must be visualized and passed only several millimeters from medial to lateral to protect the nerve.

At completion, the wound is irrigated and closed with 5-0 nylon sutures. A compression dressing is applied and the patient ambulates weight-bearing as tolerated in a removable cast boot or rehabilitative shoe for 10 to 14 days. Once the patient is comfortable, a good supportive shoe is worn and stretching and strengthening are started.[17]

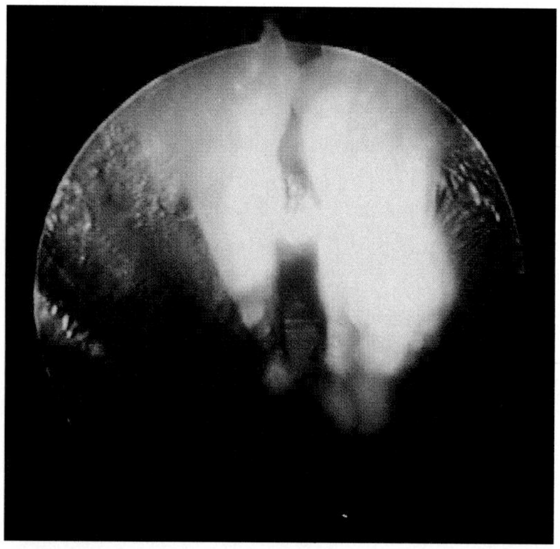

Complications

The extent of the fasciotomy varies secondary to instrumentation and anatomic variability of the plantar fascia. The learning curve is fairly steep and the expensive instrumentation can break down. Baxter and associates have noted several problems, including continued preoperative symptoms; pain in the midtarsal, calcaneocuboid, and lateral subtalar areas; and fullness at the release site.[18] In addition, they have seen several patients with postoperative nerve problems secondary to a direct injury from the release.

FIGURE 16-21.
The triangular knife blade is used to initiate the release of the lateral border of the fasciotomy.

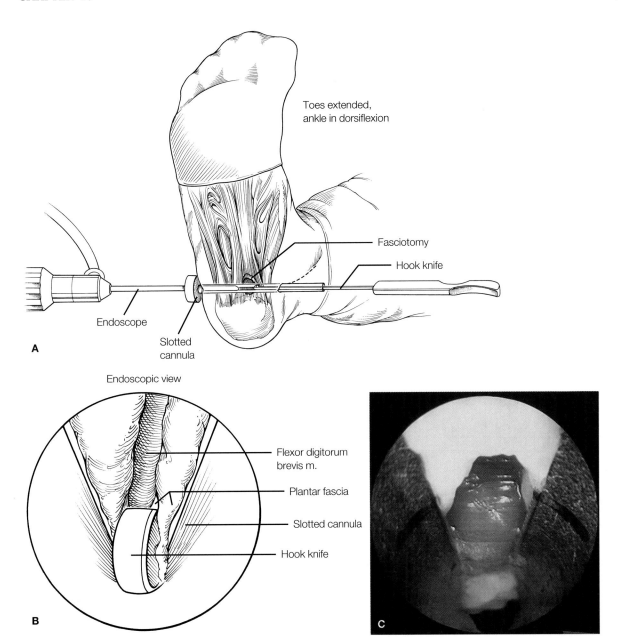

Toes extended,
ankle in dorsiflexion

Fasciotomy

Hook knife

Endoscope

Slotted
cannula

A

Endoscopic view

Flexor digitorum
brevis m.

Plantar fascia

Slotted cannula

Hook knife

B

C

FIGURE 16-22.

Endoscopic plantar fascia release. (**A**) The medial aspect of the plantar fascia is released, while the ankle is dorsiflexed and toes extended, with a hook knife from the medial portal while visualizing from the lateral portal. (**B**) When the plantar fascia is fully released, the underlying flexor digitorum brevis muscle is visualized. (**C**) The release is completed when the muscle is visualized.

Controversy

Much debate exists about the appropriateness and efficacy of this procedure.[19–21] No long-term prospective randomized studies have been done to determine its effectiveness. Dr. Lowell Scott Weil (past President of the American College of Foot and Ankle Surgeons) has termed this procedure "the rape of the plantar fascia."[20] The need for and the role of endoscopic plantar fascia release remain to be defined, and we suspect this procedure will be appropriate in only a few carefully selected patients.

SUMMARY

Endoscopic technology has revolutionized the approach to surgery in multiple specialties. Numerous arthroscopic and endoscopic procedures have been devised for orthopedic surgery. The procedures described in this chapter are not the standard of care, but do represent an increasingly widened application for arthroscopic and endoscopic technology.

REFERENCES

1. Ma GWC, Griffith TG. Percutaneous repair of acute closed ruptured Achilles tendon: a new technique. Clin Orthop 1977;128:247.
2. Hynes RA, Ma GWC. Percutaneous tendo Achilles repair. J Orthop Tech 1993;1:99.
3. Nagai H. Tunnel endoscopy. In Watanabe M, ed. Arthroscopy of small joints. Tokyo: Igaku-Shoin, 1985:162.
4. Graham CE. Painful heel syndrome: rationale of diagnosis and treatment. Foot Ankle 1983;3:261.
5. Bordelon RL. Subcalcaneal pain: a method of evaluation and plan for treatment. Clin Orthop 1983; 177:49.
6. Schepsis AA, Leach RE, Gorzyca J. Plantar fasciitis: etiology, treatment, surgical results, and review of the literature. Clin Orthop 1991;266:185.
7. Baxter DE, Pfeffer GB. Treatment of chronic heel pain by surgical release of the first branch of the lateral plantar nerve. Clin Orthop 1992;279:229.
8. Wolgin M, Cook C, Graham C, Mauldin D. Conservative treatment of plantar heel pain: long-term follow-up. Foot Ankle 1994;15:97.
9. Davis PF, Severud E, Baxter DE. Painful heel syndrome: results of nonoperative treatment. J Bone Joint Surg [Br] (in press).
10. McBryde AM Jr. Plantar fasciitis. Instr Course Lect 1984;33:278.
11. Lutter LD. Surgical decisions in athletes' subcalcaneal pain. Am J Sports Med 1986;14:481.
12. Ward WG, Clippinger FW. Proximal medial longitudinal arch incision for plantar fascia release. Foot Ankle 1987;8:152.
13. Barrett SL, Day SV, Brown MG. Endoscopic plantar fasciotomy: preliminary study with cadaveric specimens. J Foot Surg 1991;30:170.
14. Barrett SL, Day SV. Endoscopic plantar fasciotomy for chronic plantar fasciitis/heel spur syndrome: surgical technique—early clinical results. J Foot Surg 1991;30:568.
15. Kinley S, Frascone S, Calderone D, Wertheimer SJ, Squire MA, Wiseman FA. Endoscopic plantar fasciotomy versus traditional heel spur surgery: a prospective study. J Foot Ankle Surg 1993;32:595.
16. Barrett SL, Day SV. Endoscopic plantar fasciotomy: two-portal endoscopic surgical techniques—clinical results of 65 procedures. J Foot Ankle Surg 1993;32:248.
17. Graves SC. Endoscopic plantar fascia release. Presented at the American Orthopaedic Foot and Ankle Society Specialty Day, February 19, 1995, Orlando, Florida.
18. Palumbo RC, Kodros SA, Baxter DE. Endoscopic plantar fasciotomy: indications, techniques, and complications. Sports Med Arthroscopy Rev 1994;2:317.
19. Letters to the Editor. J Foot Ankle Surg 1994;33:214.
20. Weil LS. The rape of the plantar fascia. Biomechanics 1994;1:37.
21. Ten eminent practitioners respond to the July–August Biomechanics article "Rape of the plantar fasciotomy." Biomechanics 1995;2:21.

Index

The letter *f* following a page number indicates a figure; page numbers followed by *t* indicate tabular material.